# Nursing Diagnosis
## Application to Clinical Practice

**Lynda Juall Carpenito**, R.N., M.S.N.
Nursing Consultant
Mickleton, New Jersey

Formerly, Clinical Specialist in Nursing Process
Wilmington Medical Center
Wilmington, Delaware

Task Force Member
National Group for the Classification of Nursing Diagnosis

with 22 additional contributors

**J. B. Lippincott Company** ● Philadelphia

London

Mexico City

New York

St. Louis

São Paulo

Sydney

Sponsoring Editor: Diana Intenzo
Manuscript Editor: Janet H. Baker
Production Supervisor: N. Carol Kerr
Production Assistant: S. M. Gassaway
Compositor: International Computaprint Corporation
Printer/Binder: R. R. Donnelley & Sons Company

7 8 9

Library of Congress Cataloging in Publication Data

Carpenito, Lynda Juall.
  Nursing diagnosis.

  Includes bibliographies and index.
  1. Diagnosis. 2. Nursing. I. Title.
[DNLM: 1. Nursing process. 2. Patient care planning.
WY 100 C294n]
RT48.C37 1983    616.07'5'024613    82-22924
ISBN 0-397-54377-8

The author and publisher have exerted every effort to ensure that drug selection and dosage set forth in this text are in accord with current recommendations and practice at the time of publication. However, in view of ongoing research, changes in government regulations, and the constant flow of information relating to drug therapy and drug reactions, the reader is urged to check the package insert for each drug for any change in indications and dosage and for added warnings and precautions. This is particularly important when the recommended agent is a new or infrequently employed drug.

To Richard, my husband
Thank you for your steadfast support through the difficult times.


It was such a pretty day we decided
    to take a walk,
And we had not gone ten steps
    before I knew
That you and I are long past the point
    of no return.

Hand in hand we go.
Still close, still loving,
Still looking and overlooking
The flaws we hide from others.

Side by side we move,
Sometimes closer, sometimes farther apart.
Because of ways we read and talk,
Agree and disagree.

Step by step we advance
Against the cynics
Those all-knowing unknowings who
    honestly think
Marriage is dead.

—Lois Wyse, "I Still Love You"

# Contributors

**Rosalind Alfaro**, R.N., B.S.N. Graduate student, Villanova University, Villanova, Pennsylvania; Staff Nurse, Intensive Care Units, Paoli Memorial Hospital, Paoli, Pennsylvania

(Alterations in Respiratory Function, Ineffective Airway Clearance, Ineffective Breathing Patterns, Impaired Gas Exchange, Alteration in Tissue Perfusion, Diversional Activity Deficit, and selected sections of Impaired Verbal Communication, Fluid Volume Deficit and Fluid Volume Excess)

**Virginia Arcangelo**, R.N., M.S.N. Nursing Consultant, Marlton, New Jersey

(Sexual Dysfunction and selected sections of Impaired Verbal Communication)

**Cynthia Balin**, R.N., M.S.N. Clinical Specialist, Wilmington Medical Center, Wilmington, Delaware

(Alterations in Nutrition: Less Than Body Requirements, Alterations in Nutrition: More Than Body Requirements, and Powerlessness)

**Eleanor A. Bell**, R.N. Assistant Director of Nursing, Bryn Mawr Rehabilitation Hospital, Malvern, Pennsylvania

(Self-Care Deficit)

**Michelle Bockrath**, R.N., M.S.N. Instructor, College of Nursing, University of Pennsylvania, Philadelphia, Pennsylvania

(Sleep Pattern Disturbance and sections of Sensory-Perceptual Alterations)

**Christine Cannon**, R.N., M.S.N. Coordinator of Patient Education, Wilmington Medical Center, Wilmington, Delaware

(Knowledge Deficit and sections of Alterations in Cardiac Output)

**Nancy Conrad**, R.N., M.S.N. Assistant Professor, Department of Nursing, Rutgers University, Camden, New Jersey

(Fear)

**Janet Derrington**, R.N., M.S.N. Psychiatric Clinical Specialist, Wilmington Medical Center, Wilmington, Delaware

(Potential for Violence)

**Linda Goldberg**, R.N., M.A. Instructor, St. Joseph's School of Nursing, Reading, Pennsylvania

(Grieving)

**Joan W. Goloskov**, R.N., M.S.N., F.A.A.N. Pain Consultant, Psychiatry Associates, Wilmington, Delaware

(Selected sections of Alterations in Comfort)

**Elizabeth Keech**, R.N., M.S.N. Instructor, College of Nursing, Villanova University, Villanova, Pennsylvania
(Sections of Alterations in Parenting)

**Margaret Kendrick**, R.N., M.S.N. Assistant Professor, College of Nursing, Villanova University, Villanova, Pennsylvania

(Sections of Fluid Volume Deficit, Fluid Volume Excess, and Potential for Injury)

**Carol Lillis**, R.N., M.S.N. Instructor, Delaware County Community College, Media, Pennsylvania

(Alterations in Bowel Elimination)

**Janet Hoffman Mennies**, R.N., M.S.N. Nurse Practitioner, Outpatient Department, Wilmington Medical Center, Wilmington, Delaware

(Noncompliance, Ineffective Individual Coping, Alterations in Health Maintenance, and selected sections of Alterations in Family Processes)

**Kathe H. Morris**, R.N., M.S.N. Assistant Professor, College of Nursing, Villanova University, Villanova, Pennsylvania

(Rape Trauma Syndrome)

**Catherine Oblaczynski**, R.N., M.S.N. Associate Professor, College of Nursing, Villanova University, Villanova, Pennsylvania

(Alterations in Thought Processes)

**Patricia O'Brien O'Riordan**, R.N., M.S.N. Director, E. I. du Pont Division, Wilmington Medical Center, Wilmington, Delaware

(Impaired Physical Mobility)

**Mara Schwenk**, R.N., M.S.N. Assistant Professor, College of Nursing, Villanova University, Villanova, Pennsylvania

(Selected sections of Alterations in Cardiac Output)

**Laura A. Terrill**, R.N., M.S.N. Director of Nursing Education, Wilmington Medical Center, Wilmington, Delaware

(Disturbance in Self-Concept and Social Isolation)

**Mary Mishler Vogel**, R.N., M.S.N. Instructor, Helene Fuld School of Nursing, Camden, New Jersey

(Selected sections of Alteration in Patterns of Urinary Elimination)

**Julie Waterhouse**, R.N., M.S.N. Instructor, College of Nursing, University of Delaware, Newark, Delaware

(Spiritual Distress)

**Anne E. Willard**, R.N., M.S.N. Director of Nursing, Delaware State Hospital, New Castle, Delaware

(Anxiety and selected sections of Potential for Violence)

# Consultants

**Philip N. Barkins**, R.P.T. Chief, Department of Physical Therapy, Wilmington Medical Center, Wilmington, Delaware

**Daniel T. Erhard**, M.D. Department of Anesthesia, Lankenau Hospital; Associate Clinical Professor, Jefferson Medical College, Philadelphia, Pennsylvania

**Jean W. Fitzgerald**, R.N., E.T. Enterostomal Therapist, Wilmington Medical Center, Wilmington, Delaware

**Annette D. Friday**, R.N. Head Nurse, Neonatal Intensive Care Unit, Wilmington Medical Center, Wilmington, Delaware

**Margaret M. Hirst**, R.N., M.S.N. Clinical Specialist in Oncology, Wilmington Medical Center, Wilmington, Delaware

**Jacqueline W. Levett**, R.N., M.S.N. Pediatric Clinical Specialist, Wilmington Medical Center, Wilmington, Delaware

**Ledjie Roth**, B.S.N., C.R.N.A. Director, School of Anesthesia for Nurses, Lankenau Hospital, Philadelphia, Pennsylvania

**Rebecca R. Resh**, B.S., M.Ed. Spec. Ed. Art Instructor, Special Education, Devereaux Foundation, Malvern, Pennsylvania

**Carl K. Wyckoff III,** D.D.S. Private practice, Wenonah, New Jersey

# Preface

The practice of nursing often interfaces with the practices of the other health care providers.* Sometimes the nurse sees primarily the client problems that require referral for treatment and ignores or fails to detect the problems that he or she can treat independently. *Nursing Diagnosis: Application to Clinical Practice* focuses on the diagnosis and treatment of client problems that the nurse can and should treat, legally and independently. It provides a condensed, organized outline of clinical nursing practice designed to communicate creative clinical nursing. It is not meant to replace textbooks of nursing, but rather to provide nurses in a variety of settings with the information they need without requiring a time-consuming review of the literature.

From assessment criteria to specific interventions, the book focuses on nursing. It will assist students in transferring their theoretical knowledge to clinical practice; it can also be used by experienced nurses to recall past learning and to intervene in those clinical situations that previously went ignored or unrecognized.

The author believes that nursing needs a classification system to organize its functions and define its scope. Use of such a classification system would expedite research activities and facilitate communication between nurses, consumers, and other health care providers. After all, medicine took over 100 years to develop its taxonomy. Our work, at the national level, was only begun in 1973 and is still in an early stage. It is hoped that the reader will be stimulated to participate at the local, regional, or national level in the utilization and development of these diagnostic categories.

To date the nurse seeking to use nursing diagnosis has had only limited information available. Yet the difficulties nurses face in dealing with nursing diagnoses is reflected in their frequently posed questions:

- What does the label really mean?
- What kinds of assessment questions will yield nursing diagnoses?
- How do I tailor a diagnostic category for a specific individual?
- How should I intervene after I formulate the diagnostic statement?
- How do I care-plan with nursing diagnoses?

This book seeks to answer these questions.

Section I begins with a chapter on the historic etiology of nursing diagnosis and a description of the concept, with its implications for nursing.

Chapter 2 differentiates nursing diagnoses from other problems in which nurses intervene and explains the components of the diagnostic statement.

Chapter 3 focuses on the assessment and problem identification components of the nursing process, with clinical application.

---

*The model of interlocking circles on the cover depicts this relationship. The common area represents those activities on which all professionals collaborate; the rest denotes the independent dimensions for which each professional is responsible.

Chapter 4 describes the process of care planning and presents techniques for writing goals and plans. The evaluation of the plan is also described. Section I concludes with case studies to illustrate care planning.

Section II is a compilation of the nursing diagnostic categories accepted by the North American Nursing Diagnosis Association (formerly the National Group for the Classification of Nursing Diagnosis). Each diagnostic category is explained by the following components:

- Definition
- Etiological and contributing factors
- Defining characteristics
- Focus assessment criteria
- Nursing goals
- Principles and rationale for nursing care

Each diagnostic category is followed by one or more specific nursing diagnoses that relate to familiar clinical situations. These specific diagnoses are defined by subjective and objective assessment data. Outcome criteria for the diagnosis are provided with the related interventions, which represent activities in the independent domain of nursing derived from the physical and applied sciences, pharmacology, nutrition, and mental health.

This book is intended to assist nurses in addressing all the human needs of individuals, with the expectation that—as more "nursing" is added to nursing—the profession, the nurse person, and, most importantly, the client will reap the rewards.

For no other reason than to avoid awkward and redundant reading, the author has chosen to use *she* and *her* when referring to the nurse and *he, his,* and *him* when referring to the client.

The author invites comments or suggestions from readers. Correspondence can be directed to the publisher or to the author's address: 66 East Rattling Run Road, Mickleton, NJ 08056.

Lynda Juall Carpenito, R.N., M.S.N.

# Acknowledgments

A sincere thank-you to all my good friends who sustained our friendships during this demanding project. I wish also to thank my diligent typists Marion Boyle, Janet Olson, and Elizabeth Wagner for their labor at the keys. I am grateful for the professional editorial guidance of Diana Intenzo and Janet Baker at J. B. Lippincott Company.

And last, I would like to thank three special people: my son, Olen J. Carpenito, for sharing his mother; Laura A. Terrill, for her unyielding moral and professional support; and Rosalind Alfaro, who recognized the need for this book and sought to make it a reality.

# Contents

Section II
**Manual of Nursing Diagnoses** 67

Section I

# The Nursing Process

# Introduction

Nursing is "a therapeutic process involving mutual interaction of the nurse, client, and family, collaborating for the achievement of maximum health potential."* This interaction utilizes the nursing process to identify health goals, client strengths and limitations, and available resources to achieve optimal health.

Individuals are open systems who continually interact with the environment, creating individual interaction patterns. These patterns are dynamic and interact with life processes (physiological, psychological, sociocultural, developmental, and spiritual) to influence the individual's behavior and health. A person becomes a client not only when an actual or potential alteration in this interaction pattern compromises his health but also when the person desires assistance to maintain his present optimal level of health.

Nursing diagnosis describes health states or disrupted interaction patterns with which the nurse can assist the client. The nurse provides the primary assistance to clients with these alterations, just as the physician provides primary assistance for medical pathology. Nursing diagnoses focus on the human response as opposed to the cellular response.

Health is the state of wellness as defined by the client; it is no longer defined as to whether or not a biological disease is present. Health is a dynamic, ever-changing state influenced by past and present interaction patterns. The individual is an expert on himself and is responsible for seeking or refusing health care.

The use of the term *client* in place of the term *patient* to identify the health care consumer suggests an autonomous person who has freedom of choice in seeking and selecting assistance. The client is no longer a passive recipient of services but an active participant who assumes responsibility for his choices and also for the consequences of those choices. *Family* is used to describe any person or persons who serve as support systems to the client. Societal health needs have changed in the last decade; so must the nurse's view of the consumers of health care (individual, family, community).†

Nursing diagnosis provides nurses with an opportunity to pinpoint the health alterations of individuals in a concise and systematic manner while also describing the individual's unique situation.

*Carpenito LJ, Duespohl TA: A Guide to Effective Clinical Instruction, p 4. Rockville, MD, Aspen Systems Corp, 1981.
†*Ibid.*

# 1

# Nursing Diagnosis: The Beginning

Nursing diagnosis provides a useful mechanism for structuring nursing knowledge in an attempt to define the unique role and domain of nursing. The quest to define nursing and its functions began with the writings of Nightingale, who described the purpose of nursing as "to put the patient in the best condition for nature to act upon him." In the early 20th century, the attempts to differentiate nursing from medicine stemmed from the need to define each of these disciplines for legislative and educational purposes. V. Henderson in 1955 and F. Abdellah in 1960 proposed to organize nursing curriculums under nursing problems or patient needs, not medical diagnoses.

The trend to focus nursing education on the principal functions of nursing rather than on medicine continues today with the development of nursing models. During the late 1960s and '70s, nurses sought to organize nursing knowledge and practice through the construction of theoretical or conceptual frameworks. Examples of such frameworks are Roy's Adaptation Model, Johnson's Behavioral System Model, Orem's self-care concept of nursing, Rogers's Life Process Theory, and Newman's Health Systems Model. The work of these theorists helped to distinguish nursing phenomena within the broad field of health care.

Criticism of most theories and frameworks usually arises from the difficulty in applying them to clinical practice. In a critique of theory development on nursing, Kritek (p. 34) submits that most nursing theories "describe how nursing should be, not how it is in reality." She notes that the use of poorly defined or confusing terms by theorists serves only to limit professional application of these theories. Kritek advocates beginning with theory that is operational in nature, and describes "what we see and what we do," rather than with one that appears sophisticated but is obscure.

Nursing diagnosis can provide a solution to the quest of nursing because it serves to:

- Define nursing in its present state
- Classify nursing's domain
- Differentiate nursing from medicine

## The Concept of Nursing Diagnosis

In 1953 the term *nursing diagnosis* was introduced by V. Fry to describe a step necessary in developing a nursing care plan. For the next 20 years, references to nursing diagnosis appeared only sporadically in the literature. However, from 1973, when the first meeting of the National Group for the Classification of Nursing Diagnosis was held, to the present, attention in the literature has increased tenfold, and various definitions of nursing diagnosis have appeared, four of which follow. These definitions describe nursing diagnosis as problems, responses, evaluation, or judgment.

**Definitions of Nursing Diagnosis**

- The judgment or conclusion that occurs as a result of nursing assessment (Gebbie)
- An independent nursing function; an evaluation of a client's personal responses to his human experiences throughout the life cycle, be they developmental or accidental crises, illness, hardships, or other stresses (Bircher)
- Actual or potential health problems which nurses, by virtue of their education and experience, are capable and licensed to treat (Gordon)
- Responses to actual or potential health problems which nurses by virtue of their education and experience are able, licensed, and legally responsible and accountable to treat (Moritz)

## Nursing Diagnosis: Process or Outcome?

A review of the literature also reveals that nursing diagnosis has taken on two meanings. Sometimes the term is used to describe the *process of problem-solving*; at other times it means the actual *statement of the problem*. This lack of distinction has created much confusion.

When nursing diagnosis is used to define the process of analyzing data and identifying a problem, the outcome of this process can be both medical problems, which must be referred to physicians, and nursing problems, which can be treated by nurses.

After the first conference on nursing diagnosis in 1973, the term nursing diagnosis was applied to specific labels describing health states that nurses could legally and independently treat. The purpose of establishing these labels was to define and classify the scope of nursing. In this way the term came to represent an *outcome* of the process of identifying problems rather than the process itself. Thus it is important, when using the term nursing diagnosis, to clearly designate whether it represents problem identification (critical thinking) *or* a classification system of diagnostic labels such as that developed by the national conference.

Nursing diagnosis is a statement describing one specific type of problem that nurses identify. It should not be used to label all the problems nurses can ascertain, since such usage will not emphasize the unique role of the nurse. For the purpose of clarity, the use of the term in this book will be restricted to describing the problem label, or outcome. Thus nursing diagnosis is defined as follows:

Nursing diagnosis is a statement that describes a health state or an actual or potential alteration in one's life processes (physiological, psychological, sociocultural, developmental, and spiritual). The nurse uses the nursing process to identify and synthesize clinical data and to order nursing interventions to reduce, eliminate, or prevent (health promotion) health alterations which are in the legal and educational domain of nursing.

## The National Group for the Classification of Nursing Diagnosis

When the first conference on nursing diagnosis was held in 1973, its purpose was to identify nursing functions and to establish a classification system suitable for computerization. From this conference developed the National Group for the Classification of Nursing Diagnosis. This group is composed of nurses from all regions of the United States and Canada, representing all elements of the profession: practice, education, and research. From 1973 to the present, the National Group has met five times and formulated a list of 50 nursing diagnoses. These diagnostic categories are listed in the first column of Table I–1.

At its first meeting in 1973, the National Group also appointed a task force to:

1. Gather information and disseminate it through the Clearinghouse for Nursing Diagnosis.*
2. Encourage educational activities at regional and state levels to promote the implementation of nursing diagnoses. These activities include conferences to organize nurses to identify additional diagnostic labels and workshops to teach nurses about nursing diagnoses.
3. Promote and organize activities to continue the development, classification, and scientific testing of nursing diagnosis. These activities include planning national conferences, identifying criteria for accepting diagnoses, surveying current research activities, and exploring varied methods for classification.

A proposal from the task force for a more formal organization was approved at the fifth national conference. The group, renamed the North American Nursing Diagnosis Association, will continue the development of the diagnostic classification system.

## Why a Taxonomy?

Why does nursing need a classification system, or taxonomy? While perceived reasons will vary according to the individual nurse's focus, nursing in general needs a classification system to develop a sound scientific foundation to fulfill one of the criteria for a profession. A single taxonomy would benefit all nurses regardless of their orientation, whether it be practice, education, or research.

### Practice

Using a classification system to identify nursing's independent domain provides nurses with a common frame of reference. A unified system of terminology will establish a common denominator in helping direct nurses to assess selected data and identify a potential or actual client problem. Nurses can then refer to the list of terms to assist them in describing the problem. Consistent terminology facilitates oral and written communication by making it more efficient. In addition, identifying independent nursing functions will increase the nurse's accountability in assessing, identifying, and treating the diagnosis. Knowledge of the unique responsibilities of nursing will in turn stimulate nurses to acquire new knowledge and skills to intervene in solving these problems.

From the viewpoint of health care delivery, a classification of nursing diagnoses would establish a system suitable for computerization. With the potential for computer use, nursing diagnosis would:

(*text continues on page 9*)

*The Clearinghouse collects material on nursing diagnosis, publishes a newsletter, and coordinates the national conference. The address is: The Clearing House for Nursing Diagnosis, St. Louis University School of Nursing, 3525 Caroline Street, St. Louis, MO 63104.

Table I–1. **Diagnostic Categories**

| Accepted Diagnosis from the Fifth National Conference (1982) | Year Accepted | As on Amended List of Nursing Diagnoses* |
|---|---|---|
| Activity Intolerance | 1982 | |
| Airway Clearance, Ineffective | 1980 | Listed under Alterations in Respiratory Function |
| Anxiety | 1982 | |
| Bowel Elimination, Alterations in: Constipation | 1975 | |
| Bowel Elimination, Alterations in: Diarrhea | 1975 | |
| Bowel Elimination, Alterations in: Incontinence | 1975 | Combined with Bowel Elimination, Alterations in: Diarrhea |
| Breathing patterns, Ineffective | 1980 | Listed under Alterations in Respiratory Function |
| Cardiac Output, Alterations in: Decreased | 1975 | |
| Comfort, Alterations in: Pain | 1978 | |
| Communication, Impaired Verbal | 1978 | |
| Coping, Ineffective Individual | 1980 | |
| Coping, Ineffective Family: Compromised | 1980 | Combined as Coping, Ineffective Family (specify) |
| Coping, Ineffective Family: Disabling | 1980 | Compromised Disabling |
| Coping, Family: Potential for Growth | 1980 | Listed under Alterations in Health Maintenance |
| Diversional Activity Deficit | 1980 | |
| Family Processes, Alterations in | 1982 | |
| Fear (specify) | 1980 | |
| Fluid Volume Deficit, Actual | 1978 | Combined as Fluid Volume Deficit |
| Fluid Volume Deficit, Potential | 1978 | |
| Fluid Volume Excess | 1982 | |
| Gas Exchange, Impaired | 1980 | Listed under Alterations in Respiratory Function |
| Grieving, Anticipatory | 1980 | Combined as Grieving (specify) |
| Grieving, Dysfunctional | 1980 | |
| Health Maintenance, Alterations in | 1982 | |
| Home Maintenance Management, Impaired | 1978 | |

Table I-1. **Diagnostic Categories** (continued)

| Accepted Diagnosis from the Fifth National Conference (1982) | Year Accepted | As on Amended List of Nursing Diagnoses* |
|---|---|---|
| Injury, Potential for (specify) | 1980 | |
| Poisoning | | |
| Suffocation | | |
| Trauma | | |
| Knowledge Deficit (specify) | 1980 | |
| Mobility, Impaired Physical | 1980 | |
| Noncompliance (specify) | 1973, 1980 | |
| Nutrition, Alterations in: Less Than Body Requirements | 1978 | |
| Nutrition, Alterations in: More Than Body Requirements | 1978 | *Combined as* Nutrition, Alterations in: More Than Body Requirements |
| Nutrition, Alterations in: Potential for More Than Body Requirements | 1980 | |
| Oral Mucous Membrane, Alterations in | 1982 | |
| Parenting, Alterations in: Actual | 1978 | *Combined as* |
| Parenting, Alterations in: Potential | 1978 | Parenting, Alterations in |
| Powerlessness | 1982 | |
| Rape Trauma Syndrome | 1980 | Respiratory Function, Alterations in Airway Clearance, Ineffective Breathing Patterns, Ineffective Gas Exchange, Impaired |
| Self-Care Deficit: Total | 1980 | |
| Feeding | | |
| Bathing/hygiene | | |
| Dressing/grooming | | |
| Toileting | | |
| Self-Concept, Disturbance in | 1980 | |

*Where no category is given, the title is unchanged.

(continued)

Table I–1. **Diagnostic Categories** (continued)

| Accepted Diagnosis from the Fifth National Conference (1982) | Year Accepted | As on Amended List of Nursing Diagnoses * |
|---|---|---|
| Sensory-Perceptual Alterations: | 1975, 1980 | |
| Visual | | |
| Auditory | | |
| Kinesthetic | | |
| Gustatory | | |
| Tactile | | |
| Olfactory | | |
| Sexual Dysfunction | 1980 | |
| Skin Integrity, Impairment of, Actual | 1975 | Combined as Skin Integrity, Impairment of |
| Skin Integrity, Impairment of, Potential | 1975 | |
| Sleep Pattern Disturbance | 1980 | |
| Social Isolation | 1982 | |
| Spiritual Distress | 1980 | |
| Thought Processes, Alterations in | 1973 | |
| Tissue Perfusion, Alteration in: | 1980 | |
| Cerebral | | |
| Cardiopulmonary | | |
| Renal | | |
| Gastrointestinal | | |
| Peripheral | | |
| Urinary Elimination, Alteration in Patterns of | 1980 | |
| Violence, Potential for | 1980 | |

*Where no category is given, the title is unchanged.

- Provide nurses with a system to retrieve client records using nursing, not medical diagnoses
- Provide an opportunity for nurses to develop or be included in a computerized health care information system which would collect, analyze, and synthesize nursing data from practice, literature, and research
- Provide a mechanism for reimbursement of nursing activities related to nursing diagnoses, not just medical diagnoses

Clarifying nursing for nurses, employers, the public, and third-party payers can only serve to strengthen and enrich the profession.

## Education and Research

A taxonomy of nursing diagnosis would provide a framework for clinical investigation with the potential for growth in research and knowledge. Each diagnostic category—its defining characteristics as well as the related nursing interventions—should be developed and tested through research.

In education, nursing diagnosis will assist educators and students to focus on nursing phenomena rather than on medical phenomena. It challenges students to think critically rather than simply to assume that because a client has a particular medical diagnosis, certain nursing actions are always warranted.

Nurses have little difficulty in identifying problems that are directly related to medical diagnoses and with implementing the medical regime. Often the nurse focuses primarily on identifying and treating medical problems. The use of nursing diagnoses permits the nurse to go beyond the medical model and identify those problems that may or may not be related to the medical diagnoses. By relinquishing the practice of medicine to physicians, nurses can assume more completely their unique role as health care providers.

The steps that have been taken toward the development of a nursing taxonomy have been small, but at least they have been taken. The future movement on taxonomic development is linked, says Gebbie, "with the movement toward professional and scientific maturity, and each feeds on the other" (p. 12).

## The Classification Process

Classification systems for other professionals (such as physicians, biologists, and pharmacists) developed over hundreds of years; nurses have only just begun. It is a slow and difficult process. Since nursing cannot stop and wait until the classification is complete, practice must continue while the classification evolves.

Two research methods can be used to identify and validate nursing diagnosis nomenclature, the inductive and the deductive. The inductive approach moves from specific observations to generalizations; it is a generalization based on observed relationships. The nurse's observations and additional support cited from related literature serve as a basis for a tentative explanation of the relationship. A prediction can then be derived to test the association. The deductive approach, on the other hand, begins with generalizations and moves toward specific observations.

Presently, the National Group uses the inductive method to generate nursing diagnoses. Nurses with various clinical and educational experience collaborate to identify and describe health problems that nurses diagnose and treat. These nurses recall from their experiences and from the related literature those clinical phenomena that describe varied states of health. Signs and symptoms (defining characteristics) are identified to describe these states. It would be expected that this approach would initially yield fairly general diagnostic categories that could be used by most nurses. As the work continues, more clinical studies must be promoted to validate and refine the work.

Nurses using the National Group's diagnostic categories will note variations in the level of conceptualization. Some nurses have accused the list of being too broad or too restrictive, and certain diagnoses as being too medical, too abstract, or too unfamiliar. Some nurses are philosophically opposed to the use of such diagnoses as *Sensory-Perceptual Alterations* or *Noncompliance.*

In any classification system there is certain to be some disagreement over a particular item, but it has always been the individual's prerogative simply not to use that item. For example, in medicine a physician may disagree with the diagnosis *schizophrenia* and will refrain from using it in his practice. This physician does not reject the entire medical classification system, only one diagnosis. And systems change. When the medical classification system was still evolving, dropsy was listed as an accepted diagnosis; years later, it was removed.

If nursing is to become a full profession, it needs to develop and accept one classification system for those functions and responsibilities that are solely those of the nurse. Individual practitioners who are uncomfortable with the list should use only those labels that have meaning for them and add diagnoses to describe the other clinical alterations they treat. The use of the list by these nurses will help to refine and expand it. New proposed diagnostic categories can then be submitted to the National Group for consideration. (Guidelines for preparing diagnostic categories appear in Appendix II.) The task of developing additional diagnostic categories should be the responsibility of nurses from all practice and educational settings.

## Diagnostic Category Components

Each diagnostic category from the National Group has three components: the title (label), the etiological and contributing factors, and the defining characteristics.

### Title

The title, or label, offers a concise description of the state (actual, potential) of the individual's health. Qualifying terms such as *alterations, impaired, deficit,* and *ineffective* reflect a change in health status but do not label the degree of change. These terms are used in place of more subjective qualifying words such as maladaptive, poor, and inappropriate.

### Etiological and Contributing Factors

The etiological and contributing factors are those physiological, situational, and maturational factors that can cause the problem or influence its development.

### Defining Characteristics

Defining characteristics are a cluster of signs and symptoms that are observed in the person with the problem. All the defining characteristics need not be present to use the label.

To illustrate these components, let us take the nursing diagnosis *Impaired Physical Mobility* and list the etiology and the defining characteristics.

#### Impaired Physical Mobility

*Etiological and Contributing Factors*
Imposed limitations of movement within the environment

*Defining Characteristics*
Inability to move
Reluctance to attempt movement
Perceived inability to move
Goals incongruent with abilities
Altered perception of position of body part(s)
Altered perception of presence of body part(s)
Alteration in coordination of movement
Limited active range of motion
Decreased muscle strength or control
Imposed restrictions of movement

Even with defining characteristics and etiological factors for each diagnostic category, nurses continue to have difficulty utilizing nursing diagnoses, as illustrated by the questions cited in the Preface:

- What does the label really mean?
- What kinds of assessment questions will yield nursing diagnoses?
- How do I tailor a diagnostic category for a specific individual?
- How should I intervene after I formulate the diagnostic statement?
- How do I care plan with nursing diagnoses?

In order to help the nurse use nursing diagnoses, Section II of this book, Manual of Nursing Diagnoses, has been designed so that each diagnostic category is described in terms of

- Definition
- Etiological and contributing factors
- Defining characteristics
- Focus assessment criteria (subjective and objective)
- Nursing goals
- Principles and rationale for nursing care

Each diagnostic category is further described in terms of one or more specific nursing diagnoses within the category. For example, take the diagnostic category *Impairment of Skin Integrity*. A specific diagnosis under this category would be *Impairment of Skin Integrity Related to Pruritus.*
Each specific diagnosis is explained in terms of

- Assessment data (subjective and objective)
- Outcome criteria
- Clinical nursing interventions

Thus Section II provides an explanation of each diagnostic category, along with related interventions that will assist the nurse to apply nursing diagnoses in clinical practice.

## Organizational Frameworks

As previously mentioned, there are presently 50 diagnostic categories accepted by the North American Nursing Diagnosis Association. The group has arranged the list alphabetically by the operational word in each category, and it will remain as such until an organizing framework is developed.

However, for purposes of consistency, some organizational changes to the national list have been introduced in this book (see right-hand column of Table I–1). No categories have been deleted, but certain multiple diagnoses have been combined under one diagnostic category. For example, two diagnostic categories listed by the National Group as *Ineffective Family Coping: Compromised* and *Ineffective Family Coping: Disabling* have been combined into one: *Ineffective Family Coping*.

In the instance of *Alterations in Parenting: Actual* and *Alterations in Parenting: Potential*, a single diagnosis has been devised: *Alterations in Parenting*. The same approach has been taken in formulating the three diagnoses *Alterations in Fluid Volume, Alterations in Nutrition, More Than Body Requirements*, and *Impairment in Skin Integrity*. In addition, the diagnoses related to respiratory function (*Ineffective Airway Clearance, Ineffective Breathing Pattern*, and *Impaired Gas Exchange*) have been combined under the general category *Alterations in Respiratory Function*.

## Functional Health Framework

Marjory Gordon has developed a framework for organizing a nursing assessment based on function, in order to organize the diagnostic category and standardize data collection. The functional health patterns covered are:

1. Health perception–health management pattern
2. Nutritional-metabolic pattern
3. Elimination pattern
4. Activity-exercise pattern
5. Sleep-rest pattern
6. Cognitive-perceptual pattern
7. Self-perception pattern
8. Role-relationship pattern
9. Sexuality-reproductive pattern
10. Coping–stress tolerance pattern
11. Value-belief pattern

The current diagnostic categories are grouped under a functional health pattern in Table I–2.

This standardization of assessment data should not interfere with the nurse's theoretical or philosophical beliefs. It directs the nurse to the data that should be collected, not to the approach that should be used in interpreting the data or determining the interventions. Thus the nurse who subscribes to Roy's adaptation framework, Orem's self-care model, or Rogers's life process model can use the functional health pattern framework developed by Gordon (p. 80) to gather baseline data. From that point, she can continue with her individual framework after collecting the initial data.

The data base assessment guide presented in Appendix I is organized under functional health patterns. It is designed to assist the nurse to gather initial data. Should questions arise under a pattern, the nurse is instructed to gather more data about the diagnostic category by using the assessment criteria under the category. These additional data are based on a focus assessment, a procedure that will be discussed in Chapters 2 and 3.

## Summary

Nursing diagnoses provide a method for describing a client's health status in a clear and concise way to enhance communication and recognition. Difficulty in formulating diagnostic statements can be greatly reduced if the nurse uses the list of nursing diagnoses from the National Group for the majority of diagnostic statements. Those altered states that cannot be described by the current list of labels can be stated us-

Table I–2. **Nursing Diagnosis List Grouped Under Functional Health Patterns\***

| Functional Pattern | Diagnosis |
| --- | --- |
| 1. Health perception–health management | Health maintenance, alterations in<br>Noncompliance<br>Potential for injury |
| 2. Nutritional–metabolic | Fluid volume deficit<br>Fluid volume excess<br>Nutrition, alterations in, less than body require-<br>ments<br>Nutrition, alterations in, more than body re-<br>quirements<br>Oral mucous membrane, alterations in<br>Skin integrity, impairment of |
| 3. Elimination | Bowel elimination, alterations in: constipation<br>Bowel elimination, alterations in: diarrhea<br>Bowel elimination, alterations in: incontinence<br>Urinary elimination, alteration in patterns of |
| 4. Activity–exercise | Activity intolerance<br>Airway clearance, ineffective<br>Breathing patterns, ineffective<br>Cardiac output, alterations in: decreased<br>Diversional activity deficit<br>Gas exchange, impaired<br>Home maintenance management, impaired<br>Mobility, impaired physical<br>Respiratory function, alterations in<br>Self-care deficit<br>  Total<br>  Feeding<br>  Bathing/hygiene<br>  Dressing/grooming<br>  Toileting<br>Tissue perfusion, alteration in<br>  Cerebral<br>  Cardiopulmonary<br>  Renal<br>  Gastrointestinal<br>  Peripheral |
| 5. Sleep–rest | Sleep pattern disturbance |
| 6. Cognitive–perceptual | Comfort, alterations in: pain<br>Knowledge deficit (specify)<br>Sensory-perceptual alterations<br>  Visual<br>  Auditory<br>  Kinesthetic<br>  Gustatory<br>  Tactile<br>  Olfactory |

(*continued*)

Table I–2.   **Nursing Diagnosis List Grouped Under Functional Health Patterns***
(*continued*)

| Functional Pattern | Diagnosis |
|---|---|
| | Thought processes, alterations in |
| 7.  Self–perception | Anxiety |
| | Fear |
| | Powerlessness |
| | Self-concept, disturbance in |
| 8.  Role–relationship | Communication, impaired verbal |
| | Family processes, alterations in |
| | Grieving (specify) |
| | Parenting, alterations in |
| | Social isolation |
| | Violence, potential for |
| 9.  Sexuality–reproductive | Sexual dysfunction |
| | Rape trauma syndrome |
| 10.  Coping–stress tolerance | Coping, ineffective individual |
| | Coping, ineffective family |
| 11.  Value–belief | Spiritual distress |

*The functional health patterns were identified by M. Gordon in Nursing Diagnosis: Process and Application (New York, McGraw-Hill, 1982) with some minor changes by the author. This nursing diagnosis list reflects the author's adoption of the National Accepted List. The author has deleted the listing of *actual* and *potential* next to a diagnostic category, since most diagnoses can be utilized as an actual or potential label.

ing guidelines to be presented in Chapter 2. Nurses are encouraged to submit new diagnostic labels to the National Group.

The use of nursing diagnoses can stimulate nurses to explore interaction patterns that were previously ignored or unknown and to address all the human needs of individuals, with the expectation that the nurse and, most importantly, the client will reap the rewards.

## References

Bircher A: On the development and classification of nursing diagnoses. Nurs Forum 14:10–29, 1975

Fry VS: The creative approach to nursing. Am J Nurs 53:301–302, 1953

Gebbie K: Toward the theory development for nursing diagnoses classification. In Kim MJ, Moritz DA (eds): Classification of Nursing Diagnoses, p. 12. New York, McGraw-Hill, 1982

Gordon M: Historical perspective: The National Group for classification of nursing diagnoses. In Kim MJ, Moritz DA (eds): Classification of Nursing Diagnoses, p. 3. New York, McGraw-Hill 1982

Kritek PB: The generation and the classification of nursing diagnoses: Toward a theory of nursing. Image 10(2):33–40, 1978

## 2

# Differentiating Nursing Diagnosis from Other Client Problems

### The Dimensions of Nursing

Nursing can be viewed as consisting of three dimensions: dependent, interdependent, and independent. Each dimension is characterized by the level to which the nurse is involved as decision-maker.

### Dependent Dimension

The dependent dimension of nursing practice involves those problems that are the direct responsibility of the physician, who designates the interventions for the nurse to follow. The term we will use to describe such a problem is *clinical medical problem*. The nursing responsibilities in relationship to clinical medical problems are to implement the prescribed medical regimen. The dependent dimension represents interventions that the nurse cannot legally prescribe.

Examples of clinical medical problems are:

| *Treatment* | *Medical Diagnosis* |
|---|---|
| Swan–Ganz monitoring | Toxemia |
| Fetal monitoring | Diabetes mellitus |
| Medications | |

### Interdependent Dimension

The interdependent dimension of nursing refers to those problems or clinical situations that nurses and other health care professionals, most frequently physicians, collaborate to prescribe and treat. These problems will be described by the term *clinical nursing problems*. For example, hypoglycemia in a person with diabetes is both a medical and a nursing problem. However, the physician focuses on insulin dosage, while the nurse focuses on early detection and response to treatment.

Examples of clinical medical problems and their related clinical nursing problems are:

| *Clinical Medical Problem* | *Medical Order* | *Clinical Nursing Problem* | *Nursing Order* |
|---|---|---|---|
| Levin tube | Irrigate tube q 2 hours with 30 cc saline | Potential aspiration | Ascertain position of Levin tube in the stomach prior to irrigation by aspirating for gastric secretions |

15

| Clinical Medical Problem | Medical Order | Clinical Nursing Problem | Nursing Order |
|---|---|---|---|
| Diabetes mellitus | NPH Insulin 40 units S.C. o.d. in A.M. | Potential hypo- glycemia in early P.M. | Observe for signs of hy- poglycemia, especially between 2 to 4 P.M. Offer 4 oz of orange juice if signs ap- pear |

Thus, for clarity, clinical nursing problems and clinical medical problems are grouped under the term clinical problems.

## Independent Dimension

The independent dimension of nursing practice involves those clinical situations or problems that are the direct responsibility of the nurse, who selects the interventions to prevent, reduce, or alleviate the problem. These interventions can be ordered independently and legally by the nurse. The term to describe these problems is *nursing diagnosis*. To repeat the definition given in Chapter 1, nursing diagnosis is a *statement* that describes a health state or an actual or potential alteration in one's life processes (physiological, psychological, sociocultural, developmental, or spiritual). The nurse uses the nursing process *to identify and synthesize clinical data* and *to order nursing interventions* to reduce, eliminate, or prevent (health promotion) health alterations which are *in the legal and educational domain of nursing*.

## Criteria for Nursing Diagnoses

A discussion of the italicized elements of the definition helps to clarify and restrict the use of the term *nursing diagnosis*.

*Statement:* Involves the outcome of an assessment.

*To identify and synthesize clinical data:* Implies the complex problem-solving that goes into analyzing the data, followed by the systematic testing of several possible alternatives.

*To order nursing interventions:* Describes the nurse as the primary prescriber of the nursing activities needed to reduce, eliminate, or prevent the altered interaction pattern or to maintain the present health state.

*In the legal and educational domain of nursing:* Differentiates nursing diagnoses from medical diagnoses, since nurses cannot legally diagnose or prescribe for medical diagnoses.

As discussed previously, some interventions for clinical nursing problems are not ordered by physicians but are implied by the nature of the clinical medical problem. With this consideration the nurse may at first have difficulty in differentiating clinical problems from nursing diagnoses.

In order to help the nurse distinguish between clinical problems (medical or nursing) and nursing diagnoses, four criteria questions have been developed. They are listed below. In order for a problem to qualify as a nursing diagnosis, each question must be answered affirmatively.

---

**Criteria Questions**

1. Does identification or treatment of the problem require complex analysis of data or complex interventions?
2. Can the nurse identify the problem legally and educationally?
3. Can the nurse legally order the necessary interventions to treat or prevent the problem?
4. Can the nurse legally treat the problem?

---

Using these criteria, the nurse can differentiate clinical nursing problems from nursing diagnoses, as illustrated in the following case studies.

## Case Study 1

Mr. Smith is a 35-year-old male admitted for a possible concussion after a car accident, with a physician's order for

- Clear liquid diet
- Neurological assessment q 1 hour

On admission the nurse records

- Is oriented and alert
- Pupils at 6 mm, equal and reactive to light
- B.P. 120/72, pulse 84, resp 20, temp 99° F

Two hours later the nurse records

- Vomiting
- Restlessness
- Pupils at 6 cm, equal, with a sluggish response to light
- B.P. 140/60, pulse 65, resp 12, temp 99° F

*Problem:* Possible increased intracranial pressure.

## Case Study 2

Mr. Green is a 45-year-old male with a cholecystectomy incision (10 days postop). The incision is not healing, and there is continual purulent drainage. The nursing care consists of

- Inspecting and cleansing the incision and the surrounding area q 8 hours
- Applying Stomahesive and drainage pouch to contain drainage and protect skin
- Promoting optimal nutrition and hydration to enhance healing

*Problem:* Impairment in skin integrity related to draining purulent wound.

Let us now apply the four criteria questions to Case 1 and Case 2.

| Criteria Question | Case 1 | Case 2 |
|---|---|---|
| Does the identification or treatment require complex analysis or complex interventions? | Yes | Yes |
| Can the nurse identify the problem legally and educationally? | Yes | Yes |
| Can the nurse legally order the necessary interventions to treat or prevent the problem? | No | Yes |
| Can the nurse legally treat the problem? | No | Yes |

Case 1 does not meet the criteria for a nursing diagnosis and is therefore a clinical problem.

Since each individual is unique, it is difficult to develop exclusive criteria that will always differentiate nursing diagnoses from other client problems. Ultimately, the decision to use or not to use the diagnostic label will rest with the individual nurse until more refined defining characteristics for each category are developed and tested.

Learning to formulate nursing diagnoses is a skill that requires knowledge and practice. The nurse needs to familiarize herself with the diagnostic categories and their components. Certain ones such as *Alterations in Bowel Elimination* and *Alterations in Nutrition* are familiar to most nurses and thus will be easier to use. Section II provides specific information on each category to increase a working knowledge of that diagnosis.

## The Diagnostic Statement

### Two-Part Statement

The diagnostic statement should be a two-part statement consisting of the diagnostic title linked with the etiological and contributing factors. Examples include:

- Spiritual Distress related to a belief that illness is God's punishment
- Potential for Injury: Trauma related to an unstable gait secondary to arthritis
- Alteration in Bowel Elimination: Constipation related to immobility secondary to traction

### "Related to"

The use of the words *related to* reflects a relationship between the first and the second parts of the statement. It is important that the nurse not link the statements with words implying cause and effect, because such a relationship can result in legal or professional difficulty. Examples of such errors are:

- Impairment of Skin Integrity: Pressure sores caused by infrequent turning
- Potential for Injury due to the mother's frequently leaving the children at home unsupervised

On the other hand, using the diagnostic label by itself without a *related to* etiological or contributing factor would result in a vaguely stated problem that is not specific enough to direct individualized interventions.

The more specific the second part of the statement, the more specialized the interventions can be. The linking of the diagnostic category with contributing factors also assists the nurse in validating the category. For example, the diagnostic category *Noncompliance* when stated by itself usually conveys the negative implication that the client is not cooperating. When the nurse relates the noncompliance to a factor, this diagnosis can transmit a very different message. For example:

- Noncompliance with prescribed medicine regime related to the side-effects of the drug (reduced libido, fatigue)
- Noncompliance related to inability to understand the need for weekly blood pressure measurements

If the defining characteristics of a diagnostic category are present but the etiological and contributing factors are unknown, the statement can be written as:

- Fear related to unknown etiology
- Ineffective Family Coping: Manifested by anger at staff related to unknown etiology

The use of the term *unknown etiology* alerts the nurse and other members of the nursing staff to assess for contributing factors at the same time as they are intervening for the present manifestation.

Three diagnostic categories may pose an exception to the need to use the phrase *related to*. These are:

- Alterations in Cardiac Output: Decreased
- Alteration in Tissue Perfusion
- Rape Trauma Syndrome

Since a nursing diagnosis must describe a problem in the independent domain of nursing, adding *related to* to the foregoing diagnoses usually describes a situation that nurses cannot legally diagnose and treat:

- Alteration in Cardiac Output: Decreased, related to congestive heart failure
- Alteration in Tissue Perfusion: Renal, related to chronic renal failure

In order to use either of these two categories within the context of nursing diagnosis, the nurse must assess the effect of the alteration on life processes. Once identified, this effect can be linked with the label, as follows:

- Alterations in Cardiac Output: Decreased: Exercise intolerance
- Alteration in Tissue Perfusion: Renal: Fatigability and anorexia
- Alteration in Tissue Perfusion: Peripheral, secondary to peripheral arterial disease: Pain

A nurse can treat exercise intolerance, fatigability, anorexia, and pain independently, but not alterations in tissue perfusion or cardiac output.

Linking the diagnostic category *Rape Trauma Syndrome* with an etiological or contributing factor would only be repetitive (Rape Trauma Syndrome related to rape). As with the other two categories, the nurse must assess the responses of the individual's life processes after rape and link them to the category, as:

- Rape Trauma Syndrome: Difficulty in getting to sleep and remaining asleep.

However, *Rape Trauma Syndrome* can be used without a *related to*, to describe the multidimensional problems of rape.

## Actual, Potential, and Possible Nursing Diagnoses

The terms *actual*, *potential*, and *possible* describe the present state of an existing problem.

## Actual

The use of a nursing diagnosis without the word *possible* or *potential* means that the problem has been clinically validated by identifiable defining characteristics. An example of an actual nursing diagnosis is:

### Sexual Dysfunction Related to Loss of Body Part: Mastectomy

*Defining Characteristics* (present to validate)
Relates that she refused to let husband see her without undergarments
Reports no sexual activity (foreplay, intercourse) since surgery 5 months ago
Reports a previous pattern of sexual activity 5 to 7 times a month

## Potential

A potential nursing diagnosis describes an altered state that may occur if certain nursing interventions are not ordered and implemented. Defining characteristics are not present, but etiological and contributing factors are present. These interventions are preventive in nature. For example:

### Potential Impaired Gas Exchange related to
Postop immobility
Postanesthesia
Ineffective diaphragmatic movement (obesity)

*Etiological and Contributing Factors*
Somnolence (postanesthesia)
Inability to cough up secretions (pain)
Obesity (5 ft 2 in, 240 lb)

The use of the term *potential* with a nursing diagnosis can also describe a state in which health promotion activities are needed, as illustrated with:

### Potential Alteration in Nutrition: Less Than Body Requirements, related to adolescent eating patterns and lack of knowledge regarding diet during pregnancy

*Etiological and Contributing Factors*
Primagravida, 17 years old
Diet history
Breakfast: none
Lunch: sandwich, soda
Dinner: meat, vegetable, potato, soda
Snacks: potato chips, candy bars

## Possible

The word *possible* is used in nursing diagnoses to describe problems that may be present but that require additional data to be confirmed or ruled out. *Possible* serves to alert nurses to the need for additional data. Usually, defining characteristics have not been identified but the presence of factors that can contribute to the problem is confirmed. For example:

### Possible Sexual Dysfunction related to the effects of abdominal perineal surgical resection on the ability to have or sustain an erection

*Etiological and Contributing Factors*
Recent abdominal perineal resection

## Statement Variations

Although the diagnostic statement should be worded as concisely as possible, the nurse may need to resort to an expanded statement because of the number or complexity of the contributing factors. It is more important that the diagnostic statement direct specific interventions than that it be short. For example:

**Alteration in Nutrition: Less Than Body Requirements related to**
Nausea and vomiting
Stomatitis
Anorexia secondary to chemotherapy

**Potential Impairment in Skin Integrity related to**
Immobility
Dehydration
Incontinence

To direct specific interventions for each diagnosis, the nurse identifying the foregoing would probably also consider:

**Impaired Physical Mobility related to prescribed bed rest**

**Fluid Volume Deficit related to decreased fluid intake related to inability to hold a glass**

**Alterations in Oral Mucous Membrane related to impaired tissue perfusion secondary to chemotherapy**

**Alteration in Patterns of Urinary Elimination: Incontinence, related to**
Previous catheterization (post-CVA)
Dehydration

## Errors in Diagnostic Statements

The nursing diagnostic statement will reflect either some alteration in the individual's health state, related to factors that have contributed or could contribute to its development, or a healthy state that may be threatened. As with any other new skill, the writing of diagnostic statements takes practice and probably will not be completely without error. Remember to refer to the four criteria questions previously presented to help differentiate a nursing diagnosis from a clinical problem. You may formulate your own diagnostic category if one of the current categories does not accurately describe the problem. This diagnostic label should be shared with nurse colleagues to validate it.

In an attempt to increase the accuracy and usefulness of the statement (plus reduce the nurse's frustration), some common errors of diagnostic statements should be avoided.

## Common Statement Errors

Nursing diagnoses are *not*:

- Medical diagnoses—e.g., diabetes mellitus
- Medical pathology—e.g., decrease cerebral tissue oxygenation
- Treatments or equipment—e.g., hyperalimentation, Levin tube
- Diagnostic studies—e.g., cardiac catheterization

| Date | Diagnosis | Plan |
|------|-----------|------|
| 9/23 | Fear related to scheduled myelogram | 1. Allow her to share her concerns about the procedure. Correct all misconceptions. |
| | Signs and symptoms: | 2. Explain in detail: Pretest preparation |
| | Stated "I am afraid something terrible will happen." | Procedure Sensations Positions during test Medications |
| | "My neighbor had a myelogram and suffered with a headache for a month afterward." | Post-test procedure Position restrictions Fluid replacement Assessments (vital signs, motor and sensory function) |
| | | 3. Explain that water-soluble contrast agents now used are less likely to produce headaches because they are reabsorbed more readily. |

**Figure I–1.** Diagnostic label with supporting defining characteristics.

The nurse, however, may assess for the response of the individual to the above situations and may validate a nursing diagnosis as:

**Knowledge Deficit related to the relationship of activity to insulin and diet requirements in diabetes mellitus**

Nursing diagnostic statements should *not* be written in terms of:

- Cues—e.g., crying, hemoglobin level
- Inferences—e.g., dyspnea

- Goals—e.g., should perform own colostomy care
- Client needs—e.g., needs to walk every shift; needs to express fears
- Nursing needs—e.g., change dressing; check blood pressure

Avoid legally inadvisable or judgmental statements, such as:

- Fear related to frequent beatings by her husband
- Ineffective Family Coping related to mother-in-law's continual harassment of daughter-in-law
- Potential Alteration in Parenting related to low IQ of mother
- Noncompliance related to failure to return for follow-up visits

Avoid statements that cannot be supported or validated with defining characteristics. In an attempt to prevent this error, you can document the supporting defining characteristics (signs and symptoms) with the appropriate diagnostic label in the nurse's notes or on the plan of care. An example of this documentation appears in Figure I–1.

## Summary

Nursing is viewed as consisting of three dimensions—independent, interdependent, and dependent—each of which represents the level to which the nurse is involved in prescribing interventions. Nursing diagnoses represent those problems in the independent dimension that nurses are responsible to diagnose, prescribe for, and treat. The interventions for clinical medical problems are ordered by physicians, while clinical nursing problems require collaborative prescribing.

The differentiation of nursing diagnoses from clinical problems provides nurses with a framework to describe nursing practice.

# 3

# Deriving Nursing Diagnoses: Assessment and Problem Identification

Nursing diagnosis cannot be taken out of the context of the nursing process. To do so would result in a misuse of the concept and would lead to premature labeling or stereotyping. This in turn would interfere with accurate and careful observations and result in inappropriate nursing interventions.

Each client is an autonomous and precious person who interacts in a unique manner with his environment and must be assessed within the context of his uniqueness. Because nursing diagnoses are derived from these assessments and because people are continually interacting with their environment, the nurse must apply the process in a continuous round of assessment, planning, implementing, and evaluating.

## The Nursing Process

After a client has entered the health-care setting (home, office, clinic, hospital), the nurse uses systematic observational and problem-solving techniques to identify potential problems and appropriate interventions and to evaluate the effectiveness of these interventions. The nursing process describes this method, for through its five components—assessment, problem identification, planning, intervention, and evaluation—it sets the practice of nursing in motion.

The professional acknowledgment that the nursing process is pivotal to nursing is made evident by the fact that it is included in the definition of nursing in most nurse practice acts and in the conceptual framework of most curriculums. Despite this emphasis, many nurses fail to apply the process systematically in their practice. The expertise and efficiency of nursing interventions are dependent on the accurate utilization of the nursing process. A nurse who is expert in this problem-solving technique can intervene in a skillful and successful manner with clients in a variety of settings.

The depth and breadth of the knowledge of the individual nurse will directly influence the suitability and relevance of the care given. Students with a limited knowledge base can learn the nursing process by focusing initially on a selected area. As they gain more knowledge and experience, they can then increase their process skills. Experienced nurses can enhance their process skills by identifying areas that were previously avoided or misunderstood.

## Assessment

Assessment, the first phase of the nursing process, is the deliberate and systematic collection of data to determine a client's current health status and to evaluate his present and past coping patterns. Data is obtained through four methods:

- Interview
- Physical examination
- Observation
- Review of records and diagnostic reports

The purpose of collecting data is to identify the client's

- Present and past health status
- Present and past coping patterns (strengths and limitations)
- Response to present alterations
- Response to therapy (nursing, medical)
- Risk for potential alteration developments

Nurses collect data to determine nurse activities and to assist other professionals (pharmacists, nutritionists, social workers, physicians) in determining their activities. It is therefore important that health care professionals freely exchange data about their clients in order to increase the quality and the validity of health care. For example, a nurse assesses the signs of orthostatic hypotension in a client. The problem is referred to the physician to investigate the cause and determine the treatment. The nurse plans nursing activities to help the client reduce those factors that contribute to the vertigo and also to prevent injury.

Unfortunately, many nurses primarily gather physiological data for other professionals to use and ignore the other life processes, those which involve psychological, sociocultural, developmental, and spiritual considerations. From a holistic view, an understanding of the interaction patterns in all five areas is needed to identify the individual's strengths and limitations and help him achieve an optimal level of health. Ignoring any of the life processes can result in frustration and failure for all concerned.

As with the other components of the nursing process, the assessment process is dynamic and ongoing. During every nurse–client interaction, the nurse is continually processing data. The types of data gathered are dependent on the nurse's knowledge base, experience, and philosophy.

## Data Collection Formats

Data collection usually consists of two formats, the nursing data-base interview and the focus assessment, each of which can be used either alone or in conjunction with the other.

### Data-Base Interview

The data-base interview involves the collection of a predetermined set of facts during the initial contact with the client. This interview should gather data in all five life processes to determine patterns, strengths, and alterations. The assessment criteria in the data-base interview should be clear and concise in order to provide the nurse with a tool to gather data in a systematic and efficient manner. This interview should not duplicate data gathered by other professionals; the focus should clearly be nursing. Appendix I represents a sample nursing data-base interview designed for nurses in an acute care setting. It can be modified if either the setting or the client requires additional data.

### Focus Assessment

Focus assessment is the acquisition of selected or specific data as determined by the nurse and the client or family or by the condition of the client. A focus assessment can take a few minutes or a longer period of time. The nurse who assesses the condition of a new postoperative client (vital signs, incision, hydration, comfort) is performing a focus assessment.

A focus assessment can also be carried out during the initial interview if the data collected suggest a possible problem area that needs to be validated or ruled out. In Section II, each diagnostic category is described in terms of focus assessment criteria to identify specific data that may need to be collected to confirm or rule out the diagnosis. These focus assessment criteria can be used in conjunction with the data-base interview or in an isolated situation requiring additional information. Focus assessments can yield clinical problems (*e.g.*, postoperative hypovolemia) or nursing diagnoses (*e.g.*, anxiety).

## The Assessment Process

In order to perform an accurate assessment, the nurse must have the ability to:

- Communicate effectively
- Observe systematically
- Perform a nursing physical assessment
- Differentiate between cues and inferences
- Identify interaction patterns
- Validate impressions

### Communicating Effectively

All nurse–client interactions are based on communication. The term *therapeutic communication* is used to describe techniques that provide an opportunity for the client or family to share views and feelings openly. The technique incorporates verbal and nonverbal skills as well as empathy and a sense of caring. Verbal techniques include asking closed- and open-ended questions, reflecting on the answers, and summarizing the content for the client. Nonverbal techniques include active listening and the use of silence, touch, and eye contact. Active listening, which is most vital in data collection, is also the most difficult skill to learn. Few people listen objectively but tend to concentrate on their own forthcoming responses rather than on what the other person is saying.

Learning effective communication skills requires knowledge of self and of communication and learning theory as well as continuous practice. Above all, it calls for the determination to retain sensitivity, which is often lost as one develops more advanced communication skills (Ramackers).

### Observing Systematically

The ability to observe systematically is dependent on the nurse's knowledge base. With increased knowledge about human interaction, the nurse will look for specific data. Knowing what contributes to or causes a particular problem enables the nurse to explore these areas with the client. Systematic observations can be enhanced when written guidelines are used. Such guidelines are invaluable because they identify the specific types of data that need to be collected. Once you become familiar with the guidelines, you can gather the data without referring to a written guide.

For each diagnostic category listed in Section II, a focus assessment is presented to direct the nurse to gather data in order to confirm or rule out the nursing diagnosis. Each specific nursing diagnosis has its assessment signs and symptoms to further assist in diagnosing.

## Performing a Nursing Physical Assessment

Physical assessment is the collection of objective data concerning the client's physical status. The techniques used include inspection, palpation, percussion, and auscultation. Physical assessment incorporates the examination of an individual from head to toe with a focus on the body systems.

To determine the purpose of the physical exam from a nursing perspective, we must ask the following question: What can a staff nurse do with the data acquired from performing a data-base physical assessment? If the answer is only to report the findings to the physician, perhaps the nurse should leave that portion of the examination to the physician. The important thing is to stress the assessment skills that are crucial for the nurse generalist. For example, she needs to be able to assess signs of increased intracranial pressure, not necessarily to perform an entire neurological exam, but this does not mean that advanced skills should not be learned by nurses who routinely screen, case-find, and treat selected problems.

Table I–3 lists those areas of physical diagnosis in which nurses should be proficient. The examination of these areas by the nurse can yield valuable data from which nursing care can be planned. Physical diagnosis as determined by nurses should be clearly "nursing" in focus. The diagnosis of pathophysiology should be left to the physician. The individual nurse must decide how important it is to her own practice to learn to palpate livers, auscultate murmurs, or use an ophthalmoscope. By examining her philosophy and definition of nursing, she should seek to develop expertise in those areas that will enhance her nursing practice.

## Differentiating Between Cues and Inferences

In order to recognize and validate information accurately, the nurse must acquire a method of identifying that information. Little and Carnevali have identified such a process as cue identification and inferencing.

A *cue* is a fact that one acquires through the use of the five senses (taste, touch, smell, hearing, and sight). Primary sources of cues are the subjective statements of the client and the objective facts observed by the nurse. Secondary sources are family, other health care providers, and diagnostic studies. An *inference* is the nurse's judgment or interpretation of these cues. Inferences are always subjective and are influenced by the knowledge base, values, and experiences of the nurse. For example:

| *Cue* | *Corresponding Inference* |
|---|---|
| Hgb 9.1 | Abnormal |
| Crying | Possible fear, sadness |
| 5 ft 1 in, 220 lb | Obesity |

Differentiating between inferences and cues is important. Although an inference is a subjective judgment, nurses will frequently report it as a fact or fail to gather sufficient cues to confirm it or rule it out. Inferences made with little or no supporting cues can result in inappropriate and sometimes dangerous care, especially when invalid inferences are passed on to other members of the health team.

## Problem Identification

Problem identification, the second component of the nursing process, incorporates the intellectual activities that focus on identifying interaction patterns, validating

Table I-3.  **Physical Assessment by Nurse Generalists**

| Physical System | Criteria |
|---|---|
| Sensory-Perceptual | Mental status<br>Vision and appearance of eyes<br>Hearing<br>Touch<br>Taste and smell |
| Skin | Condition (color, turgor, character)<br>Lesions<br>Edema<br>Hair distribution |
| Respiratory | Rate, character<br>Breath sounds<br>Cough |
| Cardiovascular | Pulses (rate, quality, rhythm)<br>    Apical       Radial<br>    Carotid    Dorsalis pedis<br>    Brachial   Posterior tibial<br>    Femoral<br>Blood pressure<br>Circulation (mucous membranes, nail beds) |
| Neurological | Pupillary reactions<br>Orientation<br>Level of consciousness<br>Grasp strength |
| Gastrointestinal | Mouth, gums, teeth, and tongue (color and condition)<br>Gag reflex<br>Bowel sounds<br>Presence of distention, impaction, hemorrhoids (external) |
| Genitourinary | Presence of retention<br>Discharge (vaginal, urethral)<br>Uterine response (pregnancy, postpartum) |
| Musculoskeletal | Muscle tone, strength<br>Gait, stability<br>Range of motion |

the findings, and evolving a statement about the health status of the individual. As mentioned in Chapter 1, the term *nursing diagnosis* is used frequently in place of the term *problem identification* as a step in the nursing process as specified in the ANA standards of practice. However, this author will use problem identification to represent the second component of the nursing process.

## Identifying Alternatives

Problem identification involves complex thinking about the data gathered from client, family, records, and other health care providers. This thinking, combined with relevant information stored in the nurse's memory, is used to generate possible explanations for the data. These intellectual (cognitive) activities are difficult to teach and learn; many nurses who acquire expertise in assessment often flounder when asked to synthesize the data and identify a pattern. Aspinall and Tanner found (1981) that nurses take various approaches to problem identification, ranging from systematic testing of several possible explanations to the quick generation of one explanation. However, if the nurse does not take an approach that considers more than one explanation, the validity and effectiveness of the plan of care is jeopardized. According to Aspinall and Tanner, potential problems that can result when alternative explanations are not considered and tested include:

- Overvaluing the probability of one explanation
- Failing to include the accurate diagnosis in the initial hypothesis
- Failing to consider all the data because of the narrow focus
- Reaching an incorrect diagnosis because of speed, bias, or assumptions based on experience

To assist in identifying alternative explanations and in confirming or ruling out alternatives, the nurse should supplement her own memory-stored information by consulting references on the subject or by talking with other members of the health team. Unfortunately, we do not always utilize the most valuable resource available to us—other nurses.

Nursing staff conferences on client care are a nonthreatening and productive method for helping staff members to identify alternative solutions to problems and interventions. After the background of the problem has been shared with the group, the members are asked to think of possible explanations for the data. These explanations are then written on a blackboard, after which the group considers what data are needed to confirm or rule out each possibility. Explanations that have been ruled out are crossed off. The nurse caring for the client will then proceed to confirm or rule out the remaining explanations. while caring for the client.

As the nurse gains more knowledge and experience, she will need less time to think of alternative explanations. However, this step should never be eliminated. Identifying alternatives is also important when determining interventions in order to avoid failure, stereotyping, and monotony.

## Assessment Conclusions

After the data have been gathered and examined and alternative explanations tested and ruled out, the nurse will reach one of the following four conclusions:

1. No problem evident at this time; no health promotion activities indicated
2. No problem evident at this time; health promotion activities indicated
3. Actual, potential, possible clinical problem
4. Actual, potential, possible nursing diagnosis

Figure I-2 represents a schematic diagram of the problem identification phase.

### Conclusion 1

*No problem evident at this time*
*No health promotion activities indicated*

After the data have been examined and analyzed, the nurse and the client may conclude that no problem is present at this time and no health promotion activities are indicated. However, the client's present life-style and patterns will be assessed to identify any potential future problems. Planning future contacts for follow-up

**Assessment**

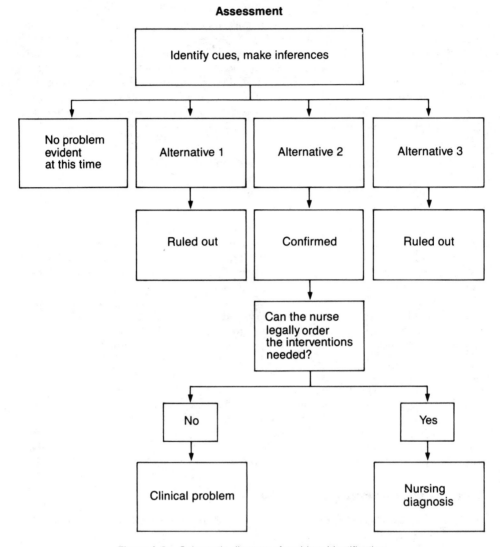

**Figure I–2.** Schematic diagram of problem identification.

assessments may be appropriate. It is more likely that this situation will exist in ambulatory settings and in private practice than in acute health care facilities.

## Conclusion 2

*No problem evident at this time*
*Health promotion activities indicated*

If, at the time of the assessment, no problem is identified but certain teaching needs are indicated to maintain the present level of wellness or to prevent health alterations, conclusion 2 is reached. The nurse, along with the client, then determines the complexity of the health promotion activities needed. If the teaching can be accomplished at the initial session without the need for the follow-up meetings, the situation remains a 2. Thus the session would probably conclude with the nurse specifying those indicators that suggest the need for future contact. This situation could occur in acute settings when a nurse has a specialized role that allows her to consult clients. Examples include enterostomal therapists, operating room nurses performing preoperative visits, clinical specialists, and nurses in private practice.

A client is admitted for surgery for a cataract removal. Since the client has a colostomy, the enterostomal therapist visits him to assess his present status. After discussing his stomal care and his postoperative expectations, the nurse concludes that follow-up visits for teaching are not indicated. The nurse instructs him to call her if needed during his hospitalization.

If the health promotion activities cannot be accomplished in one session, the nurse would then use the nursing diagnosis *Potential Alterations in Health Maintenance* and develop a teaching plan for future sessions. Other nursing diagnoses are also appropriate to describe interventions that promote health, as illustrated in the following example:

Mrs. Green is a 32-year-old woman who recently gave birth to her first child. Mrs. Green works for a large publishing company as an editor and has taken a 9-month leave of absence because of the baby. During a routine examination of her newborn in the pediatrician's office, Mrs. Green expresses concern to the nurse that she is bored and feels useless. She indicates that she has recently gained 10 pounds, is sleeping about 12 hours out of 24, and has frequent arguments with her husband. The nurse validates with Mrs. Green that these problems have developed since the birth of the baby. Since the health of the family unit is influenced by the interaction patterns of its members, the nurse identifies potential problems in the areas of parenting and coping. In analyzing the data, the nurse selects the nursing diagnosis *Disturbance in Self-Concept* to describe Mrs. Green's problem (see Section II). In order to complete the diagnosis and determine the appropriate interventions, the nurse needs to identify the contributing factors and incorporate them into the diagnosis. In the case of Mrs. Green, the complete diagnosis would appear as:

**Disturbance in Self-Concept related to change in life-style from a productive editor to the mother role**

Having made the diagnosis, the nurse can assist Mrs. Green to identify activities that will increase her productivity and improve her self-concept. Follow-up phone calls or visits should be used to evaluate progress and to reassess the situation.

## Conclusions 3 and 4

Conclusion 3 involves an actual, potential, or possible clinical problem, whereas Conclusion 4 is an actual, potential, or possible nursing diagnosis. These situations were discussed and differentiated in Chapter 2.

A clinical situation often encountered by nurses, the confused elderly client, exemplifies the dangers of incomplete assessments and impulsive problem-solving. Many nurses dismiss confusion in the elderly as an outcome of aging and fail to treat it as a signal. Before labeling a client as "confused as a result of aging associated with atherosclerosis," the nurse should assess for other explanations. The assessment criteria in Figure I-3 represent factors to be assessed when considering the history and possible contributing factors for the confusion.

| History of the Confusion | |
|---|---|
| At home and in agency | Sudden or gradual |
| Onset and duration | Continuous or intermittent |
| Acute or chronic | Time of day or night |

| History of the Individual | |
|---|---|
| Life-style (past and present) | Interests |
| | Support system |
| Work history | Coping patterns |

| Presence of Physiological Contributing Factors | |
|---|---|
| Respiratory status (blood gases) | Nutritional status (weight, hydration) |
| Renal status (output, BUN, creatinine) | Circulatory status (pulses, skin) |
| Endocrine changes (glucose) | Medication (overdose or side-effect) |
| Fluid and electrolyte balance (Na, K, specific gravity) | |

| Presence of Situational Contributing Factors | |
|---|---|
| Fear of unknown, loss | Philosophy of family and health care providers |
| Actual loss of control, income, significant others, routine, familiar objects or surroundings (house pets) | Attitude toward aging |
| | Beliefs about confusion |
| Sensory overload or deprivation | Tone, speed, volume of speech |
| | Content of communication |

**Figure I–3.** Focus assessment criteria for confusion.

## Case Study

The following case study illustrates two methods of problem solving.

Mrs. D is an 86-year-old female admitted to a medical unit because she had a blood sugar of 260. Mrs. D has intermittent periods of confusion, especially at night. In an attempt to control her outbursts (she kept screaming that she was "being held prisoner"), the nurses requested and received an order for a hypnotic at night, a sedative PRN, and a jacket restraint. Mrs. D became more agitated and confused.

**Nursing Diagnosis: Sensory-Perceptual Alterations related to cerebral arteriosclerosis (aging process)**

After noticing that Mrs. D was usually not confused when her granddaughter or daughter was present, the nurse initiated an assessment of Mrs. D's confusion by acquiring data from Mrs. D and her granddaughter, as follows:

### History of Individual

The confusion began the first night of admission. Mrs. D lives alone and is very independent. She has had a history of forgetting some facts but has not had episodes of confusion. She has strong family ties and communicates with her daughter daily via visit or phone.

### Physiological Contributing Factors

In reviewing the possible physiological factors that could contribute to confusion in Mrs. D, the nurse identified hyperglycemia and possible side-effects of hypnotic medications and sedatives.

### Situational Contributing Factors

The sudden hospitalization caused Mrs. D to lose control over her activities: her normal routine, her familiar surroundings, her significant others. All these losses contributed to her fear. Since most of the nursing staff had never known Mrs. D before her apparent confusion, their communications with her were loud and rapid, occurring primarily while they helped her with her activities of daily living (eating, ambulating, hygiene). In contrast, her family talked slowly and quietly with her about her grandchildren and about their activities. She listened carefully and responded appropriately to them. As a result, the nursing diagnosis had to be revised.

**Revised Nursing Diagnosis: Sensory-Perceptual Alterations related to unfamiliar surroundings and inability to differentiate increased incoming stimuli**

The nurse collaborated with the physician concerning the medications ordered, and both the sedative and hypnotic were discontinued. Blood glucose levels were ordered at bedtime and at 6:00 A.M. to assess the need for insulin twice a day.

A care plan was formulated with the interventions designed to:

1. Reduce unfamiliar incoming stimuli by slowly explaining procedures and activities

2. Institute reality orientation by introducing familiar objects from home, photographs, music
3. Encourage staff to talk to client about her interests: cooking, crocheting, her grandchildren

As illustrated in this case study, the deliberate search for alternative explanations for data is important to prevent problems that can be injurious to clients and frustrating to nurses.

## Summary

Data are systematically collected in the assessment phase by means of observation, examination, interviewing, and record review. Strengths and limitations of the individual and the family are considered, as are the client's patterns and perceptions. Validation of the data is sought with the client, family, nursing colleagues, other professionals, client records, and reference material.

The quality and validity of the cues and inferences are dependent on the knowledge base, experiences, and values of the nurse.

After considering several alternative explanations for the data, the nurse concludes the problem identification phase with one of the following outcomes:

- No problem
- Health promotion activities indicated
- Actual, potential, possible clinical problem
- Actual, potential, possible nursing diagnosis

## References

Aspinall MJ, Tanner C: Decision-making for Patient Care, pp 7–12. New York, Appleton-Century-Crofts, 1981

Gordon M: Nursing diagnoses and the diagnostic process. Am J Nurs 76:1298–1300, 1976

Little D, Carnevali D: Nursing Care Planning. Philadelphia, JB Lippincott, 1976

Ramackers MJ: Communication blocks revisited. Am J Nurs 79:1079–1081, 1979

Smith VN, Bass T: Communication for Health Professionals. Philadelphia, JB Lippincott, 1979

# 4

# Application
# to Care Planning

In order to become a full profession, nursing must identify its unique focus and demonstrate accountability in terms of that focus. The classification system of nursing diagnoses is a mechanism for identifying the domain of nursing, while care planning is the mechanism to demonstrate accountability. Care plans serve to communicate to the nursing staff the specific problems of the client and the prescribed interventions for directing and evaluating the care given. In order to prepare a care plan, the nurse must deliberately and systematically problem-solve.

## Care Plan Components

In order to direct and evaluate nursing care, the care plan should include the following:

- Problems (actual, possible, potential)
  Clinical problems
  Nursing diagnoses
- Outcome criteria (client goals)
- Nursing orders or interventions
- Evaluation

Some institutions restrict the use of a nursing care plan solely to nursing diagnoses without including clinical problems (medical and nursing). However, since nurses treat other problems along with nursing diagnoses, it is important that nurses have a place to record the planned interventions for these problems. Since nurses often have difficulty separating the dependent from the independent dimensions of nursing care, it would be best to use a system that requires the designation of these problems. Complex clinical problems and nursing diagnoses could be recorded with the related interventions on the care plans, while routine clinical problems would be addressed only on the Kardex. This type of documentation will be shown later in this chapter.

If the care plan is to be restricted to nursing diagnoses alone, the nurse must have another place to record nursing interventions for clinical problems. When nurses and students are directed to prepare care plans with nursing diagnoses only, they encounter the dilemma of where to write the other nursing actions, which address problems that are not nursing diagnoses. In response to this mandate, nurses tend to reword all problems as nursing diagnoses, which only serves to further confuse the problem and dilute nursing as a whole.

## Care Plan Documentation

The care planning system used in a particular setting should meet the needs of the nurses and the clients in that setting. Thus a critical care unit and a rehabilitation unit would probably not be able to utilize the same system without sacrificing effectiveness and efficiency.

All care planning systems should address the components of the nursing process: assessment, problem identification, planning, implementation, and evaluation.

## Assessment and Problem Identification

The assessment component of the nursing process is addressed in the admission data base and in the care plan. The admission data base is gathered during the nursing interview conducted during initial contact with the client. This preprinted form directs nurses to gather data in order to assess for present or potential alterations in health. This form should be organized in a manner to permit efficient data collection and with space to allow for elaboration when needed.

The assessment component is also addressed on the care plan in the intervention column, which directs the nurse to monitor or assess for a problem. For example:

*Problem*

Possible cardiogenic shock (post M.I.)

*Interventions*

Assess
  Urinary perfusion
  Level of consciousness
  Blood pressure, pulse

### Identifying Interaction Patterns

Many questions arise as the nurse gathers initial data with the data-base assessment.

1. What is the person's usual pattern?
2. What represents an altered pattern?
3. Does the person's usual pattern present a risk of contributing to an altered state?
4. When should the nurse defer the collection of data?

### What Is the Person's Usual Pattern? What Represents an Altered Pattern?

During the assessment the nurse elicits data that reflect the past and present functional patterns of the person. The nurse must be careful not to diagnose patterns with isolated data. Isolated data may be important in the content of the usual pattern, but the usual pattern must be determined before analysis can take place. The following is an example of this error.

Mrs. F is a 33-year-old woman. In response to a 24-hour recall of her diet she reports:

Breakfast: coffee (1 cup)
Morning break: coffee (1 cup)
Lunch: yogurt
Afternoon break: pound cake (1 slice)
Dinner: pizza, salad, coffee (2 cups)

The inference drawn from this data could be: Inadequate intake of basic four food groups. The nurse should ask Mrs. F, "Is this your usual daily intake?" Mrs. F's response will help the nurse determine the reason for the diet: *e.g.*, financial, lack of knowledge of nutrition, unusual circumstances.

Should the nurse determine a diagnosis of possible alteration in nutrition related to inadequate consumption of the four basic food groups, she will then look to other assessment data to validate the existence of the altered state and to contributing factors: *e.g.*, skin, bowel elimination, weight/height ratio.

If the nurse is uncertain of what data are needed to confirm the nursing diagnosis, she can refer to the specific diagnostic category in Section II for the focus assessment criteria and the defining characteristics.

### Does the Person's Usual Pattern Present a Risk of Contributing to an Altered State?

In the case of Mrs. F, if the diet recall presented is her usual state, the nurse can infer that this diet is nutritionally deficient and with additional questions can elicit contributing factors. When the nurse diagnoses the state of risk she utilizes the diagnosis of:

**Potential Alteration in Health Maintenance: Inadequate nutritional intake related to lack of knowledge of implications of inadequate diet and daily nutritional requirements, and the inconvenience of preparing meals for one person**

### When Should the Nurse Defer the Collection of Data?

A printed data-assessment form should be viewed as a guide for the nurse, not a mandate. All data-base forms should have a provision for allowing the nurse to defer the collection of selected data. (See the assessment form in Appendix I for a method of deferring.)

Before requesting information from a client, the nurse should ask herself, What am I going to do with the data? If certain information is useless or irrelevant for a particular client, then its collection is a waste of time and often distressing to clients. Asking a terminally ill man how much he smokes or drinks, for example, is inexcusable, unless the nurse has a specific goal. If a client will be NPO for an unlimited period of time, it is probably unnecessary for the nurse to collect data on nutritional patterns. The assessment will be indicated when the person resumes a diet.

If the client is extremely stressed, the nurse should collect only necessary data and defer the collection of functional patterns to another time or day. A stressed person may not be the best source of data, since often his memory is clouded. Since the initial contact with a client is stressful, as is an admission to an acute care facility, it may be advantageous to use a two-part data collection system: admission database assessment and comprehensive data-base assessment.

The admission data-base assessment is used at the time of admission to collect the information required for admission. Figure I-4 is an example of such a form.

The comprehensive data base is collected during the first 24 hours following admission. Appendix I illustrates a comprehensive data-base form.* Should the nurse determine on admission of a particular client that a comprehensive data base is desirable, it can be obtained at that time.

(*text continues on page 40*)

*This example of a comprehensive data phase represents a data collection tool that was designed to be used by itself. If the nurse or agency desired to develop a two-part admission data-base assessment, the form would need to be revised to eliminate repetition.

**Adult Nursing History
Admission Data Base**

Date_____ Arrival Time_____

Arrived via: Ambulatory Wheelchair Stretcher
Admitted: From_____ To_____
Information obtained from: Patient Family (specify)_____ Other (specify)_____
Occupation_____ Members of household (specify)_____

Deferred | I. **Communications Status**

Level of consciousness: Alert Drowsy Confused Nonresponsive
Oriented Yes No Specify_____
Cooperative Yes No Specify_____
Language spoken: English Spanish Other (specify)_____
Speech: Clear Slurred Aphasic Garbled Unable to speak
Ability to express self verbally: Yes No
Ability to communicate: Appropriate Inappropriate
Hearing: WNL Impaired Deaf Corrected Lip-reads
Vision: WNL Impaired Blind Corrected
Vertigo: Yes No Specify_____

II. **History**

Reason for admission (patient's statement) _____

What does patient expect from this hospitalization? _____

Previous hospital experience? Yes No
Existing medical problems:
  Diabetes Cardiac disease Arthritis CVA Other _____
  Hypertension Cancer Respiratory Renal _____
Allergies: None known
  Medications Yes No Specify_____Reaction_____
  Food Yes No Specify_____Reaction_____
  Other _____
Prostheses, appliances, or other devices:
  False eye Braces Dentures Eyeglasses
  Artificial limbs Hearing aid Contact lenses Cane
  Pacemaker Wig Walker Ostomy
  Other (specify) _____
Medications (prescription, over-the-counter)? Yes No If yes, list below
  Medicine Dose Reason With patient Last dose Prescribing physician

_____
_____
_____
_____
_____
_____

**Figure I–4.** Sample admission data base. (Courtesy of the Wilmington Medical Center, Wilmington, Delaware)

Deferred | III. **Functional Status**  ☐ Bedrest  ☐ BRP  ☐ Up ad lib  ☐ Immobile
☐ Right-handed  ☐ Left-handed  ☐ Ambidextrous

Motor Function:  Specify
R Arm__WNL__Amputated__Spastic__Flaccid__Paresis__Paralysis__Other_____
L Arm__WNL__Amputated__Spastic__Flaccid__Paresis__Paralysis__Other_____
R Leg__WNL__Amputated__Spastic__Flaccid__Paresis__Paralysis__Other_____
L Leg__WNL__Amputated__Spastic__Flaccid__Paresis__Paralysis__Other_____

Patient's ability to ambulate:  ☐ Independent  ☐ Assistance needed  _____
Gait:  ☐ Stable  ☐ Unstable
Bathe:  ☐ Independent  ☐ Assistance needed_____
Dress:  ☐ Independent  ☐ Assistance needed_____
Toilet:  ☐ Independent  ☐ Assistance needed_____
Eat:  ☐ Independent  ☐ Assistance needed_____
  Swallow liquids  ☐ Yes  ☐ No  Swallow solids  ☐ Yes  ☐ No
  Chew  ☐ Yes  ☐ No

Does the patient have problems/difficulty in:
Sleeping  ☐ Yes  ☐ No  Specify_____
Eating  ☐ Yes  ☐ No  Specify_____
Urination  ☐ Yes  ☐ No  Specify_____
Defecation  ☐ Yes  ☐ No  Specify_____

IV. **Physical Assessment**
Vital signs:  Temp_____BP_____Weight_____Height_____
Pulse_____Strong_____Weak_____Regular_____Irregular_____
Pedal pulse_____Deferred_____
Pupils:  ☐ Equal  ☐ Unequal

Left:  ··•••●●  Reactive to light
  Left  ☐ Yes  ☐ No  Specify_____
Right:  ··•••●●
  Right  ☐ Yes  ☐ No  Specify_____

Eyes:  ☐ Clear  ☐ Draining  ☐ Reddened  ☐ Other _____
Mouth:  Gums  ☐ WNL  ☐ White plaques  ☐ Lesions  ☐ Other _____
  Teeth  ☐ WNL  ☐ Loose  ☐ Other_____

**Skin:**
Color  ☐ WNL  ☐ Pale  ☐ Cyanotic  ☐ Ashen  ☐ Jaundice  ☐ Other _____
Temperature  ☐ Warm  ☐ Cool  Turgor:  ☐ WNL  ☐ Poor
Edema  ☐ No  ☐ Yes  Description/location _____
Lesions  ☐ None  ☐ Yes  Description/location _____
Decubitus  ☐ None  ☐ Yes  Description/location _____
Bruises  ☐ None  ☐ Yes  Description/location _____
Reddened  ☐ No  ☐ Yes  Description/location _____
Pruritus  ☐ No  ☐ Yes  Description/location _____

Respiratory rate _____
Quality:  ☐ WNL  ☐ Shallow  ☐ Rapid  ☐ Labored  ☐ Other _____
Auscultation:  Specify
Upper right lobes  ☐ WNL  ☐ Decreased  ☐ Absent  ☐ Abnormal sounds _____
Upper left lobes  ☐ WNL  ☐ Decreased  ☐ Absent  ☐ Abnormal sounds _____
Lower right lobes  ☐ WNL  ☐ Decreased  ☐ Absent  ☐ Abnormal sounds _____
Lower left lobes  ☐ WNL  ☐ Decreased  ☐ Absent  ☐ Abnormal sounds _____
Is patient aware of diagnosis?  ☐ Yes  ☐ No  ☐ Dx not established
What is the person most concerned about? _____
Summary Statement: _____
_____
_____
_____

☐ am
Date_____Time_____ ☐ pm  _____RN

**Figure I-4.**  (*continued*)

39

## Planning Conferences

Client care conferences are an excellent way to help nurses with planning care. These conferences can be daily and should be restricted to 15 to 20 minutes. If you are initiating conferences, it sometimes is advantageous to begin with weekly sessions and move gradually to daily or three-times-a-week sessions. The client or clients who are discussed can be those who are new admissions, those who have complex problems or conflicts with the staff, or those who are difficult to diagnose from a nursing diagnosis standpoint. The conference time provides nurses with an opportunity to share assessment data, feelings, problems, and knowledge (theory and practice). It can provide nurses who are reluctant to care plan with an opportunity for collaboration.

When conferences are being initiated, their success can be influenced positively if the following guidelines are considered:

- Manage the conference time judiciously by starting and ending on time
- Include all levels of nursing personnel and encourage their participation when appropriate
- Have personnel rotate covering unit during conferences
- Discourage interruptions
- Select an experienced group leader for beginning sessions
- Introduce inexperienced group leaders only after the conferences are firmly established

## The Process of Care Planning

After the actual or potential problems have been identified, the nursing activities to prevent, reduce, or eliminate the problems need to be formulated. Thus the planning phase of the nursing process is activated. The planning phase has four components:

1. Establishing priorities of care
2. Designating expected outcome criteria (client goals)
3. Setting nursing goals (process criteria)
4. Initiating the nursing care plan through the nursing orders

## Priorities of Care

Priorities of care are established to identify which nursing interventions will be directed first when an individual has multiple problems or alterations. The setting of priorities does not mean numbering problems in priority. It is a method by which the nurse and the client select which problems will be addressed on the care plan. Theoretically, some clients could have twenty nursing diagnoses on a care plan, a number which would render its use almost impossible. Often priorities are identified without collaboration when a well-intentioned nurse believes she knows what is the client's most important problem, as in the following example:

> Mrs. Gaul, a 44-year-old single parent, is admitted to the hospital because of hyperglycemia and a blood glucose level of 265. Mrs. Gaul has been an insulin-dependent diabetic for 19 years. The nurse, on reading the admitting diagnosis, asks Mrs. Gaul, "Have you been following your diet?" Her reply is "No." The nurse orders a consultation with the dietician, who spends 40 minutes with Mrs. Gaul explaining the therapeutic diet. The nurses continued to reinforce the im-

portance of adhering to the diet. After three days Mrs. Gaul shares with a nurse the discipline problems she has been having with her 15-year-old daughter. She relates that she becomes so frustrated she eats and eats.

The nurse, at the time of admission, should have assessed for the reasons why Mrs. Gaul had not been adhering to her diet, instead of inferring that she lacked knowledge about it (knowledge deficit). Questions concerning recent changes in life-style and added stressors would have supported a more accurate diagnosis:

**Ineffective Individual Coping related to indiscriminate eating when faced with discipline problems with daughter**

If the nurse had sought validation for the initial lack-of-knowledge diagnosis, valuable time and money would have not been spent on diet teaching. Any nurse can recall countless medical and nursing problems that were misdiagnosed or prioritized erroneously.

## Process Criteria vs. Outcome Criteria

Goals for nursing interventions are written to direct care, to identify desired outcomes, and to measure the effectiveness of the interventions. Goals can be process criteria goals or outcome criteria goals.

### Process Criteria

Process criteria—also called *nursing goals*—direct the nurse toward the prevention or alleviation of the altered state of wellness. Process criteria can focus on three major areas to assist the client to:

- Use his resources more effectively to facilitate an optimal level of coping
- Seek other resources to facilitate an optimal level of coping
- Modify his activities of daily living and usual life-style when resources are diminished or inadequate

In Section II, each diagnostic category lists nursing goals for that diagnosis. These goals serve to indicate what the nurse should seek to accomplish with a client. Nursing goals can be written on standards of care, but usually they are not written on care plans. Students are usually requested to write nursing goals in order to help them plan care. Practicing nurses can formulate nursing goals mentally by asking themselves:

1. What strengths of the client/family can I encourage?
2. What limitations can I assist the client/family with?
3. What resources can I direct the client/family to?

In answering these questions, the nurse will be assisted in identifying her focus.

### Outcome Criteria

Outcome criteria, or *client goals*, are the expected changes in the status of the client after he has received nursing care. Outcome criteria are utilized to:

- Direct interventions to achieve the desired changes
- Measure the effectiveness and validity of the interventions

Outcome criteria can be formulated to direct and measure positive and negative outcomes. Goals found on care plans are outcome criteria, or client goals. These goals are written in terms of what the client is expected to do, not the nurse.

*Positive outcome criteria* seek to direct interventions to provide the client with:

1. An improvement in health status by increasing comfort (physiological, psychological, social, spiritual) and coping abilities
   - Example: The client will discuss relationship between activity and carbohydrate requirements and walk unassisted to end of hall four times a day.
2. Maintenance of present optimal level of health
   - Example: The client will relate the signs, symptoms, and associated interventions for angina.
3. Optimal levels of coping with significant others
   - Example: The client will discuss with her husband her concern about returning to work.
4. Optimal adaptation to deterioration of health status
   - Example: The client will visually scan the environment while walking, to prevent injury.
5. Optimal adaptation to terminal illness
   - Example: The client will consume protein and high caloric supplements (three a day) to compensate for periods of anorexia and nausea.
6. Collaboration and satisfaction with health care providers
   - Example: The client will ask questions concerning the care of his colostomy.

*Negative outcome criteria* seek to direct interventions to prevent negative alterations in the client, such as:

1. Complications
   - Example: The client will not develop the preventable complications of imposed bed rest.
2. Disabilities
   - Example: The client will elevate left arm on pillow and exercise fingers on sponge ball to reduce edema.
3. Unwarranted death
   - Example: The client will be attached to an apnea monitor at night.

## Components of Outcome Criteria

Outcome criteria should:

- Have measurable verbs
- Be specific in content and time
- Be attainable

*Measurable verbs* are verbs that describe the exact behavior of the client/family that you expect to see when the goal has been met. The action/behavior must be such that the nurse can validate it by seeing or hearing.

Examples of verbs that are *not* measurable by sight or sound are:

| | |
|---|---|
| Accepts | Appreciates |
| Knows | Understands |

Examples of verbs that are measurable are:

| | |
|---|---|
| States | Has an increase in |
| Performs | Has an absence of |
| Identifies | Specifies |
| Has a decrease in | Administers |

The outcome criteria should describe the *specific response* planned. Three elements add to the specificity of a goal: content, modifiers, and achievement time.

The *content* area indicates what the individual is to do, experience, or learn (usually a verb), such as drink, walk, cough, or learn.

Associated with the verb are *modifiers*, which add the specifics or individual preferences to the goal. Modifiers are usually adjectives or adverbs; they explain what, where, when, and how. For example: drink (what and when), walk (where and when), learn (what), and cough (how and when).

The *time for achievement* of a goal can be added to the goal if appropriate.

- Example: Will walk 1/2 of hallway with assistance by Friday A.M.

Time may not be a factor in many goals but rather the evidence of progress to or achievement of the goal at the conclusion of the nurse/client relationship.

The outcome criteria for each nursing diagnosis in Section II are measurably stated but must be made specific to each client by adding modifiers. These outcome criteria serve to guide the nurse in the areas that need to be observed and measured. The following is an example of an outcome criterion for the diagnosis *Alterations in Comfort: Pain* that has been rewritten to reflect the goal for a particular client.

| *Outcome Criterion* | *Individualized Outcome Criteria* |
|---|---|
| The client will experience a reduction in pain and improve mobility | The client will<br>1. Complete his bath without assistance<br>2. Relate a reduction of pain and request less medication ( < 250 mg/24 hr)<br>3. Remain out of bed from 11 a.m. to 2 p.m. and 5 p.m. to 9 p.m. |

The nurse must ask herself, How will I measure that the client is experiencing less pain and has increased mobility? For this particular client, the goals stated above will serve as measurements. As this client's mobility increases, the nurse may have to revise the goals to reflect the client's changing status.

## Nursing Orders

After the problem and the outcome criteria have been stated, the nurse will focus on prescribing the care required to prevent, reduce, or eliminate the alteration. The specific directions for nursing care are called *nursing orders*. Nursing orders are composed of (Carnevali):

- Date
- Directive verb
- What, when, how often, how long, where
- Signature

The objective of the nursing order is to direct individualized care to a client. Nursing orders differ from nursing actions, which are broad interventions that can apply to any number of individuals sharing a similar problem. Examples of nursing actions are:

- Increase fluid intake
- Ambulate client
- Reassure client
- Monitor for arrhythmias

In order to translate the nursing action into a nursing order, the nurse must have data from the client to answer the following: what, when, how often, how long, and where?

The following example illustrates the translation of a nursing action to a nursing order.

| *Nursing Action* | *Nursing Order* |
|---|---|
| Increase fluid intake | Increase fluids to at least 2500 ml/24 hr |
| | 1000 ml 7–3 |
| | 700 ml 3–11 |
| | 100 ml 11–7 |
| | Likes orange and apple juice |
| | Dislikes carbonated beverages |
| | Do not count coffee or tea in the 2500 ml |

This nursing order reflects the need to hydrate an individual with tenacious secretions, considers preferences, and indicates that coffee and tea are permitted, although not as part of the measured increase since they act as diuretics.

The nursing interventions outlined in Section II for each nursing diagnosis are guidelines for the nurse. The nurse will then rewrite these interventions considering the components of a nursing order: What, when, how often, how long, and where? The example below indicates the rewriting of a nursing intervention from Section II to a nursing order.

**Nursing Diagnosis: Sleep Pattern Disturbance related to decreased activity level**

| *Nursing Action* | *Individualized Nursing Order* |
|---|---|
| Promote a well-scheduled daytime program of activity | Assist to dining room for each meal |
| | Have another resident accompany him on a daily afternoon walk around grounds |

As with outcome criteria, the nurse must have specific knowledge of an individual in order to write nursing orders. Student nurses can write care plans on clients they are yet to meet based on the information from their instructors, but it must be specified that they are writing guidelines for care, not nursing orders. After caring for the client, the student can revise the plan with specific orders.

As a nurse increases her knowledge about a client, she may need to revise the nursing orders to reflect changes or to increase the specificity. The following example illustrates a nursing order that underwent such revisions.

**Nursing Diagnosis: Fear related to uncertain future**

| | |
|---|---|
| Initial order (Day 1) | Provide opportunities to ventilate concerns |
| Order Day 2 | Encourage client to share her concerns |
| | Explore with husband his concerns for the future |
| Order Day 4 | Reinforce necessity for preserving present function (refer to problem *Impaired Physical Mobility*) |
| | Discuss a plan for increasing self-care activities |
| | Assess the communication pattern between husband and wife |
| | Provide the husband with a time to talk outside wife's room |

## Implementation

The implementation component of the nursing process comprises the skills needed to implement the nursing order. The skills and knowledge necessary for the implementation of nursing care are illustrated in Figure I–5.

---

### Primary Skills and Knowledge Needed for the Nursing Process

| Theoretical Knowledge | Communication Skills | Technical Skills | Therapeutic Use of Self |
|---|---|---|---|
| Scientific | Interviewing | Organization | Goals |
| Nursing research | Mutual sharing | Use of equipment | Past experiences |
| Pathophysiology | Writing | Knowledge of | Value system |
| Psychosocial system | Nonverbal | • technique | Limitations |
| Cultural-spiritual system | Listening | • safety | |
| Family system | | • physics | |
| Pharmocology | | • asepsis | |
| Nutrition | | | |

### Secondary Skills and Knowledge Needed for Each Component

| Assessment | Problem Identification | Planning |
|---|---|---|
| Ability to | Ability to | Ability to |
| • Differentiate cues and inferences | • Differentiate nursing diagnoses from clinical problems | • Identify goals |
| • Observe systematically | • Identify and test alternatives | • Identify interventions |
| • Perform a nursing physical assessment | • Recognize patterns | • Write nursing orders |
| • Identify patterns | • Correctly label patterns | Management skills |
| • Validate impressions | | |

| Implementation | Evaluation |
|---|---|
| Teaching skills | Knowledge of |
| Management skills | • Process criteria |
| Change theory | • Outcome criteria |

**Figure I–5.** Primary and secondary skills and knowledge needed for the nursing process.

Not only must the nurse possess these skills, she must assess, teach, and evaluate them in the nursing personnel she manages. For often the nurse is responsible for planning the care but not for its actual implementation. This requires that the nurse also possess the management skills of delegation, assertion, evaluation, and knowledge of change and motivational theory. The nurse should consult the appropriate literature on these topics.

## Evaluation

Evaluation is the final component of the nursing process. It consists of three distinct activities:

- Establishing criteria to observe and measure
- Assessing the present response for evidence
- Comparing the present response to the established criteria

Evaluation in health care facilities encompasses a quality assurance program, standards for care, and nursing audit. The individual nurse evaluates continuously with every nurse–client interaction in each component of the nursing process.

---

**Elements to Be Evaluated in Each Component of the Nursing Process**

**Assessment**
- Accuracy
- Completeness
- Validation
- Quality
- Alternatives

**Problem Identification**
- In the domain of nursing
- Clearly stated
- Accurate label
- Accurate etiology
- Validation
- Alternatives

**Planning**
- Outcome criteria
    Attainable
    Measurable
    Specific
- Nursing orders
    Clear
    Specific to individual
- Alternatives
- Validation

**Implementation**
- Client response
- Staff response
- Outcome achievement
- Alternatives
- Accurate/safe
- Validation
- Competency of care given

---

The system for evaluating care plans should be consistent with the setting in which care is provided. For example, an acute care setting might review a care plan every 3 days, while a rehabilitation unit might review plans every 2 to 4 weeks.

The problem, the goals, and the interventions all must be considered in the evaluation of the care plan.

### The Problem

- Does it still exist or does a potential for its development still exist?
- Does a new problem need to be added?

## The Goals

- Have they been resolved?
- Do they reflect the present focus of care (nurse and client)?

## Interventions

- Are they specific for the problem?
- Are they acceptable to the client?

In reviewing the problem and interventions, the nurse will record one of the following decisions in the evaluation column at the prescribed interval for evaluation.

- *Continue*: The problem still exists and the plan will continue as is
- *Revised*: The problem still exists, but the nursing orders require revision (the revisions are then written)
- *Ruled out*: A problem that had been designated as possible has been ruled out
- *Resolved*: A problem has been resolved and that portion of the care plan discontinued

Minor revisions can be made daily on a care plan by the nurse caring for or directing the care of the client. A yellow felt-tip marker (Hi-Liter) is an excellent pen with which to revise a plan, marking out those areas that are no longer being utilized. Because it is still possible to read through the yellow marking, the nurse can always refer to what was planned previously. In addition, the marking will not interfere with photo copying. (Documentation examples of evaluation are presented later in this chapter.)

Evaluation of nursing care is a process to measure the client's progress or lack of progress toward the goal. The problem list is examined for its current relevancy, and the prescribed interventions are assessed for their appropriateness and acceptance by the client.

The nursing care of individuals requires deliberate critical problem-solving and documentation of this process in a systematic manner.

## Care Planning Systems

There are numerous care planning systems, utilizing either printed guidelines or printed (or blank) care plans.

Printed guidelines are often index cards that are commercially printed to provide nurses with guidelines for writing interventions for a client with a particular problem. Most of the problems are medical diagnoses or diagnostic studies.

Printed care plans, otherwise known as standardized care plans, are care plans that have been formulated either commercially or in an institution to direct nursing care of a particular problem. These standardized care plans are typed and duplicated and are available in the units. Standardized care plans have a place in a care planning system provided they do not exclusively represent the care planning of the agency.

Figure I-6 illustrates a printed care plan. The advantages of such standardized care plans are that they:

1. Reduce the writing of routine nursing interventions
2. Instruct new staff and remind experienced staff of the interventions that are necessary

The disadvantages of standardized care plans are that they:

8. Potential Alteration in Skeletal-Muscular-Neuro Function related to surgical intervention.

   8a. Neurovascular check q 4 hr. Report any inability to dorsiflex foot.

   b. Quad setting exercises 10 × q 1 hr while awake! Knee flexion exercises 10 × q 1 hr while awake!

   c. Out of bed, to sit on elevated chair with 1 or 2 pillows. Sit with operative foot always in front of opposite foot; keep knees apart. Toe touch to partial weight bearing or may bear weight as tolerated. Operative hip flexion NO MORE THAN 75°.

   d. Ambulate with walker, with supervision t.i.d.

   e. Ambulate with crutches t.i.d.

   f. B.R.P. Use elevated toilet seat.

   g. Use knee exerciser q 1 hr.

9. Potential Alteration in Bowel Elimination: Constipation related to immobility and anesthesia effects.

   9a. Explain the causes of constipation.

   b. Urge to increase fluid intake. Include prune juice.
Specify amounts _____ 7–3
_____ 3–11
_____ 11–7
Specify likes _____
Specify dislikes _____

   c. Teach abdominal isometric exercises and encourage him to perform them 10 × q 1 hr.

   d. Discuss the need to include foods high in fiber in diet (e.g., fruit, bran)
Specify likes _____

**Figure I–6.** Section of a standardized nursing care plan for a client with a total hip replacement. Number 8 is a clinical problem and number 9 is a nursing diagnosis.

   1. May take the place of individualized nursing care plans
   2. May be placed in the client's record and never utilized

In order to help reduce the disadvantages of standardized care plans, certain strategies can be implemented. Standardized care plans should only be formulated for certain client problems that direct a set of common nursing interventions, such as a postfemoral arteriogram or total hip replacement (pre- and post-operatively).

Interposed in standardized care plans should be spaces where the nurse can add specific points to the nursing interventions. This will help avoid the problem of the staff's ignoring the printed care plans. For example, next to the intervention for increased fluid intake, space is allocated for the amount taken within a certain time span.

Increase fluid intake to: _____per 24 hours
_____ml 7a.m.–3p.m.     Likes _____
_____ml 3p.m.–11p.m.    Dislikes _____
_____ml 11p.m.–7a.m.

Also, the nurse who initiates the plan will cross out all sections that do not apply to her particular client. Requiring that the nurse individualize parts of the standardized care plan will reduce the chances of misusing it.

The documentation of implementation does not take place on a care plan but requires a separate form. This form can take several formats—flow chart, graphic chart, or prose nursing progress notes—depending on the types of data being recorded.

Flow charts are excellent formats for recording treatments, activities of daily living, selected teaching and observations. Figure I-7 is an example of a flow chart.

Flow charts should not be used to record interactions in the spiritual, cultural, social, and psychological domains. Prose progress notes are used to record these responses. Explanations and counseling given to clients and families and unusual or unexpected situations (*e.g.*, injuries, clinical emergencies) are also recorded on the nursing progress notes.

If the nurses are recording the same data over and over in the progress notes, it may be possible to adapt a flow sheet to accommodate these data more efficiently.

## Case Studies

The following two case studies and related documentation illustrate care planning.

## Case I

Mrs. Gates, a 42-year-old woman, is admitted with metastatic carcinoma of the breast (recently diagnosed).

### Medical History

Mrs. Gates went to see her medical doctor because of a lump she discovered under her left arm. After a biopsy confirmed a diagnosis of metastatic carcinoma of the breast, Mrs. Gates was admitted for further diagnostic studies. A mammogram revealed a lesion in the left breast. Mrs. Gates is scheduled for a left lower quadrant resection of the breast and node dissection on Thursday (three days away).

### Medical Plan

Present

Schedule for surgery on Thursday 6/3
Schedule bone scan, liver scan, chest x-ray
Complete blood count and urinalysis
SMA 24 blood studies
ECG

Future

Dr. Drong discussed with Mrs. Gates that approximately 3 weeks after surgery he will begin a course of chemotherapy to last 8 months, followed by radiation

### Health Status

Past

Usual childhood diseases
Appendectomy at age 21
Menarche at age 13 with a 28-day cycle

(*text continues on page 52*)

# Routine Care Record

| Date | | | | | | | | | | | | | | | | | | | | | | | | | | | | | | |
|---|---|---|---|---|---|---|---|---|---|---|---|---|---|---|---|---|---|---|---|---|---|---|---|---|---|---|---|---|---|---|

**Turn Record**
A=Abdomen
B=Back
L=Left Side
R=Right Side

(Top line Position, bottom line Initials)

| | M | 24 1 2 3 4 5 6 7 | 24 1 2 3 4 5 6 7 | 24 1 2 3 4 5 6 7 | 24 1 2 3 4 5 6 7 | 24 1 2 3 4 5 6 7 |
|---|---|---|---|---|---|---|
| | D | 8 9 10 11 12 13 14 15 | 8 9 10 11 12 13 14 15 | 8 9 10 11 12 13 14 15 | 8 9 10 11 12 13 14 15 | 8 9 10 11 12 13 14 15 |
| | E | 16 17 18 19 20 21 22 23 | 16 17 18 19 20 21 22 23 | 16 17 18 19 20 21 22 23 | 16 17 18 19 20 21 22 23 | 16 17 18 19 20 21 22 23 |

**Bladder Routine Cath. Care**

| | M | | | | | |
|---|---|---|---|---|---|---|
| | D | | | | | |
| | E | | | | | |
| | M | | | | | |
| | D | | | | | |
| | E | | | | | |
| | M | | | | | |
| | D | | | | | |
| | E | | | | | |
| | M | | | | | |
| | D | | | | | |
| | E | | | | | |

**I.V. Device Restart**

A. Infiltrated   1. Scalp
B. Phlebitis         Needle
C. Clogged      2. 1¼"
D. Routine          Angiocath.
E. Pulled Out   3. Reservoir
F. Leakage      4. 8" Intracath
G. —            5. —

| | M | | | | | |
|---|---|---|---|---|---|---|
| | D | | | | | |
| | E | | | | | |
| | M | | | | | |
| | D | | | | | |
| | E | | | | | |
| | M | | | | | |
| | D | | | | | |
| | E | | | | | |
| | M | | | | | |
| | D | | | | | |
| | E | | | | | |
| | M | | | | | |
| | D | | | | | |
| | E | | | | | |

| | | | |
|---|---|---|---|
| 1. | 6. | 11. | 16. |
| 2. | 7. | 12. | 17. |
| 3. | 8. | 13. | 18. |
| 4. | 9. | 14. | 19. |
| 5. | 10. | 15. | 20. |

**Figure I–7.** Flow chart. (Courtesy of the Wilmington Medical Center, Wilmington, Delaware)

| | | Date | | | | | |
|---|---|---|---|---|---|---|---|
| **Bath** C=Complete S=Self P=Partial | | | | | | | |
| **Oral Hygiene** R=Routine S=Special | M | | | | | | |
| | D | | | | | | |
| | E | | | | | | |
| **Food Intake** | | | | | | | |
| | B | | | | | | |
| | L | | | | | | |
| | S | | | | | | |
| **Activity** | M | | | | | | |
| | D | | | | | | |
| | E | | | | | | |
| **Special Studies or Diagnostic Procs.** | M | | | | | | |
| | D | | | | | | |
| | E | | | | | | |
| | M | | | | | | |
| | D | | | | | | |
| | E | | | | | | |
| Weight | M | | | | | | |
| **I.V. Tubing Change** | M | | | | | | |
| | D | | | | | | |
| | E | | | | | | |
| **Bowel** 1 For each B.M. O No B.M. E—Enema+Type | M | | | | | | |
| | D | | | | | | |
| | E | | | | | | |
| Evening Care by | E | | | | | | |
| Rounds | M | | | | | | |
| | M | | | | | | |
| | D | | | | | | |
| | E | | | | | | |

**Routine Care and Treatment Record**
**Medical—Surgical Units**

Asterisk After Recording Means Note Ancillary and Nursing Patient Progress Report

**Figure I-7.** (*continued*)

Present

Chronic constipation, which she treats with over-the-counter laxatives
Bowel movement q 3–4 days

## Social History

Married 22 years
No children: "I never got pregnant, so we both accepted it as God's will."
Master's degree
Works full time as a librarian
Spends most of her free time sewing, gardening, and activities with husband
    (plays, day trips)
States she signed up for an exercise dance class but will have to cancel now
Drinks 1 glass of wine with dinner
Does not smoke

## Sexual History

States that both she and her husband are very happy and satisfied with their
    sex life
Engages in intercourse approximately 5 times/month

## Sleep Patterns

Sleeps 7–8 hours a night
Retires at 11 p.m., awakens at 6 a.m.
Falls asleep easily

## Nutritional History

(24-hour diet recall)
Breakfast: 2 eggs, 1 slice toast, orange juice, coffee
Lunch: Yogurt or cottage cheese with fruit, water
Dinner: Meat, potatoes, vegetable, salad, water, 1 glass wine
Other: 2–3 cups coffee, 1–2 pieces fruit, 1 serving ice cream/cake/cookies

## Support System

Relies on husband for daily support
Married sister with 2 children (ages 12 and 14) lives 20 minutes away; they
    talk q.o.d. on phone and usually have Saturday or Sunday dinner together
Is active in her church (Lutheran) and teaches Sunday school each week

## Present Concerns

Is worried what her husband will do without her at home (*e.g.*, meals)
Stated she "hoped that their relationship would not change after the sur-
    gery"
Expressed concern about getting sick with chemotherapy
Related that her cousin, who had chemotherapy for leukemia, vomited all the
    time and lost all her hair but has been doing well for 5 years now

## Physical Examination

Height 5 ft 4 in, weight 140 lb

General appearance: well-groomed female who looks younger than stated age
Review of systems unremarkable except palpable masses in left axilla

Figure I-8 presents Mrs. Gates's preoperative nursing care plan.

Postoperatively, Mrs. Gates's care plan would include the following clinical problems and nursing diagnoses:

## Clinical Problems
Potential postoperative complications

Nausea, vomiting
Paralytic ileus
Hemorrhage

## Nursing Diagnoses

1. Alterations in Comfort: Pain Related to Surgical Incision
2. Potential Alterations in Respiratory Function Related to
   Pain
   Immobility
   Sedation (analgesics)
3. Potential Fluid Volume Excess: Edema Related to Node Dissection
4. Impairment of Skin Integrity Related to Incision
5. Potential Disturbance in Self-Concept Related to
   Loss of breast
   Threat to future
   Threat to sexuality
6. Knowledge Deficit Related to
   Wound care
   Exercises
   Restrictions
   Prosthesis
   Community resources

## Case 2

While wrestling with her 15-year-old brother, 11-year-old JS sustained a fracture to her left tibia. She was admitted to the pediatric floor and placed in Buck's extension traction with a boot.

## Medical Plan

Continuous traction for 5 weeks
Valium 2 mg p.o. q 8 hr
Demerol 50 mg p.o. q 4 hr
Regular diet

## Medical Diagnosis

Pathological fracture due to a benign cyst
Plan to discharge in 5 weeks in body cast; duration of body cast approximately 10 weeks

(*text continues on page 57*)

## Adult Patient Care Plan

### Activities of Daily Living
☐ Complete dependence ☐ Ind-Independent (No assistance needed)

Mobility:
Ability to turn self      ☒ Ind.   ☐ Assistance needed _____
Ability to sit      ☒ Ind.   ☐ Assistance needed _____
Ability to ambulate      ☒ Ind.   ☐ Assistance needed _____   Number of people _____
☐ Wheelchair ☐ Crutches    ☐ Cane ☐ Walker ☐ Braces ☐ Prosthesis   Gait: ☐ Stable ☐ Unstable
Bathing:      ☒ Ind.   ☐ Assistance needed _____
☐ Shower ☐ Sink ☐ Bathtub   ☐ Bed bath—partial, self, complete
Dressing:      ☒ Ind.   ☐ Assistance needed _____
Toileting:      ☒ Ind.   ☐ Assistance needed _____   ☐ Bathroom ☐ Commode ☐ Bed pan
Eating:      ☒ Ind.   ☐ Assistance needed _____
     Ability to:   Swallow liquids ☒ Yes   ☐ No   Chew ☒ Yes ☐ No
                Swallow solids ☒ Yes   ☐ No   Feed self ☒ Yes ☐ No

| Date | Diagnosis | Goals: The individual will: | Date | Diagnosis | Goals: The individual will: |
|---|---|---|---|---|---|
| | 1. Knowledge deficit related to pre and postop regimen and diagnostic tests (bone and liver scans) | Relate the routines concerning pre-postop care and diagnostic tests. Demonstrate postop exercises | | 4. Knowledge deficit related to preoperative skin preparation | Perform the prescribed regimen correctly and at prescribed times |
| | 2. Fear related to cancer diagnosis – Uncertain diagnosis – Uncertain future – Results of scans | Relate her concerns regarding the implications of cancer | | | |
| | 3. Alteration in family processes related to: – Uncertain future – Concern of wife that husband cannot manage household | 1. Outline for her husband specific tasks he must accomplish to manage home. 2. Share mutual concerns with her husband | | | |

**Initials / Signature**

| | | | | | | |
|---|---|---|---|---|---|---|
| 1. | | 7. | | 13. | | 19. |
| 2. | | 8. | | 14. | | 20. |
| 3. | | 9. | | 15. | | 21. |
| 4. | | 10. | | 16. | | 22. |
| 5. | | 11. | | 17. | | 23. |
| 6. | | 12. | | 18. | | 24. |

**Figure 1-8.** Care plan for Case Study 1. (Courtesy of the Wilmington Medical Center, Wilmington, Delaware)

| Date | Diagnosis | | Plan | Ints. | Evaluations |
|---|---|---|---|---|---|
| 5/30 | 1. Knowledge deficit related to pre and post operative regimens, bone and liver scans | | Discuss the details of the preoperative and postoperative experiences she can expect with client and husband preop: Physical preparation for procedure Medications NPO, skin preparation Probable size and location of incision Expected length of time of surgery Time of surgery, transportation Preanesthesia room Visit by anesthesiologist, Operating room nurse Postop Recovery room Elevated left arm Dressings and drainage devices Pain relief measures Turn, cough and deep breath routines Progressive postop period Diet, mobility, self-care Arm exercises Explain the following procedures: Bone scan (injection, fluids) Liver scan (injection, positions, time intervals) | L.C. | |

**Initials / Signature**

| | | | |
|---|---|---|---|
| 1. | 7. | 13. | 19. |
| 2. | 8. | 14. | 20. |
| 3. | 9. | 15. | 21. |
| 4. | 10. | 16. | 22. |
| 5. | 11. | 17. | 23. |
| 6. | 12. | 18. | 24. |

**Figure I-8.**  (continued)

| Date | Diagnosis | | Plan | Ints. | Evaluations |
|---|---|---|---|---|---|
| | 2. Fear related to: <br> - Cancer diagnosis <br> - Uncertain future <br> - Results of scans | | 1. Allow her to share her concerns about uncertain future <br> 2. Explore with her to ascertain her knowledge of mastectomy <br> e.g. Has she known anyone who has had a mastectomy? <br> 3. Provide information which may reduce concern about limitations if indicated at this time <br> e.g. Prosthetics <br> Reach for Recovery | | |
| | 3. Alteration in family process related to: <br> - Uncertain future and concern of wife that husband cannot manage the household alone | | 1. Assess their communication and coping patterns (previous, present) <br> 2. Ask her to write down the household chores that need to be done and when <br> 3. Explore with her the possibility of hiring a temporary housekeeper <br> 4. Suggest that a dinner meal can be ordered for him at the hospital for each evening <br> 5. Secure time with husband alone to determine: <br> - His knowledge - His concerns <br> 6. Share with each spouse separately how each may help the other | | |
| | 4. Knowledge deficit related to preoperative skin preparation | CP | Instruct her to wash operative area left of breast and under left arm with Betadine solution and rinse hs (Tuesday and Wednesday) | | |

**Initials / Signature**

| | | | |
|---|---|---|---|
| 1. | 7. | 13. | 19. |
| 2. | 8. | 14. | 20. |
| 3. | 9. | 15. | 21. |
| 4. | 10. | 16. | 22. |
| 5. | 11. | 17. | 23. |
| 6. | 12. | 18. | 24. |

**Figure I-8.** *(continued)*

## Medical History

Systems review unremarkable
1–2 episodes of upper respiratory infection a winter

## Social History

Reports
She is well-liked in school
Enjoys sports (soccer)
Likes to cook
Likes school (excels in math and science, has to work at her reading skills)

## Support System

Has a 15-year-old brother
Mother is a former librarian
Father is a pharmacist who teaches at the local university

## Diet History

Reports a usual daily intake of:
Breakfast: Pancakes or cereal, orange juice
Lunch: Sandwich, hot dog or pizza, ice cream, milk
Dinner: Meat, potatoes, vegetables (carrots, peas, corn only)
Snacks: Cookies, popcorn
Water: 4 glasses

## Sleep/Rest Pattern

Retires at 8:30 p.m. on weekdays
Awakes at 7:00 a.m.
Bedtime ritual: Bath, oral hygiene; reads a short story

## Present Status

3 days postadmission
JS experiences intermittent leg spasms that were visible the first two days.
   She continues to complain of spasms that are no longer visible. She re-
   sponds to the spasms by screaming.
JS is placed in private room at the end of the hall and the door is kept closed
   to muffle her screams.
JS's mother arrives at 10:30 a.m. and remains till 6:30 p.m. Her husband arrives at 6:30 and stays till 8:30–9:00
JS spends her day watching TV, conversing with her mother, and experiencing spasms. Her contact with the nursing staff is limited to hygiene needs
   and medications.
JS complains that her pain meds are often late and then her spasms are
   "really bad."

You are a part-time nurse caring for JS today. What are your nursing diagnoses?
Figure I-9 represents the care plan for JS.

# Adult Patient Care Plan

## Activities of Daily Living
☐ Complete dependence  ☐ Ind-Independent (No assistance needed)

Mobility:
Ability to turn self  ☐ Ind.  ☒ Assistance needed _____
Ability to sit  ☐ Ind.  ☒ Assistance needed _____  Number of People _____
☐ Wheelchair  ☐ Crutches  ☐ Cane  ☐ Walker  ☐ Braces  ☐ Prosthesis  Gait: ☐ Stable  ☐ Unstable
Bathing:  ☐ Ind.  ☒ Assistance needed _____
☐ Shower  ☐ Sink  ☐ Bathtub  ☒ Bed bath—(partial) self, complete
Dressing:  ☐ Ind.  ☒ Assistance needed *with pants*
Toileting:  ☐ Ind.  ☒ Assistance needed _____  ☐ Bathroom  ☐ Commode  ☐ Bed pan
Eating:  ☒ Ind.  ☐ Assistance needed _____
Ability to:  Swallow liquids ☒ Yes  ☐ No  Chew ☒ Yes  ☐ No
Swallow solids ☒ Yes  ☐ No  Feed self ☒ Yes  ☐ No

| Date | Diagnosis | Goals The individual will: | | Diagnosis | Goals The individual will: |
|---|---|---|---|---|---|
| 5/1 | 1. Alteration in Comfort: Pain related to muscle spasms | 1. Report less pain 2. Practice selected distraction techniques during pain episodes | 5/1 | Potential complication of Fx. tibia: Impaired circulation | Be free of complications of impaired circulation |
| 5/1 | 2. Potential impairment in skin integrity related to: -Imposed bedrest -Traction equipment | 1. Be free from skin complications of immobility | 5/1 | Potential inadequate skin traction | 1. Is positioned in free flowing, aligned traction |
| | | | 5/2 | Diversional activity deficit related to: imposed bedrest, isolation | 1. Occupy her time with activities other than TV viewing |
| 5/1 | 3. Potential alteration in bowel elimination: Constipation related to: Dietary patterns (low fiber) Embarrassment | 1. Have a daily bowel movement 2. Consume daily (at least) 3 fruit exchanges 6 vegetables 10 glasses of water | 5/4 | Potential impaired home maintenance management related to discharge with body cast to home for 10 weeks | 1. Parents will ask questions concerning home care 2. Demonstrate care of daughter's cast and other needs |

**Initials / Signature**

| | | | |
|---|---|---|---|
| 1. | 7. | 13. | 19. |
| 2. | 8. | 14. | 20. |
| 3. | 9. | 15. | 21. |
| 4. | 10. | 16. | 22. |
| 5. | 11. | 17. | 23. |
| 6. | 12. | 18. | 24. |

**Figure 1-9.** Care plan for Case Study 2. (Courtesy of the Wilmington Medical Center, Wilmington, Delaware)

| Date | Diagnosis | | Plan | Ints. | Evaluations |
|------|-----------|---|------|-------|-------------|
| 5/1 | 1. Alteration in Comfort: Pain related to muscle spasms | NDx | 1. Teach her rhythmic abdominal breathing to practice during muscle spasms<br>2. Coach her to practice breathing during episodes of spasms<br>3. Administer pain medications on time<br>4. Encourage her to use her radio with earphones during episodes of spasms and to increase the volume as the pain increases | | |
| 5/1 | 2. Potential impairment in skin integrity related to:<br>  Imposed bedrest<br>  Traction equipment | NDx | 1. Inspect back and heels at bath time, rinse soap off well<br>2. Massage skin over bony prominences<br>3. Protect heel under traction boot with a clear skin barrier dressing. Do not remove unless skin alterations are seen through dressing | | |
| 5/1 | 3. Potential alteration in bowel elimination:<br>  Constipation related to:<br>    – Dietary patterns (low fiber)<br>    – Imposed bedrest<br>    – Embarrassment | NDx | 1. Teach the relationship of activity, diet, and bowel elimination<br>2. Teach her to contract abdominal muscles several times a day<br>3. Have her keep a record of her daily intake of: Vegetables (low starch), fruits, bran, nuts, fluids, juices | | |

**Initials / Signature**

| | | | |
|---|---|---|---|
| 1. | 7. | 13. | 19. |
| 2. | 8. | 14. | 20. |
| 3. | 9. | 15. | 21. |
| 4. | 10. | 16. | 22. |
| 5. | 11. | 17. | 23. |
| 6. | 12. | 18. | 24. |

**Figure I-9.** (*continued*)

| Date | Diagnosis | | Plan | Ints. | Evaluations |
|---|---|---|---|---|---|
| | | | 4. Teach her to avoid: | | |
| | | | Bakery products | | |
| | | | Foods high in starch | | |
| | | | (corn, white bread, | | |
| | | | noodles, rice) | | |
| | | | 5. Request parents to | | |
| | | | bring in nutritious | | |
| | | | snacks (carrots, celery, | | |
| | | | apples) to keep on unit | | |
| | | | 6. Give her a bedpan | | |
| | | | after lunch | | |
| | | | − Tell her no one will in- | | |
| | | | terrupt her | | |
| | | | − Give her a room | | |
| | | | deodorizer to use | | |
| | | | − Put the TV or radio on | | |
| | | | to mask noises | | |
| 5/1 | 4. Potential complications | CP | 1. Assess limb (toes, skin | | |
| | of fractured tibia: | | around traction, popliteal | | |
| | Impaired circulation | | pulse) for temperature, color, | | |
| | | | tingling, loss of sensation | | |
| | | | Tid and hs | | |
| | | | 2. Remind her to wiggle her | | |
| | | | toes at least 10 times each hour | | |
| 5/1 | 5. Potential inadequate | CP | 1. Assure that: | | |
| | skin traction | | − Weights hang free | | |
| | | | − Ropes are away from bed | | |
| | | | − Ropes and pulleys are in | | |
| | | | straight alignment | | |
| | | | − Traction is never | | |
| | | | interrupted | | |
| | | | − She is in good align- | | |
| | | | ment and has not | | |
| | | | slipped down in bed | | |

**Initials / Signature**

| | | | |
|---|---|---|---|
| 1. | 7. | 13. | 19. |
| 2. | 8. | 14. | 20. |
| 3. | 9. | 15. | 21. |
| 4. | 10. | 16. | 22. |
| 5. | 11. | 17. | 23. |
| 6. | 12. | 18. | 24. |

**Figure I-9.** (continued)

| Date | Diagnosis | | Plan | Ints. | Evaluations |
|---|---|---|---|---|---|
| 5/2 | 6. Diversional activity deficit related to: Imposed bedrest Isolation | NDx | 1. Consult with recreational therapist for appropriate activities 2. Encourage other children on floor to visit and play cards with her 3. Encourage her to read stories to small children on unit in her room 4. Arrange for tutoring with school district 5. Try to stimulate her to do something other than watching TV e.g. Hook rug, electronic games 6. Allow her opportunities to share her feeling of loneliness | | |
| 5/4 | 7. Potential impaired home maintenance manage- ment related to Discharge with body cast to home for 10 weeks (approximate discharge date 6/10) | NDx | 1. Allow parents to share their concern about care of daughter after discharge 2. Assure them that they will have in opportunity to care for daughter under supervision in hospital 3. Discuss and teach each of the following when indicated: Cast care Hygienic measures Nutrition Elimination Diversional activities Tutoring Relief periods for parents from care | | |

**Initials / Signature**

| | | | | | | |
|---|---|---|---|---|---|---|
| 1. | | 7. | | 13. | | 19. |
| 2. | | 8. | | 14. | | 20. |
| 3. | | 9. | | 15. | | 21. |
| 4. | | 10. | | 16. | | 22. |
| 5. | | 11. | | 17. | | 23. |
| 6. | | 12. | | 18. | | 24. |

**Figure I-9.** (*continued*)

## Reference

Carnevali DL: Nursing Care Planning: Diagnosis and Management, 3rd ed, p 222. Philadelphia, JB Lippincott, 1983

## Bibliography for Section I

Aspinall MJ, Tanner C: Decision-making for Patient Care. New York, Appleton-Century-Crofts, 1981

Carpenito LJ, Duespohl TA: The nursing process. In A Guide to Effective Clinical Instruction. Rockville, Md, Aspen Systems Corp, 1981

Dickoff J, James P: A theory of theories: A position paper. Nurs Res 17:200–201, 1968

Diers D: Research in Nursing Practice, pp 44–52. Philadelphia, JB Lippincott, 1979

Ellis R: Characteristics of significant theories. Nurs Res 17:217–222, 1968

Fry VS: The creative approach to nursing. Am J Nurs 53:301–302, 1953

Griffith J, Christensen P: Nursing Process: Application of Theories, Frameworks, and Models. St Louis, CV Mosby 1982

Harris RB: A strong vote for the nursing process. Am J Nurs 81:1999–2001, 1981

Polit D, Hungler B: Nursing Research: Principles and Methods, 2nd ed. Philadelphia, JB Lippincott, 1982

### General Assessment

Communicating with patients. Am J Nurs 79:1074–1085, 1979

Dossey B: Perfecting your skill for systematic patient assessments. Nursing 9:42–45, 1979

Eggland ET: How to take a meaningful nursing history. Nursing 7(7):22–30, 1977

Mahoney EA, Verdisco L: How to Collect and Record a Health History. Philadelphia, JB Lippincott, 1982

Porter A et al: Patient needs on admission. Am J Nurs 77:112–113, 1977

### Specific Assessment

Blackburn NA, Cebenka D: Honing your respiratory assessment technique. RN 43(5):28–33, 1980

Brodish MS: Perinatal assessment. Journal of Obstetric and Gynecologic Nursing 10(1):42–46, 1981

Croushore M: Postoperative assessment: The key to avoiding the most common nursing mistakes. Nursing 9(4):47–51, 1979

Jacoby MK, Adams DJ: Teaching assessment of client functioning. Nurs Outlook 29:248–250, 1981

Jacox AK: Assessing pain. Am J Nurs 79:895–900, 1979

Jones C: Glasgow coma scale. Am J Nurs 79:1551–1553, 1979

McCaffery M: Undertreatment of acute pain with narcotics. Am J Nurs 76:1586, 1976

McCaffery M: Nursing Management of the Patient with Pain, 2nd ed. Philadelphia, JB Lippincott, 1980

McCaffery M: Patients shouldn't have to suffer—relieve their pain with injectable narcotics, Nursing 10(10):34–39, 1980

McCaffery M: Relieving pain with noninvasive techniques. Nursing 10(12):54–57, 1980

McCaffery M: Understanding your patient's pain. Nursing 10(9):26–31, 1980

Mallick MJ: Patient assessment—based on data, not intuition. Nursing Outlook 29:600–605, 1981

Margolin CP: Assessment of psychiatric patients. Journal of Emergency Nursing 10(4):30–33, 1980

Meissner JE: Evaluate your patient's level of independence. Nursing 10(9):72–73, 1980

Meissner JE: Predicting a patient's anxiety level during labor: A two-part assessment tool. Nursing 10(7):50–51, 1980

Meissner JE: Uncovering your patient's hidden psychosocial problem. Nursing 10(5):78–79, 1980

Meissner JE: Which patient on your unit might get a pressure sore? Nursing 10(6):64–65, 1980

Mortiz DA: Nursing histories: A guide yes; a form no. Oncology Nurse Forum 6(3):18–19, 1979

Pilette PC: Caution: Objectivity and specialization may be hazardous to your humanity. Am J Nurs 80:1588–1590, 1980

Salmond SW: How to assess the nutritional status of acutely ill patients. Am J Nurs 80:922–924, 1980

Spector RE: Cultural Diversity in Health and Illness. New York, Appleton-Century-Crofts, 1979

Stokes SA et al: Health assessment: Considerations for the older individual. Journal of Gerontological Nursing 6(6):328–337, 1980

Stoll RI: Guidelines for spiritual assessment. Am J Nurs 79:1574–1577, 1979

Watts RJ: Dimensions of sexual health. Am J Nurs 79:1568–1572, 1979

Whall AL: Nursing theory and the assessment of families. J Psychiatr Nurs 19:30–36, 1981

White JH et al: When your client has a weight problem. Am J Nurs 81:549–553, 1981

## Nursing Diagnosis

Aspinall MJ: Nursing diagnoses—the weak link. Nurs Outlook 24:433–437, 1976

Aspinall MJ, Jambruno N, Phoenix PS: The why and how of nursing diagnosis. Matern Child Nurs J 2:355–358, 1977

Avant K: Nursing diagnosis: Maternal attachment. Advances in Nursing Science 2(1):45–55, 1979

Bircher A: On the development and classification of nursing diagnoses. Nurs Forum 14:10–29, 1975

Bockrath M: Your patient needs two diagnoses—medical and nursing. Nursing Life 2(2):29–32, 1982

Bruce J: Implementation of nursing diagnosis: A nursing administrator's perspective. Nurs Clin North Am 14:509–515, 1979

Burgess AW, Holstrom LL: Rape trauma syndrome. Am J Psychiatry 131:981–986, 1974

Burgess AW, Holstrom LL: Assessing trauma in the rape victim. Am J Nurs 75:1288–1291, 1975

Dossey B: Nursing diagnosis. Nursing 11(6):34–38, 1981

Field L: The implementation of nursing diagnosis in clinical practice. Nurs Clin North Am 14:497–508, 1979

Fortin J, Rabinow J: Legal implications of nursing diagnosis. Nurs Clin North Am 14:555–561, 1979

Fredette S, O'Connor K: Nursing diagnosis in teaching and curriculum planning. Nurs Clin North Am 14:541–552, 1979

Gebbie K: Summary of the Second National Conference—Classification of Nursing Diagnoses. St. Louis, The Clearinghouse, St. Louis University, 1976

Gebbie K, Lavin M: Classifying nursing diagnoses. Am J Nurs 74:250–253, 1974

Gebbie K, Lavin M (eds): Classification of Nursing Diagnoses. St. Louis, CV Mosby, 1975

Gordon M: Nursing Diagnosis: Process and Application. New York, McGraw-Hill, 1982

Gordon M: Nursing diagnoses and the diagnostic process. Am J Nurs 76:1298–1300, 1976

Gordon M: The concept of nursing diagnosis. Nurs Clin North Am 14:487–495, 1979

Gordon M: Predictive strategies in diagnostic tasks. Nurs Res 29:39–45, 1980

Gordon M, Sweeney M: Methodological problems and issues in identifying and standardizing nursing diagnoses. Advances in Nursing Science 2(1):1–15, 1979

Gordon M, Sweeney M, McKeehan K: Nursing diagnosis: Looking at its use in the clinical area. Am J Nurs 80:672–675, 1980

Guzzetta C, Forsyth G: Nursing diagnostic pilot study: Psychophysiologic stress. Advances in Nursing Science 2(1):27–44, 1979

Hausman KA: The concept and application of nursing diagnosis. Journal of Neurological Nursing 12(6):76–80, 1980

Henderson B: Nursing diagnosis: Theory and practice. Advances in Nursing Science 1(1):75–83, 1978

Jones P: A terminology for nursing diagnosis. Advances in Nursing Science 2(1):65–71, 1979

Kim MJ, Moritz D: Classification of Nursing Diagnosis: Proceedings of the Third and Fourth National Conferences. New York, McGraw-Hill, 1982

Kritek PB: The generation and classification of nursing diagnosis: Toward a theory of nursing. Image 10(6):33–40, 1978

Kritek PB: Commentary: The development of nursing diagnosis and theory. Advances in Nursing Science 2(1):73–79, 1979

Leslie FM: Nursing diagnosis: Use in long-term care. Am J Nurs 81:1012–1014, 1981

McCourt AE: Measurement of functional deficit in quality assurance. Quality Assurance Update 5:1–3, 1981

McKay RP: What is the relationship between development and utilization of a taxonomy and nursing theory? Nursing Res 26:222–224, 1977

Mundinger M: Nursing diagnoses for cancer patients. Cancer Nursing 1:221–226, 1978

Popkess SA: Diagnosing your patient's strengths. Nursing 11(7):34–37, 1981

Price MR: How nursing diagnosis helps focus your care: The patient is starving . . . but why? RN 42(12):45–48, 1979

Price MR: Nursing diagnosis: Making a concept come alive. Am J Nurs 80:668–671, 1980

Rossi LP, Haines VM: Nursing diagnoses related to acute myocardial infarction. Cardiovascular Nursing 15(3):11–15, 1979

Roy C: A diagnostic classification system for nursing. Nursing Outlook 23:90–94, 1975

Soares C: Nursing and medical diagnoses: A comparison of variant and essential features. In Chaska N (ed): The Nursing Profession: Views Through the Mist. New York, McGraw-Hill, 1978

Spotts ST: A nursing diagnosis taxonomy for quality assurance and reimbursement. Pennsylvania Nurse 36(1):5–6, 1981

Weber S: Nursing diagnosis in private practice. Nurs Clin North Am 14:533–539, 1979

## Care Planning

Bailey JT, Claus KE: Decision-making in Nursing. St Louis, CV Mosby, 1975

Beck J: Standards as a guide for nursing care plans. Oncological Nursing Forum 7(4):28–30, 1980

Carnevali D: Nursing Care Planning: Diagnosis and Management, 3rd ed. Philadelphia, JB Lippincott, 1983

Duke University Hospital Nursing Services: Quality Assurance: Guidelines for Nursing Care. Philadelphia, JB Lippincott, 1980

Eichelberger KM et al: Self-care nursing plan: Helping children to help themselves. Pediatric Nursing 6(3):9–13, 1980

McCloskey JC: Nurse's orders: The next professional breakthrough. RN 43(2):99–100, 1980

Randolph D, Bernau K: Dealing with resistance in the nursing care conference. Am J Nurs 77:1955–1958, 1977

Roeder MA: Patient care plans and the evaluation of the nursing process. Supervisor Nurse 11(1):57–58, 1980

## Evaluation

American Nurses' Association: Guidelines for Review of Nursing Care at the Local Level. Washington, DC, US Government Printing Office, 1976

Barba M, Bennett B, Shaw WJ: The evaluation of patient care through use of ANA's standards of nursing practice. Supervisor Nurse 9(1):42–54, 1978

Block D: Evaluation of nursing care in terms of process and outcome: Issues in research and quality assurance. Nursing Res 24:256–263, 1975

Block D: Criteria, standards, norms—crucial terms in quality assurance. J Nurs Adm 7(9):20–30, 1977

Chow RK: Assuring the quality of care: A personal perspective—from tailoring to outcome measurement. Nursing Leadership 1(3):11–22, 1978

Hover J, Zimmer MJ: Nursing quality assurance: The Wisconsin system. Nursing Outlook 26:242–248, 1978

Hushower G, Gamberg D, Smith N: The nursing process in discharge planning. Supervisor Nurse 9(9):55–58, 1978

Laros J: Deriving outcome criteria from a conceptual model. Nursing Outlook 25:333–336, 1977

Mayers MG: A Systematic Approach to the Nursing Care Plan. New York, Appleton-Century-Crofts, 1976

Mayers MG, Norby RB, Watson AB: Quality Assurance for Patient Care: Nursing Perspectives. New York, Appleton-Century-Crofts, 1976

Phaneuf MC: The Nursing Audit: Self-Regulation in Nursing Practice. New York, Appleton-Century-Crofts, 1976

Snyder PJ: Goal setting. Supervisor Nurse 9(9):61–64, 1978

Ware A: Using nursing prognosis to set priorities. Am J Nurs 79:921–924, 1979

# Manual of Nursing Diagnoses

# Introduction

The Manual of Nursing Diagnoses consists of forty-three diagnostic categories. Each category is described with the following:
- Definition
- Etiological and contributing factors, organized according to pathophysiological, situational, and maturational factors that may contribute to or cause the altered state
- Defining characteristics, signs and symptoms of the diagnosis
- Focus assessment criteria, subjective and objective, which serve to guide the nurse to specific data collection in order to help confirm or rule out the diagnosis
- Nursing goals, statements that concisely direct nursing actions
- Principles and rationale for nursing care, statements that serve to explain the diagnosis or the rationale for assessing and intervening

Each diagnostic group is then further explained by one or more specific nursing diagnoses. These specific diagnoses were selected because of their frequency in nursing and do not in any respect represent exclusive categories. For example, *Impairment of Skin Integrity* has four specific diagnoses:

Related to pruritus
Related to immobility
Related to stoma problems
Related to pressure ulcer

But the nurse will be able to utilize this diagnosis to describe other states; for example:

**Impairment of Skin Integrity related to decreased circulation in feet secondary to diabetes mellitus**

The diagnoses listed below are not followed with specific *related to's* because of the nature of the category:

Activity Intolerance
Anxiety
Cardiac Output, Alterations in: Decreased
Comfort, Alterations in
Fear
Health Maintenance, Alterations in
Home Maintenance Management, Impaired
Knowledge Deficit
Rape Trauma Syndrome
Airway Clearance, Ineffective
Self-Concept, Disturbance in
Sleep Pattern Disturbance
Social Isolation

Instead, each of these categories has one group of interventions that focus on the treatment of the diagnostic category, regardless of the etiological and contributing factors.

Each specific nursing diagnosis is further explained with:

1. Assessment data, the subjective and objective signs and symptoms of the specific diagnosis
2. Outcome criteria, the goals for clients with the diagnosis
3. Interventions, which specifically direct the nurse to:
   - The assessment of causative and contributing factors
   - The reduction or elimination of the factors
   - The promotion of selected activities
   - Health teaching
   - Referrals

Each diagnostic category is concluded with a bibliography, containing books and periodicals in which the nurse can obtain more information about the diagnosis. Pertinent literature and organizations for the consumer are also cited when appropriate.

Readers of this manual are encouraged to become familiar with all diagnostic categories in order to incorporate them into their nursing practice. Until you become familiar with the diagnostic categories and their defining characteristics, the following guidelines are suggested:

1. Collect data, both subjective and objective, from client, family, other health care professionals, and records.
2. Validate inferences.
3. Identify a possible pattern or problem.
4. Does the problem require referral for treatment? If yes, refer (for this is a clinical problem). If no, go on to 5.
5. Look at the list of nursing diagnoses and select the possibilities.
6. Refer to Section II and examine the defining characteristics of each possible diagnosis.
7. Are they present? If yes, the diagnosis is confirmed; go on to 8. If no, refer to focus assessment criteria and gather the additional data to confirm or rule out the diagnosis.
8. Identify the etiological or contributing factors that relate to the diagnosis.

# Activity Intolerance

## Definition
Activity intolerance: A state in which the individual experiences an inability, physiologically or psychologically, to endure or tolerate an increase in activity.

## Etiological and Contributing Factors
Any factor that causes fatigue or compromises oxygen transport can cause activity intolerance. Some common factors are listed below.

## Pathophysiological
Alterations in the oxygen transport system
    Cardiac
        Congestive heart failure      Angina
        Arrhythmias      Myocardial infarction
    Respiratory
        Chronic obstructive pulmonary
          disease
    Circulatory
        Anemia
        Peripheral arterial disease
Diabetes mellitus
Chronic diseases
        Renal      Musculoskeletal
        Hepatic      Neurological
Malnourishment
Hypovolemia
Electrolyte imbalance

## Situational
Depression
Lack of motivation
Sedentary life-style
Prolonged bed rest
Stressors (*e.g.*)
        Impaired language function      Impaired motor function
        Impaired sensory function      Pain
Fatigue, caused by (*e.g.*)
        Sensory overload      Treatments
        Sensory deprivation      Treatment schedule
        Interrupted sleep      Medications
        Equipment that requires      Diagnostic studies
          strength (walkers, crutches,      Gait disorders
          braces)

## Defining Characteristics

Altered response to activity

Respiratory

Dyspnea

Shortness of breath

Pulse

Weak pulse

Decrease in rate

Excessive increase in rate

Blood pressure

Failure to increase with activity

Decrease

Weakness

Pallor or cyanosis

Confusion

Vertigo

Excessive increase in rate

Decrease in rate

Failure to return to resting rate
after 3 min

Rhythm change

Increase in diastolic 15 mm Hg

Impaired ability, related to fatigue, to

Turn in bed

Assume sitting position

Maintain alignment

Ambulate

Perform self-care activities

## Focus Assessment Criteria

Subjective data

Does person complain of

Weakness?

Fatigue?

Dyspnea?

Difficulty performing activities
of daily living?

Lack of sleep?

Objective data

1. Assess for the presence of factors that increase fatigue

Personal

Lack of incentive

History of ineffective coping

Environmental

Social isolation

Sensory overload

Disease-related

Cardiopulmonary disorders

Musculoskeletal disorders

Neurological disorders

Chronic diseases

Treatment-related

Bedrest/immobility

Medications

Treatment schedule

Diet

Diagnostic studies

Age

Lack of support system

Sensory deprivation

Insufficient rest/sleep periods

Pain

Fluid and electrolyte imbalances

Nutritional deficiencies

Assistance equipment (*e.g.*)

Crutches

Braces

Walkers

Caregivers' expectations

2. Assess response to activity*
- Take resting vital signs (see Table II–1)
  Pulse (rate, rhythm, quality)
  Blood pressure
  Respirations (rate, depth)
- Have person perform the activity
- Take vital signs immediately after activity
- Have person rest for 3 minutes; take vital signs again
- Assess for presence of

  | | |
  |---|---|
  | Pallor | Confusion |
  | Cyanosis | Disequilibrium |

## Nursing Goals

Through selected interventions the nurse will
- Identify factors in the individual that increase fatigue
- Reduce those factors when possible
- Increase the activity tolerance of the individual and decrease the signs of anoxia (abnormal pulse, blood pressure, respirations) when possible

## Principles and Rationale for Nursing Care

1. Endurance is the output of mental and physical work by the person as he seeks to accomplish a task.

Table II–1. **Physiological Response to Activity (Expected and Abnormal)**

| | Pulse | Blood Pressure | Respirations |
|---|---|---|---|
| **Resting** | | | |
| Normal | 60–90 | < 140/90 | < 20 |
| Abnormal | > 100 | > 140/90 | > 20 |
| **Immediately After Activity** | | | |
| Normal | ↑ Rate<br>↑ Strength | ↑ Systolic | ↑ Rate<br>↑ Depth |
| Abnormal | ↓ Rate<br>↓ Strength<br>Irregular rhythm | Decrease or no change in systolic | Excessive ↑<br>↓ Rate |
| **3 Min After** | | | |
| Normal | Within 6 beats of resting pulse | | |
| Abnormal | >7 beats of resting pulse or complaints of confusion, incoordination, dyspnea, pallor | | |

*Refer to Principles and Rationale for Nursing Care for interpretation of responses to activity.

2. An individual's endurance will directly influence his progress in rehabilitation.
3. The ability to maintain a given level of performance is dependent on strength, coordination, reaction time, alertness, and motivation.
4. Fatigue can result from loss of endurance, lack of motivation, pathophysiology, treatments, diagnostic studies, and medications.
5. Any stressor (personal, environmental, disease-related, or treatment-related) can reduce a person's tolerance for activity (see Etiological and Contributing Factors).
6. Any factor that compromises the cardiopulmonary, vascular, neurological, or musculoskeletal function will reduce tolerance to activity.
7. The response of the person to activity can be evaluated by pulse rate, blood pressure, and respirations (see Table II–1).
8. The daily schedule of the person must be coordinated by the nurse in order to reduce periods of excess energy expenditure.

# Activity Intolerance
## Related to (specify etiological and contributing factors)

> *Example:* **Activity Intolerance** Related to Insufficient Oxygen Transport Secondary to COPD

## Assessment

See preceding, Defining Characteristics.

---

### Outcome Criteria

The person will
- Identify factors that reduce his activity tolerance
- Progress to the highest level of mobility possible
- Exhibit a decrease in anoxic signs of increased activity (pulse, blood pressure, respirations)

---

## Interventions

The following interventions apply to most individuals with activity intolerance, regardless of the etiology.

### A. Assess for causative and contributing factors

- Disorders of oxygen transport system (see *Impaired Gas Exchange* and *Alterations in Cardiac Output: Decreased*)
- Nutritional deficiencies (see *Alterations in Nutrition: Less Than Body Requirements*)
- Fluid and electrolyte imbalances (see *Fluid Volume Deficit* and *Fluid Volume Excess*)

- Insufficient sleep or rest periods
- Pain
- Prolonged immobility
- Treatment-related considerations
  Medication
  Diagnostic studies
  Staff expectations
- Personal factors
  Lack of incentive
  Depression

## B. Reduce or eliminate contributing factors if possible

1. Inadequate rest or sleep periods
   - Plan rest periods according to the person's daily schedule (rest periods may occur between activities)
   - Encourage person to rest during the first hour following meals (rest can take the form of napping, sitting and watching TV, or sitting with legs elevated)
   - Assess nocturnal sleep (refer to *Sleep Pattern Disturbance* for additional information)
2. Pain
   - Evaluate pain and the present treatment regimen (refer to *Alterations in Comfort* for specific assessment criteria and interventions)
3. Treatment-related factors
   a. Medications
      - Assess for side-effects of medications
      - Reduce side-effects, if possible (*e.g.*, for diuretic-induced hypokalemia, teach person to increase dietary potassium—oranges, tomatoes, bananas, dried fruit; for antibiotic-induced diarrhea, teach person to consume yogurt two or three times a day if not contraindicated)
   b. Daily schedule
      - Assess the present daily schedule of the person
      - Consider treatments, diagnostic studies, etc.
      - Adjust schedule to reduce energy expenditure when possible (*e.g.*, cancel morning shower or bath when a diagnostic study is scheduled for the morning)
      - Provide rest periods between activities (*e.g.*, bath and breakfast)
4. Lack of incentive
   - Identify progress daily and encourage record keeping by patients in selected cases (*e.g.*, "Today you walked four feet farther and your pulse did not go as high as yesterday")
   - Allow person to set activity schedule and functional activity goals (if his goal is too low, contract with him: *e.g.*, "If you walk halfway up the hall, I will play three games of cards with you")
   - Plan a purpose for the ambulation, such as walking to the dayroom for a group activity or meal or walking to the hall to see grandchild
   - Promote a sincere "can do" attitude to provide a positive atmosphere to encourage increased activity; convey to the person the belief that he can improve his mobility status
   - Explore with the person and his family possible incentives; consider what the person values (*e.g.*)
     Playing with grandchild

Returning to work

Performing a task, such as a craft

- For additional interventions, refer to *Ineffective Individual Coping Related to Depression*

## C. Assess the individual's response to activity

- Take resting pulse, blood pressure, and respirations
- Consider rate, rhythm, and quality (if signs are abnormal—*e.g.*, pulse above 100 —consult with physician about the advisability of increasing activity)
- Have person perform the activity
- Take vital signs immediately after activity; take pulse for 15 seconds and multiply by 4 instead of for a full minute
- Have person rest for 3 minutes; take vital signs again
- Discontinue the activity if the individual responds to the activity with

Complaints of chest pain, dyspnea, vertigo, or confusion

Decrease in pulse rate

Failure of systolic rate to increase

Decrease in systolic blood pressure

Increase in diastolic rate 15 mmHg

Decrease in respiratory rate
- Reduce the intensity, frequency, or duration of the activity if:
  a. The pulse takes longer than 3–4 minutes to return within 6 beats of the resting pulse rate
  b. The respiratory rate increase is excessive after the activity
  c. Other signs of anoxia are present, *e.g.*, confusion, vertigo
- Prevent the complications of immobility (refer to *Alterations in Respiratory Function Related to Immobility* and *Impairment of Skin Integrity Related to Immobility*)

## D. Progress the activity gradually

1. Increase the person's tolerance for the activity by having him perform the activity more slowly, or for a shorter period of time with more rest pauses, or with more assistance. (Strenuous activity may increase the pulse by 50 beats. Such a rate is still satisfactory, as long as it returns to the resting pulse rate within 3 minutes.)
   - Encourage the person to turn and lift himself actively unless contraindicated
   - Raise the bed to a high position so that the person can slide out of the bed to a standing position rather than try to get up from a very low position
   - Provide support when the person begins to stand
   - If the person is unable to stand without buckling his knees, he is not ready for ambulation; have him practice standing in place with assistance
2. Promote optimal sitting balance and tolerance by increasing muscle strength
   - Gradually increase exercise tolerance by starting with 15 minutes, for the first time out of bed
   - Have the person get out of bed 3 times a day, increasing the time out of bed by 15 minutes each day
   - Practice transfers, having the person do as much active movement as possible
3. Promote ambulation with or without assistance devices
   - Choose a gait that is safe for the individual (If his gait appears awkward, but he has stability, allow him to continue; stay close by giving clear coaching messages: *e.g.*, "Look straight ahead, not down")

- Allow the person to gauge the rate of the ambulation
- Prevent the person from falling (Stand slightly behind him on his weaker side, one hand on his belt and one on his shoulder; *e.g.*, if the person has a weak side, your left hand should be on his left shoulder)
- Encourage person to wear comfortable walking shoes (slippers do not support the feet properly)

### E. Initiate health teaching or referrals as indicated

1. Teach the person safety precautions to prevent falls (see *Potential for Injury*)
2. Teach the person the proper use of walking aids (crutches, walkers, canes) and ensure the proper fit of such devices
3. Teach the person methods of preventing the complications of immobility
   - Encourage frequent turning and repositioning
   - Encourage exercises — range of motion, isometrics — provide bedside exercise equipment if needed
   - Encourage adequate fluid intake, 2 to 3 quarts per day
   - Encourage good dietary habits with adequate roughage
   - Encourage coughing and deep-breathing exercises (see *Alterations in Respiratory Function Related to Immobility*)
4. Consult with a physical therapist for assistance in increasing activity tolerance

### Bibliography

Allen S: Step by step: Renew a patient's initiative. Nursing 11(11):56–57, 1981

Bouman HD: An exploratory analytical survey of therapeutic exercise. Am J Phys Med 46:26–31, 1967

Licht S (ed): Therapeutic Exercise. Baltimore, Waverly Press, 1965

Louis MC, Pouse S: Aphasia and endurance: Consideration in assessment and care of the stroke patient. Nurs Clin North Am 15:265–292, 1980

Lunsford B: Clinical indicators of endurance. Phys Ther 58:704–790, 1978

Ziegler J: Physical reconditioning. Nursing 10(8):67–69, 1980

# Anxiety

## Definition

Anxiety: A state in which the individual experiences feelings of uneasiness (apprehension) and activation of the autonomic nervous system in response to a vague, nonspecific threat.*

## Etiological and Contributing Factors

### Pathophysiological

Any factor that interferes with the basic human needs for food, air, and comfort

### Situational

Actual or perceived threat to self-concept

| | |
|---|---|
| Loss of status and prestige | Failure (or success) |
| Lack of recognition from others | Loss of valued possessions |

Actual or perceived loss of significant others

| | |
|---|---|
| Death | Moving |
| Divorce | Temporary or permanent separation |

Actual or perceived threat to biological integrity

| | |
|---|---|
| Dying | Invasive procedures |
| Assault | Disease |

Actual or perceived change in environment

| | |
|---|---|
| Hospitalization | Retirement |
| Moving | |

Actual or perceived change in socioeconomic status

| | |
|---|---|
| Unemployment | Promotion |
| New job | |

Transmission of another person's anxiety to the individual

### Maturational (threat to developmental task)

Infant/child: Separation, mutilation, peer relationships, achievement
Adolescent: Sexual development, peer relationships, independence
Adult: parenting, career development, effects of aging
Elderly: sensory losses, motor losses, financial problems, retirement

## Defining Characteristics

### Physiological

| | |
|---|---|
| Increased heart rate | Insomnia |
| Elevated blood pressure | Fatigue and weakness |

*Anxiety differs from fear in that the anxious person cannot identify the threat. With fear, the threat can be identified.

Increased respiratory rate
Diaphoresis
Dilated pupils
Voice tremors/pitch changes
Tremors
Palpitations
Nausea and/or vomiting

Flushing
Dry mouth
Body aches and pains
Urinary frequency
Restlessness
Faintness
Paresthesias

## Emotional

Person states that he has feelings of

Apprehension
Helplessness
Nervousness
Fear

Lack of self-confidence
Losing control
Tension or being "keyed up"

Person exhibits

Irritability
Angry outbursts
Crying
Tendency to blame others

Criticism of self and others
Withdrawal
Lack of initiative
Self-depreciation

## Cognitive

Inability to concentrate
Lack of awareness of surroundings
Forgetfulness
Rumination
Orientation to past rather than to present or future
Blocking of thoughts (inability to remember)

## Focus Assessment Criteria

### Subjective data

1. History of the individual from client and significant others
   Life-style

   Interests
   Work history
   Coping patterns (past, present)

   Strengths, limitations
   Previous level of functioning,
   handling stress

   Support system

   Availability

   Quality of support

   History of medical problems/treatments
   Activities of daily living

   Ability to perform

   Desire to perform

2. History of unusual sensations and thought production (*e.g.*, palpitations, tingling, dyspnea, dry mouth, nausea, diaphoresis)

   Precipitating factors
   Frequency
   Duration

   Routine time of occurrence
   Description in individual's own
   words

3. Assess for presence of
   Feelings of

   Extreme sadness and worthless-
   ness
   Guilt for past actions
   Apprehension

   Harm from others
   Mind being controlled by
   external agents
   Being unable to cope

Rejection or isolation

Falling apart

Living in an unreal world

Thoughts racing

Mistrust or suspiciousness of
others

Being held prisoner

Manipulation by others

Difficulty concentrating

Senses difficulty grasping
particular circumstances or
events

States he is unable to follow
what is being said

Hallucinations (including an objective component)

Visual

Olfactory

Auditory

Tactile

Gustatory

4. Orientation

Person

"What is your name?"

"What is your occupation?"

"Tell me about yourself"

Time

"What season is it?"

"What month is it?"

Place

"Where are you?"

"Where do you live?"

5. Problem-solving ability.

"What would you do if the phone rang?"

"What is the difference between the doctor and the president?"

## Objective data

1. General appearance

Facial expression (*e.g.*, sad, hostile, expressionless)

Dress (*e.g.*, meticulous, disheveled, seductive, eccentric)

2. Behavior during interview

Withdrawm

Cooperative

Hostile

Quiet

Apathetic

3. Communication pattern

Content

Appropriate

Sexually preoccupied

Rambling

Delusions (of grandeur,

Suspicious

persecution, reference,

Denial of problem

influence, control or

Homicidal plans

bodily sensations)

Suicidal ideas

Flow of thought

Appropriate

Jumps from one topic to another

Blocking of ideas (unable to
finish idea)

Unable to come to conclusion,
be decisive

Circumstantial (unable to get to
point)

Ideas loosely connected

Rate of speech
    Appropriate                    Reduced
    Excessive                     Pressured
Nonverbal behavior
  Affect appropriate/inappropriate to verbal content
  Gestures, mannerisms, facial grimaces
  Posture

4. Interaction skills
  With a nurse
    Inappropriate             Shows dependency
    Relates well             Demanding/pleading
    Withdrawn/preoccupied with   Hostile
      self
  With significant others
    Relates with all family members   Does not seek interaction
      or with some             Does not have visitors
    Hostile toward one member/all
      members

5. Activities of daily living
  Emotionally capable of caring for self
  Physically capable of caring for self

6. Nutritional status
    Appetite                Weight (within normal limits,
    Eating patterns            decreased, increased)

7. Sleep/rest pattern
    Recent change          Early wakefulness
    Sleeps too much/too little   Insomnia

8. Personal hygiene
    Cleanliness (body, hair, teeth)   Clothes (condition,
    Grooming (clothes, hair,       appropriateness)
      makeup)

9. Motor activity
    Within normal limits
    Increased               Agitated
    Decreased             Repetitive

10. Present response to stressors
  "Acting-out" behaviors
    Derogating            Resentfulness
    Fighting              Motor restlessness
    Arguing              Pacing
    Intimidating          Physical exertion
  Paralysis and retreating behaviors
    Withdrawal           Dissociation
    Depression           Ritualistic behavior
    Denial               Blocking
  Somatizing
    Headache             Syncope
    Dyspnea
  Constructive action
    Seeking support from others
    Ventilating

## Nursing Goals

Through selected interventions the nurse will seek to
- Promote learning and problem-solving abilities in managing anxiety
- Assist the person to recognize anxiety and usual coping mechanisms
- Identify disturbed coping mechanisms
- Assist the person in identifying alternative coping mechanisms to manage anxiety when usual patterns are not adaptive
- Support the person in using adaptive coping mechanisms or implementing alternative ones
- Provide comfort and security
- Reduce severe or panic anxiety

## Principles and Rationale for Nursing Care

1. Anxiety is conceptually different from fear, in that fear has an identified stimulus. Anxiety is a feeling aroused by a vague nonspecific threat.
2. Anxiety is communicated interpersonally.
3. Anxiety varies in intensity depending on the severity of the threat, as perceived by the person, and the success or failure of his efforts to cope with his feelings.
4. The operational definition of anxiety is useful in dealing effectively with anxious individuals. Operationally, anxiety is defined as follows:
   (1) The individual has expectations and needs
   (2) These expectations or needs are not met
   (3) Discomfort (anxiety) is felt
   (4) The individual uses automatic coping mechanisms to decrease anxiety
   (5) These coping strategies are rationalized or justified rather than being explained
5. Patterns of coping with anxiety are
   (1) Acting-out: converting anxiety into anger which is either overtly or covertly expressed
   (2) Paralysis or retreating behaviors: withdrawing or being immobilized by own anxiety
   (3) Somatizing: converting anxiety into physical symptoms
   (4) Constructive action: using anxiety to learn and problem-solve (includes goal setting, learning new skills, and seeking information)
6. Coping mechanisms may be either adaptive or disturbed. This must be individually assessed.
7. Disturbed coping mechanisms are characterized by inability to make choices, conflict, repetition and rigidity, alienation, and secondary gains. Refer to *Ineffective Individual Coping* for further information.
8. The term *anxiety* is used to refer to both a response to a particular situation—state anxiety—and the differences among people in interpreting situations as threatening—trait anxiety (Spielberger).
9. Persons with relatively high levels of trait anxiety tend to perceive greater danger in situations that threaten self-esteem than do persons with lower levels. These individuals respond with higher levels of state anxiety (Spielberger).
10. The effects of anxiety on a person's abilities are as follows:

    Mild

    Perception and attention heightened; alert
    Able to deal with problem situations
    Can integrate past, present, and future experiences

Uses learning; can consensually validate; formulates meanings
Curious, repeats questions
Sleeplessness

### Moderate

Perception somewhat narrowed; selectively inattentive, but can direct attention
Slightly more difficult to concentrate; learning requires more effort
Views present experiences in terms of past
May fail to notice what is happening in a peripheral situation; will have some difficulty in adapting and analyzing
Voice/pitch changes
Increased respiratory and heart rates
Tremors, shakiness

### Severe

Perception greatly reduced; focuses on scattered details; can't attend to more even when instructed to
Learning severely impaired; highly distractable, unable to concentrate
Views present experiences in terms of past; almost unable to understand current situation
Functions poorly; communication difficult to understand
Hyperventilation, tachycardia, headache, dizziness, nausea

### Panic

Perception distorted; focuses on blown-up detail; scattering may be increased
Learning cannot occur
Unable to integrate experiences; can focus only on present; unable to see or understand situation; lapses in recall of thoughts
Unable to function; usually increased motor activity and/or unpredictable responses to even minor stimuli; communication not able to be understood
Vomiting; feelings of impending doom

11. The most common sign of anxiety in children and adolescents is increased motor activity. Signs of anxiety can be viewed developmentally and may be reflected in the following ways:

    *Birth to 9 months:* disruption in physiological functioning, *e.g.*, sleep disorders, colic

    *9 months to 4 years:* major source is loss of significant others and loss of love; therefore anxiety may be seen as anger when parents leave, somatic illnesses, motor restlessness, regressive behaviors (thumb sucking, head banging, rocking), regression in toilet training

    *4 to 6 years:* major source is fear of body damage; belief that his bad behavior causes bad things to happen *e.g.*, illness; somatic complaints of headache, stomachache

    *6 to 12 years:* excessive verbalization, compulsive behavior; *e.g.*, repeating a task over and over

    *Adolescence:* similar to 6 to 12 years plus types of negativistic behavior

12. Aggression is a response to a threat or frustration in which verbal and/or physical aggressive action offers relief to the anxiety experienced. Operationally, the steps are:

    (1) The individual experiences a threat or frustration
    (2) Anxiety is felt
    (3) Feelings of insecurity and helplessness occur
    (4) Increasing anxiety is decreased through verbal or physical aggression

13. Aggressive behavior may vary from irritation to rage and may be directed toward self, others, or objects.

14. Limits provide a sense of security. There is a need for predictability about self and environment.

15. Feelings of anger can be expressed either overtly or covertly. Examples of overt expression include hitting or fighting, nonverbal glaring, and verbal attack. Examples of covert expression of anger include somatizing, depression, and suicide.

16. Feelings of anxiety or anger may be unacceptable to the individual, and avoidance coping mechanisms may be used. Examples include denial, projection, and rationalization.

17. In managing inappropriate aggressive behavior, use the least amount of external control possible.

18. Individuals with severe or panic anxiety may be more agitated by attempts to communicate.

19. Anger is a response to frustration and anxiety.

20. Anger differs from hostility in that anger is usually short-lived and compatible in relationships. Hostility is a feeling of antagonism accompanied by a wish to hurt or humiliate others.

21. Children need opportunities and encouragement to express anger in a controlled, acceptable manner, *e.g.*, choosing not to play a particular game, choosing not to play with a particular person, slamming a door, or voicing anger. Unacceptable expressions of anger include throwing an object, hitting a person, and breaking an object.

22. Children who are not permitted to express their anger may develop hostility and perceive the world as unfriendly.

23. Hostility is usually the result of frustrated or unfulfilled needs or wishes, *e.g.*, unrealistic expectations of others, unrealistic expectations for self, low self-concept, and feelings of humiliation.

24. The hostile person may respond by repressing his hostility and withdrawing (depression), denying the hostility and overreacting with extreme compliance (politeness), or engaging in overt hostile behavior (verbal or nonverbal).

---

### Outcome Criteria

The person will
- Recognize his own anxiety and coping patterns
- Experience an increase in psychological and physiological comfort
- Use effective coping mechanisms in managing anxiety

---

## Interventions

The nursing interventions for the diagnosis *Anxiety* apply to any individual with anxiety regardless of the etiological and contributing factors.

## A. Assist the person to reduce his present level of anxiety

1. Assess level of anxiety (See Principles and Rationale for Nursing Care for specific differentiation)

|            |         |
|------------|---------|
| Mild       | Severe  |
| Moderate   | Panic   |

2. Provide reassurance and comfort
   - Stay with the person
   - Do not make demands or ask him to make decisions
   - Support present coping mechanisms, *e.g.*, allow client to walk, talk, cry; do not confront or argue with his defenses or rationalizations
   - Speak slowly and calmly
   - Be aware of your own concern and avoid reciprocal anxiety
   - Convey a sense of empathic understanding, *e.g.*, quiet presence, touch, allowing crying, talking, etc.
   - Provide reassurance that a solution can be found
3. Decrease sensory stimulation
   - Use short, simple sentences
   - Give concise directions
   - Focus on the here and now
   - Remove excess stimulation, *e.g.*, take person to quieter room; limit contact with others—patients or family—who are also anxious
   - If person is hyperventilating, have him take slow, deep breaths and breathe with him
   - Attempt to occupy person with a simple, repetitive task
   - Consult physician for possible pharmacological therapy if indicated

B. When anxiety is diminished enough for learning to take place, assist person in recognizing his anxiety in order to initiate learning or problem-solving
   - Request validation of your assessment of anxiety, *e.g.*, "Are you uncomfortable now?"
   - If person can say yes, continue in the learning process; if he is not able to acknowledge anxiety, continue supportive measures until he is able (refer to A)
   - When able to learn, determine usual coping mechanisms: "What do you usually do when you get upset?"
   - Assess for unmet needs or expectations; encourage recall and description of what the person experienced immediately prior to feeling anxious
   - Assist in reevaluation of the perceived threat by discussing the following:
     1. Were expectations realistic?
     2. Was it possible to meet his expectations?
     3. Where in the sequence of events was change possible?
   - Encourage the person to recall and analyze similar instances of anxiety
   - Explore what alternative behaviors might have been used if coping mechanisms were maladaptive
   - ~~Encourage the person to recall and analyze similar instances of anxiety~~

C. Reduce or eliminate problematic coping mechanisms
   1. Depression, withdrawal (see *Ineffective Individual Coping Related to Depression*)
   2. Violent behavior (see *Potential for Violence*)
   3. Denial
      - Develop an atmosphere of empathic understanding
      - Assist in lowering level of anxiety
      - Focus on present situation
      - Give feedback about current reality; identify positive achievements
      - Have person describe events in detail; focus on getting specifics of who, what, when, and where

4. Numerous physical complaints with no known organic base
   - Encourage expression of feelings
   - Give positive feedback when person is symptom-free
   - Acknowledge that the symptoms must be burdensome
   - Encourage interest in external environment, *e.g.*, outside activity, volunteering, helping others
   - Listen to the complaints
   - Evaluate the secondary gains the person receives and attempt to interrupt cycle; see person on a regular basis, not simply in response to somatic complaints
   - Discuss with person how others are reacting to him; attempt to have him identify his behavior when others react negatively (withdrawal? anger?)
   - Avoid "doing something" to each complaint; set limits when appropriate, *e.g.*, may refuse to call M.D. in response to a request for headache medication
   - When setting limits, provide an alternative outlet, *e.g.*, redirect to use relaxation technique (see Appendix IV, Stress Management Techniques)
5. Anger* (*e.g.*, demanding behavior, manipulation)
   a. With adults
      - Identify the presence of anger, *e.g.*, feelings of frustration, anxiety, helplessness, presence of irritability, verbal outbursts
      - Recognize your reactions to an individual's behavior; be aware of your own feelings in working with angry individuals
      - If person can verbalize feelings, assist in identifying sources of frustration and anger
      - Assist in making connections between feelings of frustration and subsequent behavior
      - Have person analyze consequences of behavior
      - Convey a sense of understanding of those things over which he has little control
      - Set limits on manipulative or irrational demands
      - State limits clearly; tell person exactly what is expected ("I cannot allow you to scream [throw objects etc.]")
      - When stating an unacceptable behavior, give an alternative, *e.g.*, suggest a quiet room, physical exertion, a chance for one-to-one communication
      - State the consequences if limits are violated
      - Develop behavior modification strategies; discuss with all personnel involved for consistency
      - When discussing a limit with the person, avoid stating it in such a way that it is perceived as a challenge
      - Give a brief explanation for the limit; if behavior continues, enforce the limit; encourage the person to express his feelings about the limit
      - Structure experiences that the person can do successfully
      - Provide positive feedback
      - Interact with the person when he is not demanding or manipulative
      - Discuss your feelings and the person's behavior with entire team; support each other and provide a consistent approach
   b. With children
      - Encourage the child to share his anger, *e.g.*, "How did you feel when

---

*Anger is a response to frustration and anxiety. Not all anger is problematic. It can be used for problem-solving.

you had your injection?" "How did you feel when Mary would not play with you?"

- Tell the child that being angry is okay, *e.g.*, "I sometimes get angry when I can't have what I want"
- Encourage and allow the child to express his anger in acceptable ways, *e.g.*, loud talking, hitting a play object, or running outside around the house

## D. Initiate health teaching and referrals as indicated

1. For patients identified as having chronic anxiety and disturbed coping mechanisms, refer for ongoing psychiatric treatment
2. Provide phone numbers for emergency intervention
   - Hotlines
   - Psychiatric emergency room
   - On-call staff if available
3. Instruct person in use of relaxation techniques (see Appendix IV)
4. Instruct person in constructive problem-solving (see Appendix VII)
5. Assist parents to respond constructively to age-related developmental needs (see Appendix VIII)

## Bibliography

Brink R: How serious is the child's behavioral problem? Matern Child Nurs J, 7:33–36, 1982

Carlson C, Blackwell B: Behavioral Concepts and Nursing Interventions, pp 128–131. Philadelphia, JB Lippincott, 1978

Decker N: Anxiety in the general hospital. In Fann W, Karacau I, Parkorny A, et al (eds): Phenomenology and Treatment of Anxiety, pp 287–298. Jamaica, NY, Spectrum Publications, 1979

Holderly R, McNulty E: Feelings, feelings: How to make a rational response to emotional behavior. Nursing 10(3):39–43, 1979

Knowles R: Dealing with feelings: Managing anxiety. Am J Nurs 81:110–111, 1981

Knowles R: Handling anger: Responding vs. reacting. Am J Nurs 81:2196–2197, 1981

Lyon G: Limit setting as a therapeutic tool. In Backer B, Dubbert P, Eisenman E: Psychiatric/Mental Health Nursing: Contemporary Readings, pp 99–111. New York, Van Nostrand, 1978

Melichar M: Using crisis theory to help parents cope with a child's temper tantrums. Matern Child Nurs J 5:181–185, 1980

Nissley B, Townes N: Guidelines for intervention in aggressive behavior. In Backer B, Dubbert P, Eisenman E: Psychiatric/Mental Health Nursing: Contemporary Readings, pp 174–180. New York, D. Van Nostrand, 1978

Silver L: Recognition and treatment of anxiety in children and adolescents. In Fann W, Karacau I, Parkorny A, et al (eds): Phenomenology and Treatment of Anxiety, pp 93–109. Jamaica, NY, Spectrum, 1979

Spielberger C, Sarason I (eds): Stress and Anxiety, vol. I. Washington, DC, Hemisphere, 1975

Stewart A: Handling the aggressive patient. Perspect Psychiatr Care, 16:5–6, 228–232, 1978

Thomas M, Baker J, Estes N: Anger: A tool for self-awareness. Am J Nurs 70:2586–2590, 1970

# Bowel Elimination, Alterations in: Constipation

*Related to* **Change in Life-Style**

*Related to* **Immobility**

*Related to* **Painful Defecation**

## Definition

Constipation: The state in which the individual experiences or is at high risk of experiencing stasis of the large intestine resulting in infrequent elimination and hard, dry feces.

## Etiological and Contributing Factors

Pathophysiological

Malnutrition

Sensory/motor disorders

| | |
|---|---|
| Spinal cord lesions | Cerebrovascular accident (stroke) |
| Spinal cord injury | Neurological diseases |

Drug side-effects

| | |
|---|---|
| Antacids | Calcium |
| Iron | Anticholinergics |
| Barium | Anesthetics |
| Aluminum | Narcotics (codeine, morphine) |

Metabolic and endocrine disorders

| | |
|---|---|
| Anorexia nervosa | Hypothyroidism |
| Obesity | Hyperparathyroidism |

Ileus

Pain (upon defecation)

Hemorrhoids      Back injury

Decreased peristalsis related to hypoxia (cardiac, pulmonary)

Megacolon

Situational

| | |
|---|---|
| Immobility | Lack of privacy |
| Pregnancy | Inadequate diet (lack of |
| Stress | roughage/thiamine) |
| Surgery | Dehydration |
| Lack of exercise | Habitual laxative use |
| Irregular evacuation patterns | Fear of rectal or cardiac pain |

Maturational

Infant: Formula

Child: Toilet training (reluctance to interrupt play)

Elderly: Decreased motility of GI tract

## Defining Characteristics

Hard, formed stool
Decreased bowel sounds
Defecation occurs less than three times a week
Reported feeling of rectal fullness
Reported feeling of pressure in rectum
Straining and pain on defecation
Palpable impaction

## Focus Assessment Criteria

### Subjective data

1. Elimination pattern
   - Usual pattern
   - Present pattern
   - Laxative use (type? how often?)
   - Enema use (type? how often?)
2. History of symptoms
   - Onset
   - Duration
   - Location
   - Description
   - Frequency
   - Precipitated by what?
   - Relieved by what?
   - Aggravated by what?
3. Associated symptoms/complaints of
   - Headache
   - Weakness
   - Lethargy
   - Anorexia
   - Thirst
   - Pain
   - Cramping
   - Weight loss/gain
4. Life-style
   - Activity level
     - Occupation
     - Exercise (what? how often?)
   - Nutrition
     - 24-hour recall of foods and liquids taken
     - Usual 24-hour intake
       - Carbohydrates
       - Fat
       - Protein
       - Roughage
       - Liquids
5. Current drug therapy
   - Antibiotics
   - Iron
   - Steroids
   - Antacids
   - CNS depressants
6. Medical-surgical history
   - Present conditions
   - Past conditions
   - Surgical history (colostomy? ileostomy?)

### Objective data

1. Stool

| Color | Odor | Consistency |
|---|---|---|
| Brown | Normal | Soft, formed |
| Yellow | Foul | Soft, bulky |
| Yellow-green | | Small, dry |
| Green | | Pasty |

| Color | Odor | Consistency |
|---|---|---|
| Black | | Diarrheal |
| Tan (clay-colored) | | Hard |
| Red | | |

| Size/shape | Components |
|---|---|
| Narrow | Blood |
| Large caliber | Mucus |
| Small caliber | Pus |
| Round | Parasites |
| | Undigested food |

2. Nutrition

| Food intake | Fluid intake |
|---|---|
| Type | Type |
| Amounts | Amounts |

3. GI motility (auscultation, light palpation)

*Bowel sounds*

| | |
|---|---|
| High-pitched, gurgling (5 per min) | Weak and infrequent |
| High-pitched frequent, loud, pushing | Absent |

*Abdominal distention*

| | |
|---|---|
| None | Moderate |
| Slight | Severe |

*Flatulence*

| | |
|---|---|
| None | Frequent |
| Occasionally | |

4. Perianal area

| | |
|---|---|
| Hemorrhoids | Irritation |
| Fissures | Impaction |

## Nursing Goals

Through selected interventions the nurse will seek to
- Promote positive lifelong dietary and health habits in an effort to facilitate adequate and regular bowel function
- Reduce present symptomatology

## Principles and Rationale for Nursing Care

General
1. Bowel patterns may be culturally determined.
2. Circadean rhythms may be utilized to assist defecation at a regular time.
3. Activity influences bowel elimination by improving muscle tone and stimulating appetite and peristalsis.

4. Factors that influence the color of stool:

| Color | Diet | Drugs | Disease |
| --- | --- | --- | --- |
| Yellow–yellow green | Breast milk | Antibiotics<br>Senna | Severe diarrhea |
| Green | Green vegetables | Mercurous chloride<br>Indomethacin<br>Calomel<br>Dithiazanine | Severe diarrhea |
| Black–dark brown | Cherries | Iron<br>Charcoal<br>Bismuth | Upper GI bleeding<br>Anticoagulants<br>Steroids and salicylates |
| Pale–whitish | Milk<br>Meat | Antacids | |
| Clay-colored | Fat | | Common bile duct<br>blockage |
| Red | Beets | Brom sulphalein<br>Tetracyclines (syrup)<br>Phenolphthalein<br>Pyridium | |

5. The odor of the stool varies with the $p$H and the amount of bacterial fermentation.
6. The normalcy of one's bowel patterns are determined by the individual.
7. Psychological discomfort and inadequate coping can produce elimination alterations.

## Physiology

1. Intestinal elimination is controlled by neural innervation from the spinal cord and by the stimulation of neural centers in the lower intestinal wall by fecal contents.
2. Bowel evacuation can be delayed by voluntarily inhibiting the urge to defecate.
3. The gastrocolic reflex and duodenocolic reflex stimulate mass peristalsis two or three times a day, most often following meals.
4. Voluntary contraction of the muscles of the abdominal wall aid in the expulsion of feces.

## Nutrition

1. Sufficient fluid intake, at least 2 liters daily, is necessary to maintain bowel patterns and promote proper stool consistency.
2. A well-balanced diet high in fiber content stimulates peristalsis. Foods high in fiber should be avoided during episodes of diarrhea. These include
   Whole grains and nuts (bran, shredded wheat, brown rice, whole wheat bread)
   Raw and coarse vegetables (broccoli, cauliflower, cucumbers, lettuce, cabbage, turnips, Brussels sprouts)
   Fresh fruits, with skins
3. Bulk and consistency of stool are influenced by dietary patterns. High vegetable diet produces soft, bulky stools. High meat diet produces small, dry, hard stools.
4. Diets high in unrefined fibrous food produce large soft stools that decrease the colon's susceptibility to disease.
5. Diets low in fiber and high in concentrated refined foods produce small hard stools that increase the colon's susceptibility to disease.

# Alterations in Bowel Elimination: Constipation
## Related to Change in Life-style

## Assessment

### Subjective data

The person reports
  Hard dry stools < three times weekly
  A change in living patterns (*e.g.*)

|  |  |
|---|---|
| Altered daily routine | Inadequate fluid intake |
| Decreased activity | Recent illness or hospitalization |
| Lack of privacy | Change in regular schedule of |
| Diet reported lacking in suffi- | elimination |
| cient roughage |  |

### Objective data

Hard formed stools
Palpable impaction

---

**Outcome Criteria**

The person will
  • Describe contributing factors when known
  • Identify methods to reduce contributing factors
  • Describe methods to prevent constipation

---

## Interventions

A. Assess for causative factors

  Stress
      Occupation
      Family responsibilities
      Financial considerations
  Sedentary life-style
  Laxative abuse
  Hospitalization
  Drug side-effect
  Debilitation
  Lack of privacy (at work or at school)
  Recent or frequent travel
  Lack of time

B. Promote corrective measures

  1. Regular time for elimination
      • Identify normal defecation pattern prior to constipation
      • Review daily routine

- Advise that time for defecation be included as part of daily routine
- Discuss suitable time (based on responsibilities, availability of facilities, etc.)
- Provide stimulus to defecation (*e.g.,* coffee, prune juice)
- Advise that an attempt to defecate should be made about an hour or so following meal and that it may be necessary to remain in bathroom a suitable length of time
- Utilize bathroom instead of bedpan if possible
- Offer bedpan or bedside commode if unable to use bathroom
- Assist into position on bedpan or commode
- Provide for privacy (close door, draw curtains around bed, play TV or radio to mask sounds, have room deodorizer available)
- Provide for comfort (reading material as diversion) and safety (call bell available)
- Allow suitable position (sitting if not contraindicated)

2. Adequate exercise
   - Review current exercise pattern
   - Provide for moderate physical exercise on a frequent basis (if not contraindicated)
   - Provide frequent ambulation of hospitalized patient when tolerable
   - Perform range of motion exercises for person who is bedridden
   - Teach exercises for increased abdominal muscle tone (unless contraindicated)
     a. Contract abdominal muscles several times frequently throughout day
     b. Do sit-ups keeping heels on floor with knees slightly flexed
     c. While supine, raise lower limbs, keeping knees straight

## C. Eliminate or reduce contributing factors

1. Untoward side-effects of current medical regimen
   - Administer mild laxative following oral administration of barium sulfate*
   - Assess elimination status while on antacid therapy (may be necessary to alternate magnesium-type antacid with other types)*
   - Encourage increased intake of high-roughage foods and increased fluid intake as adjunct to iron therapy (*e.g.,* fresh fruits and vegetables with skins; bran, nuts, and seeds; whole wheat bread)
   - Encourage early ambulation, with assistance if necessary, to counter effects of anesthetic agents
   - Assess elimination status while receiving certain narcotic analgesics (morphine, codeine) and alert physician if experiencing difficulty with defecation

2. Laxative abuse
   - Assess frequency of laxative use, type, and quantity
   - Explain long-term effects of laxative abuse on the bowel (leads to decreased peristaltic response to food and loss of intestinal tone)
   - Discourage use of laxatives unless prescribed
   - Encourage use of other supportive measures (diet, fluid intake, exercise, establishing regular habit)
   - Evaluate if other measures are ineffective; a mild laxative or stool softener may be needed temporarily
   - Encourage gradual tapering of laxatives in clients who have abused them
   - Encourage consultation with physician if problem persists

*May require a physician's order.

3. Stress
   - See Appendix II for relaxation techniques for stress reduction
4. Inadequate dietary and fluid intake: see *Alterations in Nutrition: Less Than Body Requirements*

D. Conduct health teaching as indicated
   - Explain to person and family the relationship of life-style changes to constipation
   - Explain interventions that relieve symptoms
   - Explain techniques to reduce the effects of stress and immobility

# Alterations in Bowel Elimination: Constipation
## Related to Immobility

### Assessment

Subjective data

The person reports
   Hard dry stools < three times weekly
   Inability or difficulty moving

Objective data

Immobility (*e.g.*, casts, traction, paralysis)
Altered state of consciousness
Altered body position (*e.g.*, legs elevated)

Multiple support equipment (*e.g.*, catheters, IV, arterial lines, respirator)
Body restraints
Forced bed rest

---

**Outcome Criteria**

The person will

- Describe therapeutic bowel regimen
- Relate or demonstrate improved bowel elimination
- Explain rationale for interventions
- Modify elimination routine to cope with interferences

---

### Interventions

A. Assess causative factors of immobility

Musculoskeletal (*e.g.*, fractures, sprain, contractures, hip replacement)
Reliance on life-support systems
Chronic or acute illness
Trauma (*e.g.*, burns, head injury)
Physical handicap
Inappropriate coping mechanisms
Bedrest

Psychosomatic illness
Degenerative joint changes (arthritis)
Surgery

B. Promote corrective measures

1. Balanced diet
   - Review list of foods high in bulk
        Fresh fruits with skins
        Bran
        Nuts and seeds
        Whole grain breads and cereals
        Cooked fruits and vegetables
        Fruit juices
   - Discuss dietary preferences
   - Take into account any food intolerances or allergies
   - Include approximately 800 g of fruits and vegetables (about 4 pieces of fresh fruit and large salad) for normal daily bowel movement
   - Suggest use of bran in moderation at first (may irritate GI tract, produce flatulence, cause diarrhea or blockage)
   - Gradually increase amount of bran as tolerated (may add to cereals, baked goods, etc.)
   - Consider financial limitations (encourage the use of fruits and vegetables in season)

2. Adequate fluid intake
   - Encourage intake of at least 2 liters—8 to 10 glasses—(unless contra-indicated)
   - Discuss fluid preferences
   - Set up regular schedule for fluid intake
   - Recommend a glass of hot water to be taken ½ hour before breakfast that may act as stimulus to bowel evacuation

3. Regular time for elimination
   - Identify normal defecation pattern prior to constipation
   - Review daily routine
   - Include time for defecation as part of regular routine
   - Discuss suitable time (based on responsibilities, availability of facilities, etc.)
   - Provide stimulus to defecation (*e.g.*, coffee, prune juice)
   - Suggest that person attempt defecation about an hour or so following meal and remain in bathroom suitable length of time
   - Utilize bathroom instead of bedpan if possible
   - Offer bedpan or bedside commode if unable to use bathroom
   - Assist into position on bedpan or commode
   - Provide for privacy (close door, draw curtains around bed, play TV or radio to mask sounds, make room deodorizer available)
   - Provide for comfort (reading material as diversion) and safety (call bell available)

4. Optimal position
   - Assist patient to normal semi-squatting position to allow optimum usage of abdominal muscles and effect of force of gravity
   - Assist onto bedpan if necessary and elevate head of bed to high Fowler's position or elevation permitted
   - Use fracture bedpan for comfort if preferred
   - Stress the avoidance of straining

- Encourage exhaling during straining
- Place call bell within easy reach
- Maintain safety (side rails)
- Provide privacy
- Chart results (color, consistency, amount)

## C. Eliminate or reduce contributing factors

1. Fecal impaction
   - If fecal impaction is suspected, perform digital exam of rectum: Have client assume position lying on left side. Don glove, lubricate forefinger, and insert; attempt to break up any hardened fecal mass and remove pieces
   - If impaction is out of reach of gloved finger:
     a. Administer oil retention enema to aid in removal of mass*
     b. Instruct person to retain enema at least 60 minutes or possibly over-night
     c. Follow with cleansing enema* (both enemas may need to be repeated; may need to follow with repeat attempt to break up mass digitally)
   - Make client comfortable and allow to rest
   - Client may require temporary use of stool softener or mild cathartic*
   - Maintain accurate bowel elimination record
2. Severe constipation
   - First day, insert glycerin suppository and have client attempt bowel movement through intermittent straining efforts
   - If ineffective, on second day insert glycerin suppository and follow same routine
   - If no results, on third day, request prescription for Dulcolax suppository, which if not effective should be followed by enema*
   - To aid in stimulation of reflex, suppository may be followed in 20 to 30 minutes by digital stimulation of anal sphincter
   - Return to first-day routine and follow until pattern is established (may be every 2 to 3 days)

## D. Conduct health teaching as indicated

- Explain to person and significant others the interventions required to prevent vs. treat constipation (*e.g.,* diet, exercise)
- Refer to Principles and Rationale for Nursing Care for specifics

# Alterations in Bowel Elimination: Constipation
Related to Painful Defecation

## Assessment

Subjective data

The person reports
   Pain on defecation

*May require a physician's order.

Rectal itching
Straining at stool

## Objective data
Hard consistency of stool
Hemorrhoids
Impaction palpated on rectal exam
Irritated or excoriated perirectal area

---

**Outcome Criteria**

The person will
  • Relate less pain on defecation
  • Describe causative factors when known
  • Describe rationale and procedure for treatments

---

## Interventions

A. Assess causative factors

| | |
|---|---|
| Fecal impaction/constipation | Pilonidal cyst |
| Hemorrhoids | Anorectal abscess |
| Anal fissures | Lower intestinal obstruction |
| Pregnancy | Prolonged use of cathartics and |
| Surgery that reduces ability to | enemas |
| bear down | Enlargement of prostate gland |

B. Reduce rectal pain, if possible, by instructing person in corrective measures
  • Increase fluid intake
  • Increase dietary intake of high-fiber foods
  • Increase daily exercise
  • Gently apply a lubricant to anus to reduce pain on defecation
  • Apply cool compresses to area to reduce itching
  • Take sitz bath or soak in tub or warm water (43° to 46° C) for 15-minute intervals if soothing
  • Take stool softeners or mineral oil as an adjunct to other approaches
  • Consult with physician regarding use of local anesthetics and antiseptic agents

C. Protect the surrounding skin from breakdown
  • Evaluate the surrounding skin area
  • Cleanse properly with nonirritating agent, *e.g.*, use gentle motion; use soft tissues following defecation
  • Suggest a sitz bath following defecation
  • Gently apply protective emollient or lubricant

D. Initiate health teaching if indicated
  • Teach the methods to prevent rectal pressure that contributes to hemorrhoids
  • Avoid prolonged sitting, *e.g.*, stand up every 1 hour for 5 to 10 minutes to relieve pressure

- Avoid straining at defecation
- Soften stools, *e.g.*, low roughage diet, high fluid intake (see Principles and Rationale for Nursing Care)

## Bibliography

See *Alterations in Bowel Elimination: Diarrhea*

# Bowel Elimination, Alterations In: Diarrhea

*Related to* **Untoward Side-effects**

## Definition

Diarrhea: The state in which the individual experiences or is at high risk of experiencing frequent passage of liquid stool or unformed stool.

## Etiological and Contributing Factors

### Pathophysiological

Nutritional disorders and malabsorptive syndromes

| | |
|---|---|
| Kwashiorkor | Crohn's disease |
| Gastritis | Lactose intolerance |
| Peptic ulcer | Spastic colon |
| Diverticulitis | Celiac disease (sprue) |
| Ulcerative colitis | Irritable bowel |

Metabolic and endocrine disorders

| | |
|---|---|
| Diabetes mellitus | Thyrotoxicosis |
| Addison's disease | |

Dumping syndrome

Infectious process

| | |
|---|---|
| Trichinosis | Shigellosis |
| Dysentery | Typhoid fever |
| Cholera | Infectious hepatitis |
| Malaria | |

Cancer
Uremia
Tuberculosis
Arsenic poisoning
Fecal impaction
Surgical intervention of the bowel

| | |
|---|---|
| Loss of bowel | Ileal bypass |

### Situational

Stress or anxiety
Irritating foods (fruits, bran cereals)
Tube feedings
Travel
    Change in bacteria in water
    Bacteria, virus, parasite to which no immunity is present
Hot weather
Increased caffeine consumption
Chemotherapy

Drug side-effects

|  |  |
|---|---|
| Thyroid agents | Stool softeners |
| Antacids | Antibiotics |
| Laxatives | |

## Maturational

Allergies
Infant: Breast-fed babies
Elderly: Decreased sphincter reflexes

## Defining Characteristics

Loose, liquid stools
Increased frequency (more than three a day)
Urgency
Cramping/abdominal pain
Increased frequency of bowel sounds
Increase in fluidity or volume of stools

## Focus Assessment Criteria

Refer to criteria for *Alterations in Bowel Elimination: Constipation*

## Nursing Goals

Through selected interventions the nurse will seek to
- Decrease symptomatology
- Maintain fluid and electrolyte balance
- Relieve irritation to perianal area
- Maintain optimal nutritional status

## Principles and Rationale for Nursing Care

1. Rapid transit of feces through the large intestine results in less water absorption and an unformed, liquid stool.
2. Dehydration and electrolyte imbalance occur if diarrhea continues.
3. Malabsorption results in an increase in the bulk of the colon and stimulates intestinal motility.
4. Diarrheal stool can cause excoriation of the anal area because it is usually acidic and contains digestive enzymes.
5. Hyperperistalsis is the motor response to intestinal irritants.
6. High-solute tube feedings may cause diarrhea if not followed by sufficient amounts of water.
7. Diarrhea may be related to an inflammatory process in which the intestinal mucosal wall becomes irritated, resulting in increased moisture content in the fecal mass.
8. Refer to Principles and Rationale for Nursing Care for *Constipation.*

# Alterations in Bowel Elimination: Diarrhea
Related to Untoward Side-effects

## Assessment

Subjective data

The person reports

| | |
|---|---|
| Loose stools more than three daily | Cramps |
| | Weakness |
| Pain | |

Objective data

| | |
|---|---|
| Observable signs of dehydration | Liquid stools |
| Increased bowel sounds | Frequent stools (more than three daily) |

---

**Outcome Criteria**

The person will
- Describe contributing factors when known
- Explain rationale for interventions
- Experience less diarrhea

---

## Interventions

A. Assess causative factors

Tube feedings
Dietary indiscretions
Food allergies

B. Eliminate or reduce contributing factors

1. Administration of tube feeding
   - Control infusion rate (depending on delivery set)
   - Administer smaller, more frequent feedings*
   - Change to continuous-drip tube feedings*
   - Administer more slowly if signs of GI intolerance occur
   - Control temperature
   - If refrigerated, warm in hot water to room temperature
   - Dilute strength of feeding temporarily*
   - Follow standard procedure for administration of tube feeding
   - Follow tube feeding with specified amount of water to assure hydration
   - Be careful of contamination/spoilage (unused but opened formula should not be used after 24 hours; keep unused portion refrigerated)

*May require a physician's order.

2. Dietary indiscretions and food allergies
   a. For adults, teach to avoid
      - Foods with usually irritating GI effect
      - Large caffeine intake (greater than 300 mg per day)
      - Foods that produce known allergic response
      - Coarse foods (high fiber)
      - See Principles and Rationale for Nursing Care for specific foods
   b. For breast-fed infants
      - Discontinue solids
      - Offer clear liquid supplements
      - Continue breast-feeding
   c. For formula-fed infant or milk-fed child
      - Discontinue formula, milk products, and solid foods
      - Offer small amounts of clear fluids (sweetened diluted tea, diluted cola, ginger ale, sugar water, diluted Jell-O water) 15 ml to 30 ml each ½–1 hour for first 8 hours
      - Increase amount to 60 ml to 90 ml every 1–2 hours if number of stools has lessened
      - Add plain solids (Jell-O, bananas, rice, cereal, crackers) after 24 hours, if improved
      - Gradually return to regular diet (except milk products) after 36–48 hours; after 3–5 days gradually add milk products (half-strength skim to skim milk to half-strength whole milk to whole milk)
      - Gradually introduce formula (half-strength formula to full-strength formula)

## C. Replace fluids and electrolytes

- Increase oral intake to maintain a normal urine specific gravity
- Encourage liquids (water, apple juice, flat ginger ale)
- Children, may need administration of commercially prepared solution (*e.g.,* Pedialyte)*
- Encourage fluids high in potassium and sodium (orange and grapefruit juices, bouillon)
- Caution against use of very hot or cold liquids
- See *Fluid Volume Deficit* for additional interventions

## D. Conduct health teaching as indicated

- Explain to client and significant others the interventions required to prevent future episodes
- Explain the effects of diarrhea on hydration

## Bibliography

Aman RA: Treating the patient, not the constipation. Am J Nurs 80:1634–1635, 1980

Brill EL, Kilts DF: Foundations for Nursing, pp 535–562. Appleton-Century-Crofts, New York, 1980

Chow M et al: Handbook of Pediatric Primary Care, pp 632–638. New York, John Wiley & Sons, 1979

Hickey J: The Clinical Practice of Neurological and Neurosurgical Nursing, pp 221–222, 279–280. Philadelphia, JB Lippincott, 1981

*May require a physician's order.

John RL: Giardiasis and amebiasis. RN 44(4):52–57, 1981

Krause MV, Mahan LK: Food, Nutrition, and Diet Therapy, pp 485–496. Philadelphia, WB Saunders, 1979

Rodman MJ: Diarrhea: Think twice before giving meds. RN 43(10):73–84, 1980

Rodman MJ, Smith DW: Pharmacology and Drug Therapy in Nursing, pp 928–935. JB Lippincott, Philadelphia, 1979

Shelter MG: Stool specimens: Key to detecting intestinal invaders. RN 43(10):50–53, 1980

Sorensen K, Luckmann J: Basic Nursing, pp 693–721. Philadelphia, WB Saunders, 1979

Watson J: Medical-Surgical Nursing and Related Physiology, pp 538–544. Philadelphia, WB Saunders, 1979

Wolff L, Weitzel M, Furst E: Fundamentals of Nursing, pp 479–494. Philadelphia, JB Lippincott, 1979

# Cardiac Output, Alterations In: Decreased (specify)

## Definition

Alterations in cardiac output, decreased: A state in which the individual experiences a reduction in the amount of blood pumped by the heart, resulting in compromised cardiac function.

**Note:** The use of this diagnostic category will not cover the treatment of decreased cardiac output (which is a clinical problem) but will focus on the functional abilities of the individual that are compromised because of decreased cardiac output. To represent this relationship, the diagnosis will be linked with the compromised functional abilities by means of a colon (:) and not by the phrase *related to*. Using the phrase *related to*, as in *Alterations in Cardiac Output Related to Congestive Heart Failure*, would refer to a clinical situation that is more the realm of medicine than nursing. Because the nurse can diagnose and treat *responses* to decreased cardiac output, the diagnosis can be structured as: *Alterations in Cardiac Output: Decreased: Activity Intolerance Secondary to Myocardial Ischemia.*

## Etiological and Contributing Factors

### Pathophysiological

Cardiac factors

| | |
|---|---|
| Bradycardia | Congestive heart failure |
| Tachycardia | Cardiogenic shock |
| Heart block | Valvular stenosis or insufficiency |
| Reduced stroke volume | Hypertension |
| Myocardial infarction | |

Pulmonary disorders

| | |
|---|---|
| Chronic obstructive pulmonary disease | Congestive heart failure |
| COR pulmonale | |

Endocrine disorders

| | |
|---|---|
| Adrenocortical insufficiency | Diabetes mellitus |
| Hypothyroidism | |

Hemotological disorders

| | |
|---|---|
| Polycythemia | Clotting alterations |
| Anemia | |

Fluid and electrolyte imbalances

| | |
|---|---|
| Hypo- or hypercalcemia | Hypo- or hypervolemia |
| Hypo- or hyperkalemia | |

### Situational

Shock
Vagal stimulation

Starvation
Sepsis
Hypo- or hyperthermia
Stress
Dialysis
Surgery, anesthesia
Medications

| | |
|---|---|
| Diuretics | Vasoconstrictors |
| Antihypertensives | Vasodilators |

Allergic response

## Maturational

Newborn/infant

| | |
|---|---|
| Tetrology of Fallot | Valvular defects |
| Septal defects | Coarctation of the aorta |
| Patent ductus arteriosus | |

## Defining Characteristics

| | |
|---|---|
| Low blood pressure | Dysrhythmia |
| Rapid pulse | Oliguria |
| Restlessness | Fatigability |
| Cyanosis | Vertigo |
| Dyspnea | Edema (peripheral, sacral) |
| Angina | |

## Focus Assessment Criteria

### Subjective data

1. History of symptoms

| | |
|---|---|
| Onset and duration | Precipitated by what? |
| Location | Relieved by what? |
| Description | Aggravated by what? |

2. Presence of

| | |
|---|---|
| Pain | Vertigo |
| Fatigue | Anorexia |
| Dyspnea | Nausea |

3. History (medical-surgical, family)
4. Current drug therapy

### Objective data

Heart

| | |
|---|---|
| Rate | Presence of gallops, murmurs |
| Rhythm | |

Blood pressure

| | |
|---|---|
| Normal | Widening pulse pressure |
| Elevated | Narrowing pulse pressure |
| Decreased | |

Respiratory system

| | |
|---|---|
| Rate | Presence of cough, rales |
| Rhythm | |

Pulse

> Apical
> Peripheral (bilateral, rate,
> > amplitude)

Neck veins (lying, sitting)

> Distended                                     Flat

Skin

> Color                                          Presence of edema
> Temperature

## Principles and Rationale for Nursing Care

### General

1. All living cells require oxygen. The degree of oxygenation of cells is dependent on the functions of the heart, lungs, and circulatory systems in the presence of adequate atmospheric oxygen.
2. Cardiac output is the amount of blood (liters) that is pumped by the heart per minute and is calculated by:

> heart rate × stroke volume = cardiac output

Units can be beats/min; ml/min; liters/min.

3. Stroke volume is the amount of blood ejected with each contraction of the heart.
4. Cardiac output increases with an increase in filling of the ventricles, up to a certain point. When "overfilling" of the ventricles occurs, as in congestive heart failure (CHF), myocardial fibers are overstretched and lose some of their contractility, thus ultimately reducing cardiac output.
5. Cardiac output is affected by the heart rate, the amount of ventricular filling during diastole, the contractility of the myocardial fibers, and the degree of peripheral resistance.
6. Decreased cardiac output affects the body systems. Decreased cardiac output results in early compensatory mechanisms of selected vasoconstriction (which serve to provide oxygen to the vital organs by shunting blood from the abdominal organs and peripheral areas (arms, legs, skin) to the brain and heart. The results of this shunting are cold clammy skin and reduced urine output.

> The heart responds by increasing its rate (tachycardia), as does the respiratory system (tachypnea), in an attempt to increase the amount of circulating oxygen.

> If cardiac output continues to decline, anoxia of brain tissue will produce restlessness, then coma, and the heart will indicate ischemia with angina and dysrhythmias.

> Sustained tissue hypoxia results in anaerobic metabolism, producing metabolic acidosis and eventual death if not corrected.

7. Exercise and physical activity increase cardiac output, heart rate, and blood pressure. Regular exercise, leading to physical fitness, makes the heart more efficient so that stroke volume increases and heart rate is not greatly altered with exercise. Warning signs that the heart is not able to meet demands placed on it by exercise include chest pain, dyspnea, dizziness, and pulse and blood pressure alterations that do not return to normal resting rates 3 minutes after the activity has ceased.
8. The heart is required to work harder following the ingestion of larger meals, as

opposed to smaller meals. Intake of large amounts of fluid increases blood volume and, in turn, blood pressure, especially when sodium intake is high.

9. The two main sources of pain in low cardiac output states are (a) ischemia resulting from diminished oxygenation and (b) venous congestion and engorgement caused by the backup of blood that enters the heart.
10. The effects of reduced cardiac output are:
    Physical symptoms (pain, fatigue, edema, weight loss)
    Alterations in life-style (occupational, social, sexual, financial, role responsibilities)
    Alterations in self-concept
11. Required reduction in the level of personal activity may result in role identification conflict and, in the case of married couples, may disrupt the division of labor among the partners.

## Nutritional

1. Dietary management of persons with decreased cardiac output varies with the amount of decompensation present. Restrictions may be placed on calories (weight reduction), sodium (edema reduction), fluids (edema reduction), and fat (lipid reduction).
2. Individuals on sodium-restricted diets must be monitored for hyponatremia resulting from sodium restrictions in the presence of renal insufficiency. Hypokalemia (potassium loss) can result from the loss of potassium with certain diuretics.
3. The four levels of sodium restriction diets are severe (250 mg daily), strict (500 mg daily), moderate (1000 mg daily), and mild (2000–3000 mg daily).
4. Food restrictions occur at each level (these restrictions do not apply to persons also on low-fat diets).

|  | *Severe* | *Strict* | *Moderate* | *Mild* |
|---|---|---|---|---|
| Milk | Low-sodium 2 cups | 2 cups | 2 cups | 2 cups |
| Low-salt meat/eggs | Meat 4 oz Eggs 3 wk | 6 oz daily | moderation | moderation |
| Fruits | 2–3 | 2–3 | 2–3 | 2–3 |
| Bread (slices) | 4 salt-free | 4 salt-free | 2 | 4 |
| Vegetables | Low-sodium | Low-sodium | Moderate use of high-sodium types | No restrictions; limit canned vegetables |
| Table salt | None | None | None | 1/4 tsp |

5. A high intake of sodium causes increased retention of water.
   Foods with high sodium content include salted snacks, bacon, cheddar cheese, pickles, soy sauce, processed luncheon meats, MSG (monosodium glutamate), canned vegetables, catsup, mustard; also, Some over-the-counter drugs such as bicarbonate of soda, antacids, cough suppressants, and many oral hygiene products
   Foods with moderate sodium content include eggs, milk, hamburger, canned corn, and canned tomato juice
   Foods with low sodium content include fruits, chicken, liver, fresh vegetables, unsalted bread, and unsalted crackers

6. Foods with a high potassium content include bananas, dates, raisins, oranges, puffed wheat cereal, potatoes, liver, Pepsi, and Gatorade.

---

**Outcome Criteria**

The person will
  • Identify factors that increase cardiac workload
  • Describe adaptive techniques needed to perform activities of daily living
  • Demonstrate cardiac tolerance to increased activity (*e.g.*, stable pulse, respirations, and blood pressure)

---

## Interventions

The nursing interventions for this diagnostic category represent interventions for individuals with decreased cardiac output regardless of the etiological and contributing factors.

### A. Assess for causative and contributing factors that increase cardiac workload

Activity
Stress
Smoking
Edema
Overweight/obesity

### B. Reduce or eliminate causative factors if possible

1. Activity
   a. Plan nursing strategies to promote rest, incorporating them into the care plan
      • Organize care to minimize unnecessary disturbances
      • Provide scheduled periods for rest and sleep when no one is permitted to disturb patient (except in emergencies)
      • Acknowledge the importance of visitors but assist the family to meet the needs of the individual without compromising sleep/rest patterns
      • Encourage increases in activity and ambulation to prevent a sudden increase in cardiac workload
      • Minimize activity prior to planned periods that require exertion, such as treatments, ambulation, meals
   b. Decrease fatigue at mealtime
      • Encourage a light meal in the evening to promote a more comfortable night's rest
      • Initially provide easily digestible and chewable foods
      • Schedule meals to avoid intervention with other activities
      • Offer food preferences, avoiding dislikes
      • Consider sociocultural influences
   c. Teach the person energy conservation methods for activities
      • Take rest periods during activities, at intervals during the day, and 1 hour after meals

- Sit rather than stand when performing activities, unless this is not feasible
- When performing a task, rest every 3 minutes for 5 minutes to allow the heart to recover
- Stop an activity if fatigue or signs of cardiac anoxia are present (*e.g.*, ↑ pulse, dyspnea, chest pain)

d. Instruct the person to avoid certain exercises
- Isometric exercises, *e.g.*, using arms to lift himself up; lifting objects (slide them instead)
- Valsalva maneuver; *e.g.*, bending from the waist, straining during a bowel movement

e. Monitor the person's response to increased activity in the hospital or teach him to monitor (see Principles and Rationale for Nursing Care)
- Take a resting pulse
- Take a pulse immediately after or during activity
- Take a pulse 3 minutes after
- Instruct him to report
    Rate decreases on activity
    Rates > 110
    Irregular pulse
    Pulses that do not return with six beats of resting pulse after 3 min
    Dyspnea
    Cyanosis
    Chest pain
    Palpitations

2. Stress
a. Assist the person to identify stressors (home, work, social)
b. Discuss his usual response to stressors (*e.g.*, anger, depression, avoidance, discussion)
c. Explain the effects of stress on the cardiovascular system (*e.g.*, increased heart rate, increased blood pressure, increased respirations)
d. Discuss various methods for stress reduction
- Deliberate problem-solving (see Appendix VI)
    What is the problem?
    Who/what is responsible for the problem?
    What are the options?
    What are the advantages of each option?
    What are the disadvantages and risks of each option?
- Relaxation techniques (see Appendix IV)
- Yoga, biofeedback
- Regular exercise (30 min at least 3 times a week)*
e. See *Ineffective Individual Coping* for additional assessment and intervention information

3. Smoking
a. Discuss with the person the effects of smoking on his cardiovascular system (*e.g.*, vasoconstriction increases workload of the heart)
b. Teach person when not to smoke: before an activity and after an activity
c. Discuss methods that can help reduce the amount of cigarettes smoked

*May require a physician's order.

    d.  Refer person to programs that can assist him to stop smoking if he desires

4. Edema

    a.  Assess for the presence of edema in ankles and sacral area

    b.  See *Fluid Volume Excess* for interventions for edema

5. Overweight/obesity

    a.  Assess whether the person is overweight or obese by securing height and weight of person and comparing these findings with a standardized weight/height chart, or use anthropometric measurements (See *Alteration in Nutrition: More Than Body Requirements* for charts of weight for heights and anthropometric norms)

    b.  If weight reduction is indicated and the person has validated an interest to lose weight refer to *Alterations in Nutrition: More Than Body Requirements*

C. Discuss with the person his perceived effects that his condition will have on role responsibilities (social, home, sexual), occupation, and finances

D. Provide the family with an opportunity to share their concerns
- Assess their knowledge of the condition, treatment, and prognosis
- Encourage them to share their concerns about the future and about role responsibilities

E. Initiate health teaching and referrals if indicated
- Instruct the person to consult his physician and physiatrist for a long-term exercise program, or to contact the American Heart Association for names of cardiac rehabilitation programs
- Explain the diet restrictions to the person and his family (*e.g.*, give them written instructions, or refer them to pertinent literature on preparation of food for restricted diets)
- Explain the prescribed drug therapy (*e.g.*, diuretics, vasodilators, dosage, side-effects, administration, and storage
- Refer to one or more selected nursing diagnoses, if indicated, for additional information
*Activity Intolerance*
*Alterations in Bowel Elimination*
*Diversional Activity Deficit*
*Sexual Dysfunction Related to Change/Loss of Body Part*
*Alterations in Family Processes Related to Ill Family Member*
*Grieving Related to a Perceived Loss*
*Alterations in Respiratory Function*
*Ineffective Individual Coping*

## Bibliography

Adler J: Patient assessment: Pulses. Am J Nurs 79:115–132, 1979

Alexy BJ: Monitoring cardiovascular status with noninvasive techniques. Nurs Clin North Am 13:423–435, 1978

Arlin M: Controversies in nutrition: A brief review. Nurs Clin North Am 14:199–214, 1979

Cole C, Levin EM, Whitley JO et al: Brief sexual counseling during cardiac rehabilitation. Heart Lung, 8:124–129, 1979

Coyle N: Analgesics at the bedside. Am J Nurs 79:1554–1557, 1979

Jordan J: Your fingers on the pulse: Evaluating what you feel. Nursing 10(11):33–39, 1980

McGurn W: People with Cardiac Problems: Nursing Concepts. Philadelphia, JB Lippincott, 1981

Oehler JM: Family Centered Neonatal Nursing Care, pp 221–242, Philadelphia, JB Lippincott, 1981

Sacksteder S et al: Common congenital cardiac defects. Am J Nurs 78:266–272, 1978

Sedlock S: Cardiac output: Physiologic variables and therapeutic interventions. Critical Care Nurse, 1(2):14–22, 1981

Williams, RB, Gentry WD (eds.): Psychological Aspects of Myocardial Infarction and Coronary Care. St. Louis, CV Mosby, 1975

## Pertinent Literature for the Consumer

Booklets for low-cholesterol low-sodium diets
American Heart Association Cookbook
Weight Reduction
Nutrition Labeling

Available from local chapters of the American Heart Association or the National Center, 7320 Greenville Avenue, Dallas, Texas 75231.

# Comfort, Alterations in:

**Acute Pain**

**Chronic Pain**

**Pain in Children**

## Definition

Alterations in comfort: pain—A state in which the individual experiences an uncomfortable sensation in response to a noxious stimulus.

## Etiological and Contributing Factors

Any factor can contribute to alterations in comfort. The most common are listed below.

### Pathophysiological

Musculoskeletal disorders

       Fractures                      Arthritis

       Contractures              Spinal cord disorders

       Spasms

Visceral disorders

       Cardiac                    Intestinal

       Renal                      Pulmonary

Cancer

Vascular disorders

       Vasospasm             Phlebitis

       Occlusion             Vasodilation (headache)

Inflammation

       Nerve                     Joint

       Tendon                  Muscle

       Bursa

### Situational

Trauma (surgery, accidents)

Diagnostic tests

       Venipuncture           Biopsy

       Invasive scanning (*e.g.,* IVP)

Immobility/improper positioning

Overactivity

Pressure points (tight cast, Ace bandage)

Pregnancy (prenatal, intrapartem, postpartum)

## Defining Characteristics

The person reports pain (may be the only defining characteristic present)

Autonomic response in acute pain
    Blood pressure increased
    Pulse increased
    Respirations increased
    Diaphoresis
    Dilated pupils
Guarded position
Facial mask of pain
Crying, moaning

## Focus Assessment Criteria

**Note:** This nursing assessment of pain is designed to acquire data in order to assess the individual adaptation to pain, not to determine the cause of the pain or whether it exists.

### Subjective data

1. "Where is your pain located; does it radiate?" (Ask child to point to place)
2. "When did it begin?"
3. "Can you relate the cause of this pain?" or "What do you think is the cause of your pain?"
4. Ask person to describe the pain and its pattern
   Time of day
   Duration
   Frequency (constant, intermittent, transient)
   Quality/intensity
5. Ask person to rate his pain using a scale of 0 to 10 (0 = absence of pain; 10 = worst pain ever experienced)
   Rate at its best
   Rate after pain relief measures
   Rate at its worst
6. "How do you usually react to pain (crying, anger, silence)?"
7. "Are there any other symptoms associated with your pain (nausea, vomiting, numbness)?"
8. "What helps you when you have pain (medications [what, dosage, how often], heat, cold, activity, rest)?"
9. "Do you talk to others about your pain (spouse, friends, doctor, nurse)?"
10. Have person indicate the effect of each of the following factors on his pain by noting if there is an increase, a decrease, or no effect*

| | | |
|---|---|---|
| Liquor | Vibration | Defecation |
| Stimulants (*e.g.,* | Pressure | Tension |
|   caffeine) | No Movement | Bright lights |
| Eating | Movement/activity | Loud noises |
| Heat | Sleep, rest | Going to work |
| Cold | Lying down | Intercourse |
| Damp | Distraction (*e.g.,* TV) | Mild exercise |
| Weather changes | Urination | Fatigue |
| Massage | | |

*Adapted from the McGill Pain Questionnaire.

11. Ask person what effect pain has had on the following areas or what effect is anticipated
> Work/activity pattern (work/home activities, leisure/play)
> Sleep pattern (difficulty falling asleep/staying asleep)
> Eating pattern (appetite, weight gain/loss)
> Elimination patterns (bowel, constipation/diarrhea, bladder)
> Menses
> Sexual pattern (libido, function)

## Objective data

1. Behavioral manifestations

| *Mood* | *Eye movements* |
|---|---|
| Calmness | Fixed |
| Moaning | Searching |
| Crying | Open |
| Grimacing | Closed |
| Pacing | Perception |
| Restlessness | Oriented to time and place |
| Withdrawn | |

2. Musculoskeletal manifestations

| *Mobility of painful part* | *Muscle tone* |
|---|---|
| Full | Spasm |
| Limited/guarded | Tenderness |
| No movement | Tremors (in effort to hide pain) |

3. Dermatologic manifestations

| Color (redness) | Moisture/diaphoresis |
|---|---|
| Temperature | Edema |

4. Cardiorespiratory manifestations

| *Cardiac* | *Respiratory* |
|---|---|
| Rate | Rate |
| Blood pressure | Rhythm |
| Palpations present | Depth |

5. Neurologic manifestations
Sensory alterations
> Paresthesia
> Dysesthesias

6. Cognitive manifestations
Thought processes

| Appropriate | Combative |
|---|---|
| Inappropriate | Confused |
| Cooperative | |

## Nursing Goals

Through selected interventions the nurse will seek to assist the individual to
- Reduce pain and improve mobility
- Identify techniques that decrease the pain experience and improve coping mechanisms
- Identify and reduce factors that precipitate or aggravate pain
- Decrease dependency on analgesics by using alternate pain relief measures

## Principles and Rationale for Nursing Care

### General

1. Each individual experiences and expresses pain in his own manner, utilizing various sociocultural adaption techniques.
2. All pain is real, regardless of its causes. Pure psychogenic pain is probably rare, as is pure organic pain. Most bodily pain is a combination of mental events (psychogenic) and physical stimuli (organic).
3. Pain tolerance is the duration and intensity of pain that an individual is willing to endure. Pain tolerance differs in individuals and may vary in one individual in different situations.
4. Personal factors that influence pain tolerance are:
   Knowledge of pain and its cause
   Meaning of pain
   Ability to control pain
   Energy level (fatigue)
   Stress level
5. Social and environmental factors that influence pain are:
   Interactions with others
   Response of others (family, friends)
   Secondary gains
   Sensory overload or deprivation
   Stressors
6. If a person must try to convince health care providers that he has pain, he will experience increased anxiety that increases the pain. Both of these are energy depleting.
7. Persons who are prepared for painful procedures by explanations of the actual sensations that will be felt experience less stress than individuals who receive vague explanations of the procedure.
8. Drug tolerance is a physiological phenomenon in which, after repeated doses, the prescribed dose begins to lose its effectiveness.
9. Addiction is a psychological phenomenon, involving the regular use of narcotics for emotional reasons, not medical ones.
10. Studies have shown that the human brain secretes endorphins, which have opiate-like properties that relieve pain. The release of endorphins may be responsible for the positive effects of placebos and noninvasive pain relief measures.
11. Studies have shown that diagnosed physiological pain does respond to placebos, so a positive response to placebos cannot be used to diagnose pain as psychogenic.
12. The use of noninvasive pain relief measures (*e.g.*, relaxation, massage, distraction) can enhance the therapeutic effects of pain relief medications.

## Acute pain compared to chronic pain

1. Pain can be classified as acute or chronic pain, according to cause and duration, not intensity.
2. Acute pain is an episode of pain that has a duration of one second to less than six months. The cause is usually organic disease or injury. With healing, the pain subsides and eventually disappears.
3. Chronic pain is a pain experience that lasts for six months or longer. Chronic pain can be described as limited, intermittent, or persistent. *Limited pain* is pain caused by known physical pathology, and an end of the pain will come (*e.g.,* burns). *Intermittent pain* is pain that provides the person with pain-free periods. The cause may or may not be known (*e.g.,* headaches). *Persistent pain* is pain that usually occurs daily. The cause may or may not be known and is usually not a threat to life (*e.g.,* low back pain).
4. The visible signs of pain (physical and behavioral) are determined by the individual's pain tolerance and the duration of the pain, not the pain intensity.
5. The person may respond to acute pain physiologically and behaviorally: physiologically by diaphoresis, an increased heart rate, an increased respiratory rate, and increased blood pressure; behaviorally by crying, moaning, or anger.
6. The person with chronic pain usually has adapted to pain, both physiologically and behaviorally, so that visible signs of pain may not be present.
7. The inability to manage pain produces feelings of frustration and inadequacy in the health care providers.
8. The person with chronic pain may respond with withdrawal, depression, anger, frustration, and dependency, all of which can affect the family in the same way.

## Children

1. The response to pain in children is influenced by maturational age, cultural-ethnic background, previous experience with pain, and response from others to the pain.
2. The child's maturational and chronological age will inflence this response to pain.

    A child less than 3 years old responds with tense body posture, irritability, rolling of the head, rubbing or pulling the affected body part, and physical resistance to painful procedure.

    A preschool child responds in the same way as a younger child and may verbalize about location of pain.

    A school-age child is influenced by cultural and parental influences. He can control the pain response, can clearly describe the pain, and may conceal or exaggerate pain for personal gain.
3. Verbal communication is usually not sufficient or reliable for explaining pain or painful procedures to children under 7. The nurse can explain by demonstrating with pictures or dolls. The more senses that are stimulated in the explanations to children, the greater the communication.
4. Even though children usually respond more openly to pain when their parents are present, the parents should be encouraged to be present in order to promote trust.
5. The weight of the child, not the age, should be considered when calculating analgesic relief.

## Medications

1. The preventive approach to pain is to a regular schedule for medication administration to treat the pain before it becomes severe rather than follow the PRN approach.
2. The preventive approach may reduce the total 24-hour dose as compared to PRN approach, provides a constant blood level of the drug, reduces craving for the drug, and reduces the anxiety of having to ask and wait for PRN relief.
3. The oral route of adminstration is preferred when possible. Liquid medications can be given to individuals who have difficulty swallowing.
4. If frequent injections are necessary, the IV route is preferred because it is not painful and absorption is guaranteed, but the side-effects ($\downarrow$ respirations, $\downarrow$ B.P.) may be more profound.

# Alterations in Comfort: Acute Pain

Acute pain is pain that can last from one second to as long as 6 months. It subsides with healing or when the stimulus is removed.

## Assessment

### Subjective data

The person reports
    Pain (may be the only sign of pain)
    Fear of pain
    Inability to concentrate

### Objective data

Guarded positioning
Muscle spasm
Increase in pulse, blood pressure, and respiration
Evidence of inflammation (redness, heat, swelling)
Rubbing or pulling of body part
Tense body posture

---

**Outcome Criteria**

The person will
- Receive validation that the pain exists
- Relate that he feels more comfortable

---

## Interventions

A. Assess for factors that decrease pain tolerance

Disbelief on the part of others
Lack of knowledge
Fear (*e.g.,* of addiction or loss of control)
Fatigue
Monotony

B. Reduce or eliminate factors that increase the pain experience

1. Disbelief on the part of others
   a. Relate to the individual your acceptance of his response to pain
      - Acknowledge the presence of his pain
      - Listen attentively to him concerning his pain
      - Convey to him that you are assessing his pain because you want to better understand it (not determine if it is really present)
   b. Assess the family for the presence of misconceptions about pain or its treatment
      - Explain the concept of pain as an individual experience
      - Discuss the reasons why an individual may experience increased or decreased pain, *e.g.,* fatigue (increased) or presence of distractions (decreased)
      - Encourage the family to share their concerns privately, *e.g.,* fear that the person will use his pain for secondary gains if they give him too much attention
      - Assess whether the family doubts the pain and discuss the effects of this on the person's pain and on the relationship
      - Encourage the family to give attention also when pain is not exhibited
2. Lack of knowledge
   - Explain causes of the pain to the person, if known
   - Relate how long the pain will last, if known
   - Explain diagnostic tests and procedures in detail by relating the discomforts and sensations that will be felt and approximate the length of time involved (*e.g.,* "During the intravenous pylogram you might feel a momentary hot flash through your entire body")
   - Allow person to see and handle equipment if possible
3. Fear
   a. Provide accurate information to reduce fear of addiction
      - Explore with him the reasons for the fear
      - Explain the difference between drug tolerance and drug addiction (refer to Principles and Rationale for Nursing Care)
   b. Assist in reducing fear of losing control
      - Provide him with privacy for his pain experience
      - Attempt to limit the number of health care providers who provide care to him
      - Allow him to share how intense his pain is and express to him how well he tolerated the pain
   c. Provide information to reduce fear that the medication will gradually lose its effectiveness
      - Discuss drug tolerance with him
      - Discuss the interventions for drug tolerance with the physician (*e.g.,*

changing the medication, increasing the dose, decreasing the interval)
• Discuss the effect of relaxation techniques on medication effects

4. Fatigue
   • Determine the cause of fatigue (sedatives, analgesics, sleep deprivation)
   • Explain that pain contributes to stress, which increases fatigue
   • Assess the person's present sleep pattern and the influence of his pain on his sleep
   • Provide him with opportunities to rest during the day and with periods of uninterrupted sleep at night (must rest when pain is ↓)
   • Consult with physician for an increased dose of pain medication at bedtime
   • Refer to *Sleep Pattern Disturbance* for specific interventions to enhance sleep

5. Monotony
   a. Discuss with the person and family the therapeutic uses of distraction, along with other methods of pain relief
   b. Emphasize that the degree an individual can be distracted from his pain is not at all related to the existence of or the intensity of the pain
   c. Explain that distraction usually increases pain tolerance and decreases pain intensity, but after the distraction ceases the individual may experience increased awareness of pain and fatigue
   d. Vary the environment if possible. If on bed rest:
      • Encourage personnel to wear seasonal pins and bright-colored apparel
      • Encourage family to decorate room with flowers, plants, pictures
      • Provide the person with music
      • Consult with recreational therapist for an appropriate task
   e. If at home:
      • Encourage individual to plan an activity for each day, preferably outside the home
      • Discuss the possibility of learning a new skill (*e.g.*, a craft, a musical instrument)
   f. Teach a method of distraction during an acute pain (*e.g.*, painful procedure) that is not a burden; *e.g.*, count items in a picture, count anything in the room (such as patterns on wallpaper) or count silently to self; breathe rhythmically; listen to music and increase the volume as the pain increases

C. Collaborate with the individual to determine what methods could be utilized to reduce the intensity of his pain
   a. Consider the following prior to selecting a specific pain relief method:
      • The individual's willingness to participate (motivation), ability to participate (dexterity, sensory loss), preference, support of significant others for method, contraindications (allergy, health problem)
      • The method's cost, complexity, precautions, and convenience
   b. Explain the various noninvasive pain relief methods to the individual and his family and why they are effective (see Appendix V)

D. Collaborate with the individual to initiate the appropriate noninvasive pain relief measures (refer to Appendix V for specific instructions on each method)
   1. Relaxation
      • Instruct on techniques to reduce skeletal muscle tension, which will reduce the intensity of the pain

- Utilize pillows and blankets to support the painful part to reduce the amount of muscle tension
- Promote relaxation with a back rub, massage, or warm bath; *e.g.*, for a person with a fractured limb, rub the opposite limb over the fractured site
- Teach a specific relaxation strategy, *e.g.*, slow rhythmic breathing or deep breath—clench fists—yawn
- Enlist the aid of the family as coaches

2. Cutaneous stimulation
- Discuss with the person the various methods of skin stimulation and their effects on pain (see Appendix V)
- Discuss the use of heat applications*: their therapeutic effects and when indicated
- Discuss each of the following methods and the precautions
  Hot water bottle
  Electric heating pad
  Warm tub
  Moist heat pack
  Hot summer sun
  Thin plastic wrap over painful area to retain body heat (*e.g.*, knee, elbow)
- Discuss the use of cold applications*: their therapeutic effects and when indicated
- Discuss each of the following methods and the precautions
  Cold towels (wrung out)
  Cold-water immersion for small body parts
  Ice bag
  Cold gel pack
  Ice massage
- Explain the therapeutic uses of menthol preparations and massage/back rub

E. Provide the person with optimal pain relief with prescribed analgesics
- Determine preferred route of administration: p.o., I.M., IV, rectal (refer to Principles and Rationale for Nursing Care)
- Assess vital signs, especially respiratory rate, prior to administering medication
- Consult with pharmacist for possible adverse interactions with other medications (*e.g.*, muscle relaxants, tranquilizers)
- Use a preventive approach
  a. Medicate prior to an activity (*e.g.*, ambulation) to increase participation, but evaluate the hazard of sedation
  b. Instruct the person to request PRN pain medication before the pain is severe
  c. Collaborate with physician to order meds on a 24-hour basis rather than PRN (refer to Principles and Rationale for Nursing Care for information on the preventive approach)

F. Assess the response to the pain relief medication
- After administering a pain relief medication, return in ½ hour to assess effectiveness
- Ask person to rate the severity of his pain, prior to the medication, and the amount of relief received

*May require a physician's order.

- Ask him to indicate when the pain began to increase
- Consult with physician if a dosage or interval change is needed

## G. Reduce or eliminate common side-effects of narcotics

1. Sedation
   - Assess if the cause is the narcotic, fatigue, sleep deprivation, or other drugs (sedatives, antiemetics)
   - Inform person that drowsiness usually occurs the first 2 to 3 days and then subsides
   - If drowsiness is excessive, consult with physician to try a slight dose reduction
2. Constipation
   - Explain the effect of narcotics on peristalsis
   - Consult with physician on the use of a stool softener with long-term drug use
   - Refer to *Alterations in Bowel Elimination: Constipation* for additional interventions
3. Nausea and vomiting
   - Instruct person that nausea will usually subside after a few doses
   - Refrain from withholding narcotic doses because of nausea; rather, secure an order for an antiemetic
   - Instruct individual to take deep breaths and to voluntarily swallow to decrease vomiting reflex
   - If nausea persists, consult with physician for the appropriate antiemetic or for a change of narcotic that produces less nausea (*e.g.*, morphine)
4. Dry mouth
   - Explain that narcotics decrease saliva production
   - Instruct person to rinse mouth often, suck on sugarless sour candies, eat pineapple chunks or, watermelon, if permissible, and drink liquids often
   - Explain the necessity of good oral hygiene and dental care

## H. Assist the family to respond positively to the individual's pain experience

- Assess the family's knowledge of and response to the pain experience
- Give accurate information to correct family misconceptions (*e.g.*, addiction, doubts about pain)
- Provide individuals with opportunities to discuss their fears, anger, and frustrations in private; acknowledge the difficulty of the situation
- Incorporate the family in the pain relief modality if possible (*e.g.*, stroking, massage)
- Praise their participation and their concern

## I. Assist the person with the aftermath of pain

- Inform him when the cause of the pain has been removed or decreased (*e.g.*, spinal tap)
- Encourage him to discuss his pain experience
- Praise him for his endurance and convey to him that he handled his pain well, regardless of how he behaved
- Allow person to keep souvenir of his pain, if desired (*e.g.*, gallstones), or a record of repeated procedures (*e.g.*, venipunctures)

J. Initiate health teaching as indicated
  - Discuss with the person and the family noninvasive pain relief measures (relaxation, distraction, massage)
  - Teach the techniques of choice to the person and his family
  - Explain the expected course of the pain (resolution) if known (*e.g.*, fractured arm, surgical incision)

# Alterations in Comfort: Chronic Pain

Chronic pain is persistent or intermittent pain that lasts for more than six months.

## Assessment

### Subjective data
The person reports that the following signs have existed for more than 6 months
  Pain (may be the only assessment datum present)
  Discomfort
  Anger, frustration, depression

### Objective data
Facial mask of pain
Anorexia, weight loss
Insomnia
Guarded movement
Muscle spasms
Redness, swelling, heat
Color changes in affected area
Reflex abnormalities

---

### Outcome Criteria
The person will
  - Receive validation that the pain exists
  - Practice selected noninvasive pain relief measures to manage his pain
  - Relate improvement of pain and an increase in daily activities

---

## Interventions

A. Assess the person's pain experience; determine the intensity of the pain at its worst and best
  - Ask person to rate his pain using a scale of 0–10 (0 = absence of pain; 10 = worst pain)

Rate it at its best
Rate it after a pain-relief measure
Rate it at its worst
- Collaborate with the individual to determine what methods could be utilized to reduce the intensity

## B. Assess for factors which decrease pain tolerance

Disbelief on the part of others
Fear
Fatigue
Monotony

## C. Reduce or eliminate factors that increase the pain experience

1. Disbelief of others
   a. Relate to the individual your acceptance of his response to pain
      - Acknowledge the presence of his pain
      - Listen attentively to him concerning his pain
      - Convey to him that you are assessing his pain because you want to better understand it, not determine if it is really present
   b. Assess the family for the presence of misconceptions about pain or its treatment
      - Explain the concept of pain as an individual experience
      - Discuss the reasons why an individual may experience increased or decreased pain, *e.g.*, fatigue (increased) or presence of distractions (decreased)
      - Encourage family to share these concerns privately, *e.g.*, fear that the person will use his pain for secondary gains if they give him too much attention
      - Assess if the family doubts the pain
      - Discuss the effects of this on the person's pain and on the relationship
      - Encourage family to give him attention also when he does not exhibit pain
2. Provide person with accurate information to reduce his fears
   a. Fear of addiction
      - Explore with him the reasons for the fear
      - Explain the difference between drug tolerance and drug addiction (refer to Principles and Rationale of Nursing Care)
   b. Fear of losing control
      - Provide privacy for his pain experience
      - Attempt to limit the number of health care providers who provide care to him
   c. Fear that the medication will gradually lose its effectiveness
      - Discuss drug tolerance with him
      - Explain the use of combining noninvasive pain relief measures with medications
   d. Fear of family that the person will use his pain for secondary gains
      - Encourage family to share these concerns privately
      - If the family doubts the pain, discuss the effects of this on the person's pain experience and on their relationship
      - Encourage family to give him attention when he does not exhibit pain also

3. Fatigue
   - Determine the cause of fatigue (sedatives, analgesics, sleep deprivation)
   - Explain that pain contributes to stress, which increases fatigue
   - Assess the person's present sleep pattern and the influence of pain on his sleep
   - Provide opportunities to rest during the day and periods of uninterrupted sleep at night
   - Refer to *Sleep Pattern Disturbance* for specific interventions to enhance sleep
4. Monotony
   a. Discuss with the person and family the therapeutic uses of distraction, along with other methods of pain relief
   b. Emphasize that the degree to which an individual can be distracted from his pain is not at all related to the existence of or the intensity of the pain
   c. Explain that distraction usually increases pain tolerance and decreases pain intensity, but after the distraction ceases the individual may experience increased awareness of pain and fatigue
   d. Vary the environment if possible. If on bed rest:
      - Encourage personnel to wear seasonal pins and bright-colored apparel
      - Encourage family to decorate room with flowers, plants, pictures
      - Provide the person with music
      - Consult with recreational therapist for an appropriate task
   e. If at home:
      - Encourage individual to plan an activity for each day, preferably outside the home
      - Discuss the possibility of learning a new skill (*e.g.*, a craft, a musical instrument)

D. **Assess the effects of chronic pain on the individual's life, utilizing the person and his family**

Performance (job, role responsibilities)
Social interactions
Finances
Activities of daily living (sleep, eating, mobility, sexuality)
Cognition/mood (concentration, depression)
Family unit (response of members)

E. **Assist the person and his family to reduce the effects of depression on life-style**
   - Encourage verbalization of individual and family concerning difficult situations
   - Listen carefully
   - Explain the relationship between chronic pain and depression
   - See *Ineffective Individual Coping Related to Depression* for additional interventions

F. **Consult with the individual to determine what methods could be utilized to reduce the intensity of his pain**
   - Before selecting a specific noninvasive pain relief method, consider the person's
     Willingness to participate (motivation)
     Ability to participate (dexterity, sensory loss)
     Preference

Support of significant others for method
Contraindications (allergy, health problem)
- Consider the method's cost, complexity, precautions, and convenience
- Explain the various noninvasive pain relief methods to the individual and his family and why they are effective (Appendix V)

G. Collaborate with the individual to initiate the appropriate noninvasive pain relief measures (refer to Appendix V for specific instructions on each method)
1. Relaxation
   - Instruct on techniques to reduce skeletal muscle tension that will reduce the intensity of the pain
   - Utilize pillows and blankets to support the painful part to reduce the amount of muscle tension
   - Promote relaxation with a back rub, massage, or a warm bath,* *e.g.,* for a person with a fractured limb, rub the opposite limb over the fractured site
   - Teach a specific relaxation strategy, *e.g.,* slow rhythmic breathing or deep breath—clench fists—yawn
   - Enlist the aid of the family as coaches
   - Discuss other techniques that can be learned (meditation, yoga, biofeedback, guided imagery)
2. Cutaneous stimulation
   - Discuss with the person the various methods of skin stimulation and their effects on pain (Appendix V)
   - Discuss the use of heat applications,* their therapeutic effects and when indicated
   - Discuss each of the following methods and the precautions
     Hot water bottle
     Electric heating pad
     Electric light bulb
     Warm tub
     Moist heat pack
     Hot summer sun
     Thin plastic wrap over painful area to retain body heat (*e.g.,* knee, elbow)
   - Discuss the use of cold applications,* their therapeutic effects and when indicated
   - Discuss each of the following methods and the precautions
     Cold towels (wrung out)
     Cold-water immersion for small body parts
     Ice bag
     Cold gel pack
     Ice massage
   - Explain the therapeutic uses of
     Menthol preparations
     Massage/back rub
     Pressure
     Vibration
     Transcutaneous electric nerve stimulation (TENS)

*May require a physician's order.

3. Discuss with the person and the family the therapeutic uses of distraction along with other methods of pain relief
  - Emphasize that the degree to which an individual can be distracted from his pain is not at all related to the existence or intensity of the pain
  - Explain that distraction usually increases pain tolerance and decreases pain intensity, but after the distraction ceases the individual may experience increased awareness of pain and fatigue
  - If possible, use modalities that stimulate one or more of the major senses in a rhythmic manner
      a. Hearing: music, counting silently to self, being read to
      b. Vision: TV, counting items in a picture or patterns on wallboard, reading (or telling) a story
      c. Touch and movement: massage, rocking, rhythmic breathing, stroking
  - Encourage the person to participate in activities that are pleasurable and time-consuming (*e.g.*, arts and crafts)

H. Provide the individual pain relief with prescribed analgesics*

1. Determine preferred route of administration: p.o., I.M., IV, rectal (refer to Principles and Rationale for Nursing Care)

2. Assess the response to the medication
  a. For admitted persons
      - After administering a pain relief medication, return in ½ hour to assess effectiveness
      - Ask him to rate the severity of his pain prior to the medication and the amount of relief received
      - Ask him to indicate when the pain began to increase
      - Consult with the physician if a dosage or interval change is needed
  b. For outpatients
      - Ask him to keep a record of when he takes his medication and what kind of relief was received
      - Instruct him to consult his physician with questions concerning medication dosage

3. Encourage the use of p.o. medications as soon as possible
  - Consult with physician for a schedule to change from I.M. to p.o.
  - Explain to individual and family that oral medications can be as effective as I.M.
  - Explain how the transition will occur:
      a. Begin p.o. medication at a larger dose than necessary (loading dose)
      b. Continue PRN I.M. medication
      c. Gradually reduce p.o. medication dose
      d. Use the person's account of pain to regulate doses
  - Consult with the physician for the possibility of adding aspirin or acetaminophen to the medication regime

I. Reduce or eliminate common side-effects of narcotics

1. Sedation
  - Assess if the cause is the narcotic, fatigue, sleep deprivation, or other drugs (sedatives, antiemetic)

*May require a physician's order.

- Inform individual that drowsiness usually occurs the first 2 to 3 days, then subsides
- If drowsiness is excessive, consult with physician to try a slight dose reduction

2. Constipation
   - Explain the effect of narcotics on peristalsis
   - Consult with physician for the use of a stool softener with long-term drug use
   - Instruct person to always use the toilet or commode to have a bowel movement, in order to assume the correct position for defecation
   - Teach to increase roughage in diet, *e.g.*, add 1 to 2 teaspoons of bran to food and increase fruit, whole grain breads, and cereal in diet
   - Encourage to drink 8 to 10 glasses (8 oz) of liquids each day
   - Encourage daily exercises, *e.g.*, walking; teach isometric exercises to individuals in bed
   - Refer to *Alterations in Bowel Elimination: Constipation* for additional interventions

3. Nausea and vomiting
   - Consult with physician for the appropriate antiemetic or for a change of narcotic that produces less nausea (*e.g.*, morphine)
   - Instruct person that nausea will usually subside after a few doses
   - Refrain from withholding narcotic dose because of nausea; rather, secure an order for an antiemetic
   - Encourage small, frequent amounts of ice chips or cool, clear liquids (dilute tea, Jell-O water, flat ginger ale, or Coke) unless vomiting continues (*e.g.*, adults, 30 cc to 60 cc q ½–1 hour; children, 15 cc to 30 cc q ½–1 hour)
   - Consider giving medications by suppository rather than by mouth
   - Decrease the stimulation of the vomiting center by reducing unpleasant sights and odors and providing good mouth care after vomiting
   - Instruct person to
     Practice deep breathing and voluntary swallowing to suppress the vomiting reflex
     Sit down after eating but not lie down
     Eat smaller meals; eat slowly
     Restrict liquids with meals to avoid overdistending the stomach; avoid drinking fluids 1 hour before and after meals
     If possible, avoid the smell of food preparation
     Try eating cold foods because they have less odor
     Avoid sweets and fried or fatty foods
     Eat salty foods if not contraindicated
     Loosen clothing
     Sit in fresh air

4. Dry mouth
   - Explain that narcotics decrease saliva production
   - Instruct to rinse mouth often, suck on sugarless sour candies, eat pineapple chunks or watermelon, and drink liquids often
   - Explain the necessity of good oral hygiene and dental care

## J. Assist the family to respond optimally to the individual's pain experience

- Assess the family's knowledge of pain and of responses to the pain experience
- Give accurate information to correct family misconceptions (*e.g.*, addiction, doubt about pain)

- Provide individuals with opportunities to discuss their fears, anger, frustrations in private; acknowledge the difficulty of the situation
- Incorporate the family in the pain relief method if possible (*e.g.*, coaching relaxation, massaging)
- Encourage family to seek assistance if needed for specific problems, such as coping with chronic pain: family counselor; financial and service agencies (*e.g.*, American Cancer Society)

K. Promote optimal mobility
- Discuss the value of exercise to strengthen and stretch muscles, decrease stress, and promote sleep
- Assist individual to plan daily activities when pain is at its lowest level

L. Initiate health teaching and referrals as indicated; discuss with the individual and family the various treatment modalities available:

Family therapy
Group therapy
Behavior modification
Biofeedback
Hypnosis
Acupuncture
Exercise program

# Alterations in Comfort: Pain in Children

## Assessment

Subjective data

| | |
|---|---|
| Whimpering | Reduced appetite (poor feeder) |
| Crying | Does not want to be left alone |
| Moaning | Inability to be comforted |

Objective data

| | |
|---|---|
| Tense body posture | Rubbing or pulling body part |
| Irritability | Refusal to move body part |
| Restlessness | Strained facial expression |

---

**Outcome Criteria**

The child will, according to age and ability
- Identify the source of his pain
- Identify activities that increase and decrease pain
- Receive comfort from others during the pain experience

---

## Interventions

### A. Assess for causative or contributing factors

1. Assess the child's pain experience
   - Determine the child's concept of the cause of the pain, if feasible
   - Ask child to point to the area that hurts
   - Determine the intensity of the pain at its worst and best (may not be useful for children under 5)
   - Ask child to rate his pain using a scale of 0 to 10 (0=no pain and 10=worst pain)

     "What number is your pain when it hurts the least?"

     "What time of day (morning, afternoon, evening)?"
   - Ask the child what makes the pain better and what makes it worse
   - Assess if fear or loneliness are contributing to pain

2. Assess the child and his family for the presence of misconceptions about pain or its treatment
   - Explain the pain source to the child using verbal and sensory (visual, tactile) explanations, *e.g.*, allow child to handle equipment or perform treatment on doll (refer to Appendix III for specific techniques of play therapy)
   - Explicitly explain and reinforce to the child that he is not being punished
   - Explain to the parents the necessity of good explanations to promote trust
   - Explain to the parents that the child may cry more openly when they are present but that their presence is important for promoting trust

### B. Reduce causative or contributing factors if possible

1. Promote open, honest communications
   - Tell the truth; explain

     How much it will hurt

     How long it will last

     What will help the pain
   - Do not threaten, *e.g., do not* tell the child, "If you don't hold still you won't go home"
   - Explain to the child that the procedure is necessary so he can get better and it is important to hold still so it can be done quickly
   - Discuss with the parents the importance of truth telling; instruct parents to

     Tell child when they are leaving and when they will return

     Relate to the child that they cannot take away his pain but that they will be with him (except in circumstances when parents are not permitted to remain)
   - Allow the parents opportunities to share their feelings about witnessing their child's pain and their helplessness

2. Prepare the child for a painful procedure
   - Discuss the procedure with the parents; determine what they have told the child
   - Explain the procedure in words suited to the child's age and developmental level (see Appendix VII for age-related needs)

     Allow a 2-year-old to watch you taking out sutures from a doll or stuffed animal

     Permit the child to hold instruments
   - Relate the discomforts that will be felt, *e.g.*, what the child will feel, taste, see or smell

"You will get an injection that will hurt for a little while and then it will stop"

Be sure to explain when an injection will cause two discomforts: the prick of the needle and the absorption of the drug

- Encourage the child to ask questions before and during the procedure; ask the child to share with you what he thinks is going to happen and why
- Share with the child (who is old enough: $> 3\frac{1}{2}$) that

  You expect that he will hold still and that it will please you if he can

  It is all right to cry or squeeze your hand if it hurts
- Arrange to have parents present for procedures (especially for children 18 months to 5 years)

3. Reduce the pain during treatments when possible

   a. If restraints must be utilized, have sufficient personnel available in order not to delay the procedure

   b. When administering injections
      - Expect the child (over $2\frac{1}{2}$ or 3) to hold still
      - Have the child participate by holding the Band-Aid for you
      - Tell the child how pleased you are that he helped
      - Pull the skin surface as taut as possible (for I.M.)
      - Comfort the child after the procedure
      - Tell child step-by-step what is going to happen right before it is done

   c. Explain to the child that he can be distracted from the procedure if he wants (the use of distraction without the child's knowledge of the impending discomfort is not advocated because the child will learn to mistrust)
      - Tell a story with a puppet
      - Ask the child to name or count objects in a picture
      - Ask the child to look at the picture and to locate certain objects ("Where is the dog?")
      - Ask child to tell you about his pet
      - Ask child to count your blinks

   d. Avoid rectal temperatures in preschoolers; if possible, use electronic oral probes

   e. Provide the child with privacy during the painful procedure; utilize a treatment room rather than the child's bed
      - The child's bed should be a "safe" place
      - No procedures should be done in the playroom or schoolroom

4. Provide the child optimal pain relief with prescribed analgesics
   - Medicate child prior to painful procedure or activity (*e.g.,* ambulation)
   - Assess for visual signs of pain, since child may not request pain medication because of fear of needle

5. Reduce or eliminate the common side-effects of narcotics

   a. Sedation
      - Assess if the cause is the narcotic, fatigue, sleep deprivation, or other drugs (sedatives, antiemetics)
      - If drowsiness is excessive, consult with physician to try a slight dose reduction

   b. Constipation
      - Explain to older children why pain medications cause constipation
      - Increase roughage in diet (*e.g.,* ask child what fruits he likes; sprinkle 1–2 teaspoons of bran on cereal)
      - Encourage child to drink eight to ten (8 oz) glasses of liquids each day

- Teach child how to do abdominal isometric exercises if activity is restricted, *e.g.*, "Pull in your tummy; now relax your tummy; do this 10 times each hour during the day"
- Instruct child to keep a record of his exercises, *e.g.*, make a chart with a star sticker placed on it whenever the exercises are done
- Refer to *Alterations in Bowel Elimination: Constipation* for additional interventions

c. Dry mouth

- Explain to older children that narcotics decrease saliva production
- Instruct to rinse mouth often, suck on sugarless sour candies, eat pineapple chunks and watermelon, drink liquids often
- Explain the necessity of brushing his teeth after every meal

6. Assist the child with the aftermath of the pain
- Tell the child when the painful procedure is over
- Pick up the small child to indicate it is over
- Encourage the child to discuss his pain experience (draw or act out with dolls)
- Allow the child to perform the painful procedure using the same equipment on a doll under supervision (See Appendix III for specific interventions)
- Praise the child for his endurance and convey to him that he handled the pain well regardless of how he behaved (unless he was violent to others)
- Give the child a souvenir of his pain (Band-Aid, badge for bravery)
- Teach the child to keep a record of painful experiences and to place a star next to those he held still for, *e.g.*, gold stars on a paper for each injection or venipuncture

7. Collaborate with child to initiate appropriate noninvasive pain relief modalities
- Encourage mobility as much as indicated, especially when pain is at its lowest level
- Discuss with child and parents activities that are liked and incorporate them in daily schedule (*e.g.*, clay modeling, painting)
- Discuss with the child (over 7) that the pain can be less if the child thinks about something else and demonstrate the effects
  a. Ask child to count to 100 (or count your eye blinks)
  b. As child is counting, apply gentle pressure to Achilles tendon (pinch back of heel)
  c. Gradually increase the pressure
  d. Ask child to stop counting but keep pressure on the heel
  e. Ask child if he can feel the discomfort in his heel now and if he felt it when he was counting
- Refer to guidelines for noninvasive pain relief measures (Appendix V)

8. Assist the family to respond optimally to the child's pain experience
- Assess the family's knowledge of and response to the pain experience, *e.g.*, does the parent support the child who has pain?
- Assure the parents that they can touch or hold their child (if feasible), *e.g.*, demonstrate that touching is possible even in the presence of tubes and equipment
- Give accurate information to correct misconceptions, *e.g.*, the necessity of the treatment even though it causes pain
- Provide parents with opportunities to discuss their fears, anger, frustrations in private
- Acknowledge the difficulty of the situation

- Incorporate the parents in the pain relief modality if possible, *e.g.*, stroking, massage, distraction
- Praise their participation and their concern

## C. Initiate health teaching and referrals if indicated
- Provide child and family with ongoing explanations
- Utilize the care plan to promote continuity of care for hospitalized child
- Refer parents to pertinent literature for themselves and children (See Bibliography and Appendix VII)

## Bibliography

Anderson J: Nursing management of the cancer patient in pain: A review of the literature. Cancer Nursing 5:33–41, 1982

Barber J: Hypnosis as a psychological technique in the management of cancer pain. Cancer Nursing 1:361–363, 1978

Beyerman K: Flawed perceptions about pain. Am J Nurs 82:302–304, 1982

Copley IJ: No matter what you call it, it's still pain to the patient. RN 41(2):64, 1978

Davis AJ: Brompton's cocktail: Making good-byes possible. Am J Nurs 78:610–612, 1978

Evans M, Hansen B: Administering injections to different-age children. Matern Child Nurs J 6:194–199, 1981

Fagerbaugh S, Strauss A: How to manage your patient's pain . . . and how not to. Nursing 10(6):44–47, 1980

Hansen B, Evans M: Preparing a child for procedures. Matern Child Nurs J 6:392–397, 1981

Jacox AK (ed): Pain: A Source Book for Nurses and Other Professionals. Boston, Little, Brown, 1977

Jacox AK: Assessing pain. Am J Nurs 79:895–900, 1979

Klisch ML: The Simonton method of visualization. Cancer Nursing 3:295–300, 1980

Krieger D: Therapeutic touch: The imprimatur of nursing. Am J Nurs 75:784–787, 1975

Lasagna L: The influences of age on analgesic pain relief. JAMA 218:1831–1833, 1971

Leuner H: Guided affective imagery. Am J Psychother 23:4–22, 1969

Lipman AJ: Drug therapy in cancer pain. Cancer Nursing 10:26–31, 1980

McCafferty M: Understanding your patient's pain. Nursing 10(4):26–31, 1980

McCafferty M: Nursing Management of the Patient with Pain, 2nd ed. Philadelphia, JB Lippincott, 1980

Perry S, Heidrich G: Placebos. Am J Nurs 81:721–725, 1981

Saunders C: Care of the dying: Control of pain in terminal cancer. Nursing Times 72:1133–1135, 1976

Silman J, Diblasi M, Washburn CJ: The management of pain. Am J Nurs 79:74–78, 1979

Storlie F: Pointers for assessing pain. Nursing 8(3):37–39, 1978

Wilson R, Elmassian B: Endorphins. Am J Nurs 81:722–725, 1981

# Communication, Impaired Verbal

*Related to* **Impaired Ability to Speak Words**

*Related to* **Aphasia**

*Related to* **Foreign Language Barriers**

## Definition

Impaired verbal communication: The state in which the individual experiences, or could experience, a decreased ability to speak appropriately or understand the meaning of words.

## Etiological and Contributing Factors

### Pathophysiological

Cerebral impairment
    Expressive or receptive aphasia
    Cerebrovascular accident
    Brain damage (*e.g.*, birth/head trauma)
    CNS depression/increased intracranial pressure
    Tumor (of the head, neck, or spinal cord)
    Mental retardation
    Chronic hypoxia/decreased cerebral blood flow
Neurologic impairment
    Quadriplegia
    Nervous system diseases (*e.g.*, myasthenia gravis, multiple sclerosis)
    Vocal cord paralysis
Respiratory impairment (*e.g.*, shortness of breath)
Auditory impairment (decreased hearing)
Laryngeal edema/infection

### Situational

Surgery
    Endotracheal intubation
    Tracheostomy/tracheotomy/laryngectomy
    Surgery of the head, face, neck, or mouth
Pain (especially of the mouth or throat)
Drugs (*e.g.*, CNS depressants, anesthesia)
Oral deformities
    Cleft lip or palate
    Malocclusion or fractured jaw
    Missing teeth
Speech pathology
    Stuttering
    Lisping

Ankyglosia ("tongue-tie")
Voice problems
Language barrier (unfamiliar language or dialect)
Psychological barrier (*e.g.*, fear, shyness)
Lack of privacy
Lack of support system

## Defining Characteristics

Stuttering
Slurring
Problem in finding the correct word when speaking
Weak or absent voice
Shortness of breath, ineffective breathing pattern
Decreased auditory comprehension
Deafness or inattention to noises or voices
Articulation or motor planning problems (*i.e.*, difficulty forming words, making
   sentences)
Inappropriate speech
Confusion
Inability to speak dominant language

## Focus Assessment Criteria

### Subjective data

1. Note the usual pattern of communication as described by the person or his
   family

   | | |
   |---|---|
   | Very verbal | Speaks only when spoken to |
   | Sometimes verbal | Does not speak |

   - Does the person feel he is communicating normally today?
   - If not, what does he feel may help him to communicate better?
   - Is there a specific person he would like to talk with or have present to help
     him express ideas?
2. Does the person feel he can usually express himself well?
3. Does the person feel there are barriers hindering his ability to communicate?
   Lack of privacy
   Fear of uncertain origin
   Fear of being inappropriate or "stupid"
   Not enough time to gather his thoughts and ask questions
   Need for presence of significant other or familiar face
   Language, dialect, or cultural barrier (specify)
   Lack of knowledge of subject being discussed
   Pain or stress

### Objective data

1. Describe the person's ability to form words

   | | |
   |---|---|
   | Good | Weak (whisper) |
   | Slurred | Absent |
   | Lisping | Language barrier |
   | Stuttering | Difficulty breathing and talking |
   | Slow | |

2. Describe the person's ability to comprehend
    Understands simple commands or ideas
    Able to follow complex instructions or ideas
    Sometimes able to follow instructions or ideas
    Not able to follow simple instructions or ideas
3. What is the person's developmental age?

| | | |
|---|---|---|
| Infant | Child | Adult |
| Toddler | Adolescent | Aged |

4. Describe the person's ability to make sentences

| | | |
|---|---|---|
| Good | Unclear ideas | Can make short |
| Slow | Nonsensical or |   simple sentences |
| Weak |   confused | Language barrier |

5. How does the person's affect or manner appear to you?

| | | |
|---|---|---|
| Nervous | Fearful | Pained |
| Anxious | Withdrawn | Uncomfortable |
| Attentive | Flat | Comfortable |

6. Does the person maintain eye contact?

| | | |
|---|---|---|
| Good | Occasional | None |

7. Are there contributing factors that may inhibit the person's ability to communicate?
    Alterations in thought processes (*e.g.*, memory deficit psychosis)
    Pain or stress
    Oral, facial, or neck deformity (or surgery)
    Breathing impairment
    Auditory impairment
    Visual impairment
    CNS depression
    Vocal cord paralysis
    Muscle paralysis
    Expressive aphasia
    Receptive aphasia

## Nursing Goals

Through selected nursing interventions, the nurse will seek to
- Create an atmosphere conducive to communication
- Promote optimal communication by encouraging the person to use adaptive devices for speech and hearing if necessary (*e.g.*, hearing aid, artificial larynx)
- Provide alternative methods of communicating (*e.g.*, pad and pencil, pictures, alphabet)
- Encourage the person to express himself in whatever way he can

## Principles and Rationale for Nursing Care

### General

1. Speech is man's fundamental way of expressing needs, desires, and feelings. Poor communication can cause feelings of frustration, anger, hostility, depression, fear, confusion, and isolation.
2. Communication is affected by eye contact, loudness and intonation of voice, facial expression, and proximity of the communicators.
3. Communication may be hampered by lack of privacy.

4. Good communicators are also good listeners, who listen for both facts and feelings.
5. Silence may signify either acceptance, defiance, a delay in wishing to comment, or a needed break to gather thoughts. Allowing silence may enhance communication.
6. To be sure a message is understood, one should have the receiver repeat what has been said. A reply of "Yes" or "I understand" may not be enough.
7. People should overcome the human tendency to shout or "talk down" to a person who is verbally handicapped. Impaired verbal speech does not necessarily signify impairment of intelligence or of the ability to hear and understand.
8. Dysarthria is a disturbance in the voluntary muscular control of speech caused by conditions such as Parkinson's disease, multiple sclerosis, myasthenia gravis, cerebral palsy and CNS damage. The same muscles are used in eating and swallowing. Persons with dysarthria usually do not have problems with comprehension.

## Aphasia

1. Aphasia is an altered ability to communicate because of cerebral damage. The alterations can be verbal, gestural, visual, or graphic.
2. Expressive aphasia is a disturbance in the ability to speak, write, or gesture understandably.
3. Receptive aphasia is a disturbance in the ability to comprehend written and spoken language.
4. The person with receptive aphasia may have intact hearing but cannot process or is unaware of his own sounds.
5. Aphasic persons may have difficulty with retention and memory recall. Old memories may return first, with memory recall of recent events returning last.
6. Emotional lability (swings between crying and laughing) is common to persons with aphasia. This behavior is not intentional and declines with recovery.

## Cultural or foreign language barriers

1. Knowledge of a foreign language depends upon four elements: The knowledge of how to speak the language in conversation, the ability to understand the language in conversation, the ability to read the language, and the ability to write the language.
2. An answer of "yes" from a foreigner may be an effort to please rather than a sign of understanding what has been said.
3. Even though the nurse cannot speak another's language, she can convey a climate of acceptance by talking in a pleasant tone of voice and using actions to demonstrate meaning (*e.g.*, smiling and motioning to sit down, while saying, "Sit down, please").
4. An attempt on the nurse's part to communicate over a language barrier encourages a foreign individual to do the same.
5. People should overcome the human tendency either to ignore or shout at people who do not speak the dominant language.
6. Appropriate distance between communicators varies from culture to culture. Some may normally stand face to face, while others must stand several feet apart to be comfortable.

7. Communicating through the use of touch or holding varies from culture to culture. For example, some cultures view touching as an extremely familiar gesture, some cultures shy away from touching a given part of the body (a pat on the head may be offensive), and some cultures consider it appropriate for men to kiss each other and for women to hold hands.

# Impaired Verbal Communication
## Related to Impaired Ability to Speak Words

### Assessment

#### Subjective data
The person reports inability or difficulty in pronouncing words

#### Objective data
Difficulty in pronouncing words due to apparent physiologic problem, *e.g.,*

| | |
|---|---|
| Parkinson's syndrome | Myasthenia gravis |
| Multiple sclerosis | Cerebral palsy |

Inability to speak

| | |
|---|---|
| Postlaryngectomy | Tracheostomy |
| Intubation | |

---

**Outcome Criteria**

The person will
- Demonstrate improved ability to express self
- Relate decreased frustration with communication

---

### Interventions

#### A. Identify a method by which person can communicate his basic needs

1. Assess ability to comprehend, speak, read, and write
2. Provide alternative methods of communication
   - Use pad and pencil, alphabet letters, hand signals, eye blinks, head nods, bell signals
   - Make flash cards with pictures or words depicting frequently used phrases (*e.g.,* "Wet my lips," "Move my foot," glass of water, bedpan)
   - Encourage the person to point, use gestures, and pantomime
   - Consult with speech pathologist for assistance in acquiring flash cards

## B. Identify factors that promote communication

1. For individuals with dysarthria

   - Reduce environmental noise to increase the caregiver's ability to listen to words (*e.g.*, radio, TV)
   - Do not alter your speech or messages, since his comprehension is not affected; speak on an adult level
   - Encourage the person to make a conscious effort to slow down his speech and to speak louder (*e.g.*, "Take a deep breath between sentences")
   - Ask him to repeat words that are unclear; observe for nonverbal cues to help understanding
   - If he is tired, ask questions that require only short answers
   - If speech is unintelligible, teach the person to use gestures, written messages, and communication cards

2. For individuals who cannot speak (*e.g.*, endotracheal intubation, tracheostomy)

   - Reassure that his speech will return, if it will
   - If not, explain what alternatives are available (*e.g.*, esophageal speech, sign language)
   - Do not alter your speech, tone, or type of message, since the person's ability to understand is not affected; speak on an adult level
   - Read lips for cues

## C. Promote continuity of care to reduce frustration

1. Observe for signs of frustration or withdrawal

   - Verbally address the problem of frustration over inability to communicate, and explain that patience is needed for both the nurse and the person who is trying to talk
   - Maintain a calm, positive attitude (*e.g.*, "I can understand you if we work at it")
   - Use reassurance (*e.g.*, "I know it's hard, but you'll get it")
   - Maintain a sense of humor
   - Allow tears (*e.g.*, "It's OK. I know it's frustrating. Crying can let it all out")
   - For the person who has a limited ability to talk (*e.g.*, can make simple requests, but not lengthy statements), encourage writing letters or keeping a diary to ventilate feelings and share concerns
   - Anticipate needs and ask questions that need a simple yes or no answer

2. Maintain a specific care plan

   - Write the method of communication that is used (*e.g.*, "Uses word cards," "Points to night stand for bedpan")
   - Record directions for specific measures to reduce communication problems (*e.g.*, allow him to keep urinal in bed)

## D. Initiate health teaching and referrals as indicated

- Teach significant others techniques and repetitive approaches to improve communications
- Encourage the family to share feelings concerning communication problems
- Seek consultation with a speech pathologist early in treatment regime

# Impaired Verbal Communication
## Related to Aphasia

Aphasia is a communication impairment—a difficulty in expressing, a difficulty in understanding, or a combination of both—resulting from cerebral deficits.

---

**Outcome Criteria**

The person will
- Demonstrate increased ability to understand
- Demonstrate improved ability to express himself
- Relate decreased frustration with communication

---

## Assessment

### Subjective data

The person reports
  An inability to express self
  A difficulty in responding verbally
  History of
      Cerebral vascular accident
      Tumor
      Cerebral trauma

### Objective data

  Slurred speech
  Unintelligible speech
  Inappropriate responses to questions

## Interventions

A. Identify a method the person can use to communicate basic needs

  1. Assess ability to comprehend, speak, read, and write
  2. Provide alternative methods of communication
     - Use pad and pencil, alphabet letters, hand signals, eye blinks, head nods, bell signals
     - Make flash cards with pictures or words depicting frequently used phrases (*e.g.,* "Wet my lips," "Move my foot," glass of water, bedpan)
     - Encourage person to point, use gestures, and pantomime
     - Consult with speech pathologist for assistance in acquiring flash cards

B. Identify factors that promote communication

  1. Create atmosphere of acceptance and privacy
  2. Provide a non-rushed environment
     - Use normal loudness level and speak unhurriedly, in short phrases
     - Encourage the person to take his time talking and to enunciate words carefully with good lip movements

- Decrease external distractions
- Delay conversation when the person is tired

3. Assess the individual's frustration level and don't push beyond it
   - Estimate 30 seconds of passed time before providing the individual with the word he may be trying to find (except when the person is frustrated or needs the request immediately *e.g.,* bedpan)
   - Provide cues through pictures or gestures

4. Utilize techniques to increase understanding
   - Face the individual and establish eye contact if possible
   - Use uncomplicated one-step commands and directives
   - Have only one person talk (it's more difficult to follow a multisided conversation)
   - Encourage the use of gestures and pantomime)
   - Match words with actions; use pictures
   - Terminate conversation on a note of success (*e.g.,* move back to an easier item)

## C.  Utilize techniques that enhance verbal expression

1. Make a concerted effort to understand when the person is speaking
   - Allow enough time to listen if the person speaks slowly
   - Rephrase his message aloud to him in order to validate it
   - Respond to all attempts at speech even if they are unintelligible (*e.g.,* "I do not know what you are saying. Can you try to say it again?")
   - Acknowledge when you understand, and do not be concerned with imperfect pronunciation at first
   - Ignore mistakes and profanity
   - Don't pretend you understand if you don't
   - Observe the person's nonverbal cues for validation (*e.g.,* he answers yes and shakes his head no)
   - Allow the person time to respond; do not interrupt; supply words only occasionally

2. Teach techniques to improve speech
   - Ask the person to slow speech down, and say each word clearly, while providing the example
   - Encourage the person to speak in short phrases
   - Explain to the person that his words are not clearly understood (*e.g.,* "I can't understand what you are saying")
   - Suggest a slower rate of talking, or taking a breath prior to speech
   - Encourage the person to take his time and concentrate on forming his words
   - Ask the person to write down his message, or to draw a picture, if verbal communication is difficult
   - Encourage the person to speak in short phrases
   - Ask questions that can be answered with a yes or no
   - Focus on the present; avoid topics that are controversial, emotional, abstract, or lengthy

## D.  Acknowledge the individual's frustration

1. Verbally address the problem of frustration over inability to communicate, and explain that patience is needed for both the nurse and the person who is trying to talk

2. Maintain a calm, positive attitude (*e.g.,* "I can understand you if we work at it")
3. Use reassurance (*e.g.,* "I know it's hard, but you'll get it"); use touch if acceptable
4. Maintain a sense of humor
5. Allow tears (*e.g.,* "It's OK. I know it's frustrating. Crying can let it all out")
6. For the person who has a limited ability to talk (*i.e.,* can make simple requests, but not lengthy statements), encourage writing letters or keeping a diary to ventilate feelings and share concerns
7. Give the person opportunities to make decisions about his care ("Do you want a drink? Would you rather have orange juice or prune juice?")
8. Provide alternative methods of self-expression
   Humming/singing
   Dancing/exercising/walking
   Writing/drawing/painting/coloring
   Helping (tasks such as opening mail, choosing meals)

E. Identify factors that promote comprehension

1. Assess hearing ability and use of functioning hearing aids
2. Assess ability to see, and encourage the person to wear his glasses
   - Explain to the person that seeing better will increase understanding of what is happening around him
   - Even if the person is blind, look at him when talking to "throw" voice in his direction
3. Provide sufficient light and remove distractions (see *Sensory-Perceptual Alterations*)
4. Speak when the person is ready to listen
   - Achieve eye contact, if possible
   - Gain the person's attention by a gentle touch on the arm and a verbal message of "Listen to me" or "I want to talk to you"
5. Modify your speech
   - Speak slowly, enunciate distinctly
   - Use common adult words
   - Do not change subjects or ask multiple questions in succession
   - Repeat or rephrase requests
   - Do not increase volume of voice unless person has a hearing deficit
   - Match your nonverbal behavior with your verbal actions—to avoid misinterpretation (*e.g.,* do not laugh with a co-worker while performing a task)
   - Try to use the same words with the same task (*e.g.,* bathroom vs. toilet; pill vs. medication)
   - Keep a record at bedside of the words to maintain continuity
   - As the person improves, allow him to complete your sentences (*e.g.,* "This is a ———— [pill]")
6. Utilize other methods of communication besides verbal
   - Use pantomime
   - Point
   - Use flash cards
   - Show him what you mean (*e.g.,* pick up a glass)
   - Write key words on a card, so he can practice them while you show the object (*e.g.,* paper, toilet)

F. Show respect when providing care

1. Avoid discussing the person's condition in his presence; assume he can understand despite his deficits
2. Monitor other health care providers
3. Talk to the person whenever you are with him

G. Initiate health teaching and referrals if indicated

1. Teach techniques to significant others and repetitive approaches to improve communications
2. Encourage the family to share feelings concerning communication problems
   - Explain the reasons for labile emotions and profanity
   - Explain the need to include the person in family decision-making
3. Seek consultation with a speech pathologist early in treatment regime

# Impaired Verbal Communication
## Related to Foreign Language Barriers

### Assessment

#### Subjective data

The person states
   "I don't understand———[name of language]"
   "I don't speak———[name of language]"

#### Objective data

Foreign accent
Absence of speech
Body language only means of communication (person only nods or gestures)

---

**Outcome Criteria**

The person will
- Be able to communicate basic needs
- Relate feelings of acceptance, reduced frustration and isolation

---

### Interventions

A. Assess the individual's ability to communicate in English*

1. Assess what language the person speaks best
2. Assess the person's ability to read, write, speak, and comprehend English

*English will be used as an example of the dominant language.

B. Identify factors that promote communication through a language barrier when a translator is not present
1. Face the person and give a pleasant greeting, in a normal tone of voice
2. Talk clearly and somewhat slower than normal (don't overdo it)
3. If the person does not understand or speak (respond), use alternative method of communication
   - Try writing down message
   - Use gestures or actions
   - Use pictures or drawings
     Make flash cards that translate words or phrases
4. Encourage the person to also use the aforementioned methods of communication (try to overcome shyness)
5. Encourage the person to teach others some of the words or greetings of his own language (this helps to promote a feeling of acceptance and a willingness to learn)

C. Be cognizant of possible cultural barriers
1. Be careful when touching the person, for it may not be appropriate in some cultures
2. Be aware of the different ways that men and women are expected to be treated (cultural differences may influence whether a man speaks to a woman about certain matters, or vice versa)
3. Make a conscious effort to be nonjudgmental about another's cultural differences
4. Make note of what seems to be a comfortable distance from which to speak

D. Initiate referrals when needed
1. Use a *fluent* translator when discussing matters of importance (such as taking a health history or signing an operation permit)
2. If possible, allow the translator to spend as much time as the person wishes (be flexible with visitor's rules and regulations)
3. If a translator is not available, try to plan a daily visit from someone who has some knowledge of the person's language (many hospitals and social welfare offices keep a "language" bank with names and phone numbers of people who are willing to translate)

## Bibliography

Bartnick W: Health care and counseling skills. The Personal and Guidance Journal 58:666–667, 1980

Collins M: Communications in Health Care. St. Louis, CV Mosby, 1977

Conture E: Stuttering. Englewood Cliffs, NJ, Prentice-Hall, 1982

DeVilleous L: What to do when you just can't communicate. Nursing Life 2(2):34–32, 1982

Dreher B: Overcoming speech and language disorders. Geriatric Nursing 2:345–349, 1981

Jungman L: When your feelings get in the way. Am J Nurs 79:1074–1075, 1979

Kyes J: Pseudocommunication is the nurse-patient game. Nursing Life: 2(1):50–54, 1982

Ragnakers MJ: Communications blocks revisted. Am J Nurs 79:1079–1081, 1979

Santopietro M: How to get through to a refugee patient. Nursing 11(1):43–48, 1981

Smith B: Communications for Health Professionals. Philadelphia, JB Lippincott, 1979

Van Riper C: Speech Correction 6 E, Englewood Cliffs, NJ, Prentice-Hall, 1982

Weinhouse I: Speaking to the needs of your aphasic patient. Nursing 11(3):34–36, 1981

# Coping, Ineffective Individual

*Related to* **Depression in Response to Identifiable Stressors**

## Definition
Ineffective individual coping: A state in which the individual experiences or is at risk of experiencing an inability to manage internal or environmental stressors adequately due to inadequate resources (physical, psychological, or behavioral).

## Etiological and Contributing Factors

Pathophysiological

Changes in body integrity
    Loss of body part
    Disfigurement secondary to trauma or surgery
    Altered appearance due to drugs, radiation, or other treatment
Altered affect caused by changes in body chemistry
    Tumor (brain)
    Hormonal treatment
    Injection of mood-altering substance
Physiological manifestations of persistent stress

Situational

Changes in physical environment
        War                      Seasonal work (migrant worker)
        Natural disaster        Poverty
        Relocation
Disruption of emotional bonds due to
        Death                  Relocation
        Separation or divorce    Hospitalization
        Desertion           Incarceration
Unsatisfactory support system
Institutionalization
        Jail                   Nursing home
        Foster home        Educational institution
        Orphanage          Maintenance institution for disabled

Sensory overload
        Critical care unit      Urbanization: crowding, noise
        Factory environment      pollution, excessive activity
Inadequate psychological resources
        Poor self-esteem       Helplessness
        Excessive negative beliefs about   Lack of motivation to respond
          self

Culturally related conflicts with life experiences

Premarital sex

Abortion

Need for medical intervention
(*e.g.*, Christian Scientist)

## Maturational

Child

Developmental tasks
(independence vs. dependence)

Entry into school

Competition among peers

Peer relationships

Adolescent

Physical and emotional changes

Independence from family

Heterosexual relationships

Sexual awareness

Educational demands

Career choices

Young adult

Career choices

Educational demands

Leaving home

Marriage

Parenthood

Middle adult

Physical signs of aging

Career pressures

Child-rearing problems

Problems with relatives

Social status needs

Aging parents

Elderly

Physical changes

Changes in financial status

Change in residence

Retirement

Response of others to older
people

## Defining Characteristics

Verbalization of inability to cope

Distortion or confusion of roles

Inability to meet basic needs

Inability to make decisions

Inability to ask for help

Destructive behavior toward self or others

Change in usual communication patterns

Inappropriate use of defense mechanisms

Frequent illness

High rate of accidents

## Focus Assessment Criteria

Ineffective coping can be manifested in a variety of ways. A person or family may respond with an alteration in another life process (*i.e.*, spiritual distress, alteration in parenting, potential for violence). The nurse should be aware of this and use assessment data to ascertain the dimensions affected.

### Subjective data

Self-concept

"How would you describe yourself?"

"What do you like (dislike) about yourself?"

Support system

"To whom do you turn or usually go for help when you have a problem?" (See *Alterations in Family Processes* for additional data)

Emotional status
  "How would you describe your usual emotional state?"
  "What can cause a change in your usual state of mind?"
  "How would you describe your current life situation?"
Problem-solving abilities
  "When you have a problem, how do you usually deal with it?"

## Objective data

Appearance
           Altered affect (flat; "poker face")          Poor grooming
           Appropriate                                  Inappropriate dress
Behavior
           Calm                                         Tearful
           Hostile                                      Sudden mood swings
           Withdrawn
Cognitive function
   Altered orientation to time, place, person
   Impaired concentration
   Altered ability to problem-solve
Presence of stress-related symptoms

  *Cardiovascular*                              *Gastrointestinal*

  Headaches                                     △Nausea
  △Fainting                                     Vomiting
  Tachycardia                                   △Abdominal pain or cramps
  △Palpitations                                 △Change in appetite
                                                Constipation
                                                Diarrhea
  *Respiratory*

  Tachypnea                                     *Genitourinary*
  Bronchospasm
  △Shortness of breath                          Menstrual disturbance
                                                Urinary frequency hesitancy
                                                Sexual disturbances
  *Musculoskeletal*                             △Anorgasmia
                                                Impotence
  △Pain                                         △Painful intercourse
  △Headache                                     △Altered libido
  △Backache
  △Fatigue
  Tremors
△= subjective symptoms

Abusive behaviors
   To self
       Excessive smoking
       Excessive alcohol intake
       Excessive food intake
       Drug abuse
       Reckless driving
   To others
       Doesn't care
       Neglects needs of dependent family members
       Is unwilling to listen
       Doesn't communicate
       Imposes physical harm on family member (bruises, burns, broken bones)

## Nursing Goals

Through selected interventions, the nurse will seek to
- Determine etiology(ies) of ineffective coping
- Assess competency of the person's coping strategies
- Facilitate the person's insight into sources and consequences of prolonged stress in his or her environment
- Support the person's coping strengths and collaborate to determine alternative strategies for dysfunctional efforts

## Principles and Rationale for Nursing Care

### Concepts related to the nature of coping

1. Coping refers to psychological and behavioral activities made to master, tolerate, or minimize external or internal demands and conflicts (Lazarus).
2. Coping effectively requires successful management of many tasks: maintenance of self-concept, maintenance of satisfying relationships with others, maintenance of emotional balance, and management of stress.
3. There is no one way to cope with all situations.
4. There are two basic types of coping behavior (Lazarus): problem-focused—manipulation of the persons and environmental factors inducing stress—and emotion-focused—the management of stress-related emotions. Examples follow.

| *Problem-focused* | *Emotion-focused* |
|---|---|
| 1. Make appointment with the boss to discuss pay raise | 1. Play basketball three times per week |
| 2. Write out time schedule for homework and adhere to it | 2. Allow myself to cry when I get home |
| | 3. Practice yoga daily |

5. Appraisal is the thought process that evaluates the situation. Constructive realistic appraisal strategies can be facilitated with the following questions: What is at stake? What are the choices? Where is there help?

### Stress

1. Stress may be defined as the nonspecific response of the body to any demand (Selye).
2. Stress has physiological manifestations.

*Cardiovascular*

Migraine headache
Fainting
Tachycardia
Palpitations

*Gastrointestinal*

Irritable colon
Change in appetite
Nausea
Vomiting
Abdominal pain or cramps
Bowel irregularity

*Respiratory*

Tachypnea
Bronchospasm with shortness of breath

*Genitourinary*

Menstrual disturbance
Urinary frequency or hesitancy
Painful intercourse
Anorgasmia
Impotence
Delayed or premature ejaculation

*Musculoskeletal*

Pain secondary to sustained muscle tension
Headache
Backache
Fatigue
Tremors

*Skin*

Pruritus
Urticaria
Excessive perspiration

## Depression

1. Reactive depression occurs as a response to a situational stressor.
2. Endogenous depression, possibly somatic in origin, is a maladaptive response to often unidentifiable causes.

### Reactive vs. Endogenous Depression

| Element | Reactive Depression | Endogenous Depression |
|---|---|---|
| Precipitating event | Identifiable | Unclear |
| Family history | Unrelated | Familial tendency |
| Symptoms | Related to grief and anxiety; worse at night | Seemingly unrelated to events; worse in morning |
| Activity | Diminished motor and cognitive behavior | Agitated, restless |
| Emotion | Client feels sad | Alternates between sadness and manic gaiety |
| Cognitive abilities | May be slightly diminished | Retarded psychomotor performance |
| Orientation | Oriented and responsive to environment | May not be oriented or responsive |
| Treatment | Responds well to counseling and environmental change | Requires somatic treatment |

# Ineffective Individual Coping
## Related to Depression in Response to Identifiable Stressors

## Assessment

### Subjective data

The person verbalizes feelings of

Failure ("I should have ———)
Sadness, blues
Loneliness
Worry, fear

Vague confusion
Helplessness ("I can't ———")
Hopelessness, apathy
Preoccupation with self

The person describes symptoms of

Fatigue
Constipation or diarrhea
Insomnia or excessive sleep
Anorexia

General pain
Stiffness
Menstrual changes
Dizziness, numbness

|                | |
|----------------|--|
| Headache       | Frequent crying episodes |
| Dry mouth      | (or desire to cry) |

## Objective data
Physical symptoms

|                              | |
|------------------------------|--|
| Rashes                       | Lusterless eyes |
| Tachycardia                  | Weight changes |

Emotional symptoms

|                              | |
|------------------------------|--|
| Distressed, tearful, sad     | Altered affect |

Altered cognitive ability

|                              | |
|------------------------------|--|
| Inability to concentrate     | Difficulty with problem-solving |
| Poor memory                  | Inability to make decisions |

Physical appearance

|                              | |
|------------------------------|--|
| Poor personal hygiene        | Poor nutrition |
| Lack of grooming             | |

---

**Outcome Criteria**

The person will
- Verbalize feelings related to his emotional state
- Identify his coping patterns and the consequences of the behavior that results
- Identify personal strengths and receive support through the nursing relationship
- Make decisions and follow through with appropriate actions to change provocative situations in personal environment

---

## Interventions

### A. Assess causative and contributing factors
- Negative self-concept
- Moral or ethical conflict (see *Spiritual Distress*)
- Disapproval by others
- Inadequate problem-solving
- Loss-related grief (see *Grieving*)
- Sudden change in life pattern
- Recent change in health status of self or significant other
- Inadequate support system

### B. Assess individual's present coping status
1. Determine onset of feelings and symptoms and their correlation with events and life changes
2. Assess ability to relate facts
3. Listen carefully as client speaks, to collect facts and observe facial expressions, gestures, eye contact, body positioning, tone and intensity of voice
4. Determine risk of client's inflicting self-harm and intervene appropriately
   a. Assess for signs of potential suicide
      - History of previous attempts or threats (overt and covert)
      - Changes in personality, behavior, sexual life, appetite, sleep habits

- Preparations for death (putting things in order, making a will, giving away personal possessions, acquiring a weapon)
- A sudden elevation in mood

b. Demonstrate to client that you believe him and desire to help
  - Avoid challenging him, minimizing his feelings, arguing, or trying to reason with him
  - Listen attentively and stay close until the danger has passed or help is secured

c. Offer support as client talks
  - Reassure him that the feelings he has must be difficult
  - When client is pessimistic, attempt to provide a more hopeful, realistic perspective

d. See *Potential for Violence* for additional information on suicide prevention

## C. Teach constructive problem-solving techniques

1. Assist the person to problem-solve in a constructive manner
   - What is the problem?
   - Who or what is responsible for the problem?
   - What are his options? (Make a list)
   - What are the advantages and disadvantages of each option?
2. Discuss possible alternatives; *i.e.,* talk over the problem with those involved, try to change the situation, or do nothing and accept the consequences
3. Assist the individual to identify problems that he cannot control directly and help him to practice stress-reducing activities for control (*e.g.,* exercise program, yoga); see Appendix VI for problem-solving techniques
4. Instruct client in relaxation techniques; emphasize the importance of setting 15 to 20 minutes aside each day to practice relaxation. Write down the following guidelines (see Appendix IV for additional relaxation techniques)
   - Find a comfortable position in chair or on floor
   - Close eyes
   - Keep noise to a minimum (only very soft music is desired)
   - Concentrate on breathing slowly and deeply
   - Feel the heaviness of all extremities
   - If muscles are tense, tighten then relax each one from toes to scalp

## D. Assist client to develop appropriate strategies based upon his personal strengths and previous experiences

1. Have client describe previous encounters with conflict and how he managed to resolve them
2. Encourage client to evaluate own behavior
   - "Did that work for you?"
   - "How did it help?"
   - "What did you learn from that experience?"
3. Be supportive of functional coping behaviors
   - "Your way of handling this situation two years ago worked well for you then, can you do it now?"
   - Give options; however, the decision-making must be left to the client
4. Mobilize the client into a gradual increase in activity
   - Identify activities that were previously gratifying but have been neglected: personal grooming or dress habits, shopping, hobbies, athletic endeavors, arts and crafts

- Encourage client to include these activities in daily routine for a set time span ("I will play the piano for 30 minutes every afternoon")
- Stress importance of activity in helping one recover from depression; state that depression is immobilizing and that client must make a conscious effort to fight it in order to recover

5. Find outlets that foster feelings of personal achievement and self-esteem
   - Make time for relaxing activities (*e.g.*, dancing, exercising, sewing, woodworking)
   - Find a helper to take over responsibilities from time to time (get a babysitter)
   - Learn to compartmentalize (don't carry problems around with you all the time; enjoy free time)
   - Take longer vacations (not just a few days here and there)
   - Provide opportunities to learn and use stress management techniques (*e.g.*, jogging, yoga; see also Appendix IV)
6. Correct lack of support systems
   - Establish a network of people who understand your situation
   - Decide who is best able to act as a support system (don't expect empathy from people who themselves are overwhelmed with their own problems)
   - Make time to share personal feelings and concern with coworkers (encourage ventilation; frequently people who share the same circumstances are helpful to one another)
   - Maintain a sense of humor
   - Allow tears

## E. Initiate health teaching and referrals as indicated
   - For depression-related problems beyond the scope of nurse generalists, refer to appropriate professional (marriage counselor, psychiatric nurse therapists, psychologist, psychiatrist)

## Bibliography

### General

Bennett A: Recognizing the potential suicide. Geriatrics 22(3):175–181, 1967

Carlson C, Blackburn B: Behavioral Concepts and Nursing Interventions. Philadelphia, JB Lippincott, 1978

Donnelly G: Can self-hypnosis conquer stress? RN 68(1):63–64, 1981

Dorin A: Adolescent sexuality, adolescent depression. Pediatric Nursing 3(4):49–50, 1978

Fontana AF, Dowds BN, Marcus JL et al: Coping with interpersonal conflict through life events and hospitalization. Nerv Ment Dis 162:88–98, 1976

Halton C: Suicide: Assessment and Intervention. New York, Appleton-Century-Crofts, 1977

Lazarus R, Folkman S: An analysis of coping in a middle-aged community sample. J Health Soc Behav 21:219–239, 1980

Martin RA, Poland EY: Learning to Change: A Self-Management Approach to Adjustment. New York, McGraw-Hill, 1980

Maxwell M: Cancer and suicide. Cancer Nursing 3(2):33–38, 1980

Pender N: Health Promotion in Nursing Practice, Part 3. New York, Appleton-Century-Crofts, 1982

Rosenbaum M: Depression: What to do, what to say. Nursing 10(8):64–66, 1980

Selye H: Stress Without Distress. Philadelphia, JB Lippincott, 1974

Tobachnick N, Farberow N: The assessment of self-destructive potentiality. In Farberow NL, Shneidman ES (eds): The Cry for Help, pp 61–77. New York, McGraw-Hill, 1961

## Substance Abuse

Finley B: Counseling the alcoholic client. J Psychiatr Nurs 19(6):32–34, 1981

Kurose K, Anderson T, Bull W et al: A standard care plan for alcoholism. Am J Nurs 81:1001–1006, 1981

Leporatic N, Chychula L: How you can really help the drug-abusing patient. Nursing 12(6):46–49, 1982

Marks VL: Health teaching for recovering alcoholic patients. Am J Nurs 80:2058–2061, 1980 81:755–757, 1981

Richard E, Shepard AC: Giving up smoking: A lesson in loss theory. Am J Nurs 81:755–757, 1981

Wieczorek R, Natapoff J: Alcoholism–drug abuse. In A Conceptual Approach to the Nursing of Children, pp 1239–1251. Philadelphia, JB Lippincott, 1981.

Wilson J: The plight of the elderly alcoholic. Geriatrics 2(2):114–118, 1981

## Pertinent Literature and Organizations

### Books

Kuntzleman CT: The Complete Book of Walking. New York, Simon and Schuster, 1979

Girdano D, Everly G: Controlling Stress and Tension. Englewood Cliffs, NJ, Prentice Hall, 1979

Selye H: Stress Without Distress. Philadelphia, JB Lippincott, 1974

Newman M, Berkowitz B: How to Be Your Own Best Friend. Ballantine Books, New York, 1971

Mace D, Mace V: How to Have a Happy Marriage. Nashville, Festival Books, 1977

Simonton OC, Simonton S, Creighton J: Getting Well Again. New York, St. Martin's Press, 1978

### Organizations

Drug and Alcohol Nursing Association, Inc., Box #371, College Park, Maryland 20740

Alcohol, Drug Abuse and Mental Health Administration, Office of Communications and Public Affairs, 5600 Fishers Lane, Room 6C-15, Rockville, Maryland 20857

National Clearinghouse for Mental Health Information, Public Inquiries Section, 5600 Fishers Lane, Room 11A-21, Rockville, Maryland 20857

American Cancer Society, 777 3rd Avenue, New York, New York 10017

American Heart Association, 7320 Greenville Avenue, Dallas, Texas 75231

American Lung Association, 1740 Broadway, New York, New York 10019

National Interagency Council on Smoking and Health, 291 Broadway, Room 1005, New York, New York, 10007

# Coping, Ineffective Family

*Related to* **Domestic Violence**

## Definition
Ineffective family coping: The state in which a family demonstrates destructive behavior in response to an inability to manage internal or external stressors due to inadequate resources (physical, psychological, cognitive, and/or behavioral).*

## Etiological and Contributing Factors
The following describes those individuals or families who are at high risk for contributing to a family's destructive coping behavior.

| *Parent(s)* | *Child* |
|---|---|
| Single | Of unwanted pregnancy |
| Adolescent | Of undesired sex |
| Abusive | With undesired characteristics |
| Emotionally disturbed | Physically handicapped |
| Alcoholic | Mentally handicapped |
| Drug addict | Hyperactive |
| Terminally ill | Terminally ill |
| Acute disability/accident | Adolescent rebellion |

Situational

| | |
|---|---|
| Separation from nuclear family | Relationship problems |
| Lack of extended family | Marital discord |
| Lack of knowledge | Divorce |
| Economic problems (inflation, unemployment) | Separation |
| | Step-parents |
| Change in family unit (*e.g.*, new child, relative moves in) | Live-in boy/girl friend |
| | Relocation |

Other

History of ineffective relationship with own parents
History of abusive relationships with parents
Unrealistic expectations of child by parent
Unrealistic expectations of self by parent
Unrealistic expectations of parent by child
Unmet psychosocial needs of child by parent
Unmet psychosocial needs of parent by child

*The nursing diagnosis *Ineffective Family Coping* describes a family that has a history of demonstrating destructive behavior. This diagnosis differs from *Alteration in Family Processes,* which describes a family that usually functions constructively but is challenged by a stressor that has altered or may alter its function.

## Defining Characteristics

Neglectful care of the client in regard to basic human needs and/or illness-
related treatments

Neglect of other family members (abandonment, desertion)

Distortion of reality regarding the client's health problem, including prolonged
denial

Unresolved emotions of anger, depression, hostility, and aggression

Verbalization of abuse by spouse

Hyperactivity

Helpless, inactive dependency of client

## Focus Assessment Criteria

Owing to the complexity and variability of this diagnostic category, the nurse must
determine the type and extent of the assessment needed with each family.

1. Individual coping patterns of adult members: refer to assessment criteria for *Ineffective Individual Coping*
2. Family coping patterns: refer to assessment criteria for *Alterations in Family
Processes*
3. Parenting patterns: refer to assessment criteria for *Alterations in Parenting*

## Nursing Goals

Through selected interventions, the nurse will seek to

- Determine etiology(ies) of coping difficulty
- Identify family strengths and weaknesses
- Assess competency of family's coping and problem-solving abilities
- Facilitate communication and mutually supportive behaviors among family
  members
- Maintain therapeutic nursing relationship with family for duration of profession-
  al interaction

## Principles and Rationale for Nursing Care

### General

Refer to *Alterations in Family Processes* for principles of the family

### Spouse abuse

1. Spouse abuse in the form of beatings occur in 1% all families. Fifteen percent of
   all homicides are spouse killings; 50% of the victims are women. Women usually
   kill their husbands with guns and knives, while husbands usually beat wives to
   death.
2. Studies have reported that violence usually results from social conflicts (*e.g.*,
   money, jealousy).
3. Violent episodes
   Escalate in frequency and severity over time
   Require less and less provocation to trigger them
   Include verbal as well as physical abuse
   Are made more brutal by alcohol use
4. Battering has a distinct cycle, as indicated in Figure II–1.
5. Women who attempt to defend themselves during the tension-building phase
   often are successful in preventing the beating, while women who attempt to
   defend themselves during the assaultive phase often sustain a more brutal
   beating.
6. The abuser's ability to control his spouse directly increases his feelings of

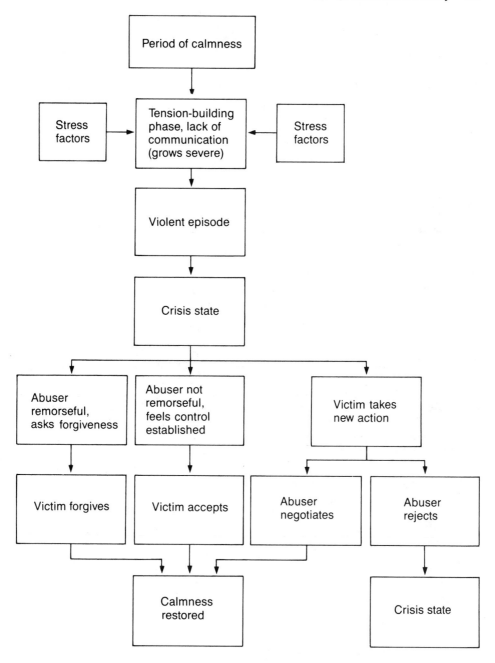

**Figure II–1.** Escalation of violence.

autonomy and esteem. Therefore, the fear of loss (and control) of his spouse directly influences his feelings about himself.

7. Battered women who did not witness abuse as children usually remain in the marriage twice as long as women who witnessed abuse as children.

8. Factors contributing to a battered woman's remaining in the marriage are

    Belief that children need a two-parent family

    Lack of financial support

    Lack of a place to go

    Belief that the abuse will stop

    Fear for her life or her children's lives

    Fear of unknown future

9. Personal characteristics of the abuser

    No dominant ethnic or socioeconomic characteristics

    History of abuse from caregivers or witnessed abuse as a child

    Blames outside factors for everything that goes wrong; blames wife for causing him to get angry

    Denies the violence or minimizes its severity

    Impulsive

    Excessively dependent on and jealous of spouse (spouse is usually the only significant relationship he has)

    Fears losing her, which can contribute to suicide, homicide, depression, or anger

    When not hitting, is often a good loving husband

10. Personal characteristics of the battered woman

    Low self-esteem

    Easily upset

    Belief that she has incited her husband to beat her and is to blame

    Raised in families that restricted emotional expression (*e.g.*, anger, hugging)

    Subscribes to the feminine sex role stereotype

    Frequently marries to escape restrictive, confining family

    Becomes extremely resourceful and self-sufficient in order to survive

    Usually was not abused as a child and did not witness abuse

    Views herself as a victim with no option but to try to appease her spouse

11. The likelihood of a woman seeking and utilizing assistance for abuse is increased if (Sammons)

    She has been in the relationship less than 5 years

    She is employed

    She has friends or relatives who live nearby (within a few miles)

    She discusses the abuse with others

    The abuse is frequent (daily, weekly), severe (requires medical treatment/hospitalization), or increasing in frequency

# Ineffective Family Coping
## Related to Domestic Violence

Domestic violence is defined as any deliberate physical assault by a man on his partner*

## Assessment

### Subjective data
The person relates
> Punishments that inflict physical or emotional harm
> Statements indirectly suggesting abuse
>> "I need help"
>> "I can't go home"
>> "I need a friend"
> A family history of violence

### Objective data
Bruises or welts
> On face, buttocks, thighs, or upper body
> May appear patterned (by rope, belt, or palm)
> May be different colors from different episodes
> Incompatible with normal injuries

Burns
> From cigarettes (on palms, soles, hands, back, or buttocks)
> Oval-shaped (from immersion in scalding liquids)
> From rope (around neck or extremity)

Fractures or dislocations
Lacerations and abrasions
Miscellaneous injuries
> Nausea and abdominal swelling (from being punched in abdomen)
> Bald patches (from having hair pulled)
> Poisoning
> Gunshot wound

---

### Outcome Criteria

The person will
- Discuss the physical assaults
- Identify factors that contribute to violence
- Relate community resources available when help is desired

---

*Even though men can be victims of domestic violence, this diagnosis will focus on violence to women.

## Interventions

The interventions needed to address the complexity and the magnitude of the problems inherent in domestic violence are usually out of the scope of a nurse generalist. The interventions provided here are to assist the nurse who has a short-term interaction with the individual.

A. Assess for the presence of factors that inhibit the battered woman from seeking aid

1. Personal beliefs
    Fear for safety of self or children
    Fear of embarrassment
    Low self-esteem
    Guilt (punishment justified)
    Myths ("It is normal"; "It will stop")
2. Lack of knowledge of
    The severity of the problem
    Community resources
    Legal rights
3. Lack of financial independence
4. Lack of support system

B. Reduce or eliminate factors if possible

1. Personal beliefs
    • Provide an opportunity for the woman to validate abuse and talk about her feelings (if the acutely injured woman is accompanied by her spouse, who is persistent about staying with her, make an attempt to see the woman alone, *e.g.*, tell her you need a urine specimen and accompany her to the bathroom).
    • Provide the woman with options but allow her to make a decision at her own pace
    • Encourage a realistic appraisal of the situation; dispel guilt and myths
        Violence is not normal for most families
        Violence may stop but it usually becomes increasingly worse
        She is not responsible for the violence
2. Lack of knowledge
    • Provide a list of community agencies available to her and her husband (emergency and long-term)
        Hotlines
        Legal services
        Shelters
        Counseling agencies
    • Discuss the availability of the social service department for assistance
3. Lack of financial independence
    • Refer to social service (agency or community)
4. Lack of support system
    • Assess the availability and quality of her support system (relatives, neighbors)
    • Discuss the importance of regular social contacts to provide her with opportunities to share and to prevent isolation

C. Initiate health teaching and referrals if indicated

1. Teach the community about the problem of wife abuse
    Parent-school organiations
    Women's clubs
    Programs for schoolchildren
2. Refer the abuser to the appropriate community service (only refer men who have asked for assistance or admitted their abuse, for revealing the wife's confidential disclosure may trigger more abuse)
3. To secure additional information, contact
    National Clearinghouse on Domestic Violence
    P.O. Box 2309
    Rockville, Maryland 20852

## Bibliography

Allen J, Allen B: Violence in the family. Family and Community Health 4(2):19–33, 1981

Harris C: Women and violence. In Fogel C, Woods N: Health Care of Women: A Nursing Perspective, pp 139–145. St. Louis, CV Mosby, 1981

Fleming J: Stopping Wife Abuse. Garden City, NY, Doubleday & Co, 1979

Friedman MM: Family Nursing: Theory and Assessment. New York, Appleton-Century-Crofts, 1981

Greenland C: Violence and the family. Can J Public Health 71(1):19–24, 1980

Hall JE, Weaver BR: Nursing of Families in Crisis. Philadelphia, JB Lippincott, 1974

Hymovich D, Barnard M (eds): Family Health Care, 2 Vols. New York, McGraw-Hill, 1979

Lieberknecht K: Helping the battered wife. Am J Nurs 78:654–656, 1978

Martin D: Battered Wives. San Francisco, Glide Publications, 1976

Roy M (ed): Battered Women: A Psychosociological Study of Domestic Violence. New York, Van Nostrand Reinhold, 1977

Sammons L: Battered and pregnant. Matern Child Nurs J 6:246–250, 1981

Star B: Battered Women. In McNall LK: Contemporary Obstetric and Gynecologic Nursing, pp 121–135. St. Louis, CV Mosby, 1980

Steinmet S: Violence between family members. Marriage Family Review 1:1–16, 1978

Walker L: The Battered Woman. New York, Harper & Row, 1979

# Diversional Activity Deficit

*Related to* **Monotony of Confinement**

*Related to* **Post-Retirement Inactivity (Change in Life-Style)**

## Definition

Diversional activity deficit: The state in which the individual experiences or is at risk of experiencing an environment that is devoid of stimulation or interest.

## Etiological and Contributing Factors

### Situational

Monotonous environment
Long-term hospitalization or confinement
Lack of motivation, with signs of depression
Loss of ability to perform usual or favorite activities
Frequent lengthy treatments
Excessively long hours of stressful work
No time for leisure activities
Career changes (*e.g.*, teacher to housewife, retirement)
Children leaving home ("empty nest")

## Defining Characteristics

### Statements of boredom

Constant expression of unpleasant thoughts or feelings
Yawning or inattentiveness
Flat facial expression
Body language (shifting of body away from speaker)
Restlessness/fidgeting
Immobile (on bedrest or confined)
Weight loss or gain
Hostility

## Focus Assessment Criteria

### Subjective data

Perception of person's current activity level
   Overly busy (not enough time for relaxing activities)
   Busy but able to find time to do relaxing activities
   Bored, trapped, wishes there was more recreational activity
Past activity patterns (type, frequency)
   Work
   Leisure

Activities the person desires
>>Availability
>>Feasibility

Assistance needed
Support system

## Objective data

Developmental age

Motivation
>>Interested
>>Disinterested

Withdrawn
Hostile

Presence of barriers to recreational activities

>Physical
>>Mobility
>>Altered level of consciousness
>>Fatigue
>>Altered hand mobility

Pain
Sensory deficits (visual, auditory)
Equipment (traction, IVs)

>Psychological/cognitive
>>Lack of motivation
>>Lack of knowledge

Depression
Embarrassment

>Socioeconomic
>>Lack of available support system
>>Previous patterns of inactivity

Financial limitations
Transportation difficulties

## Nursing Goals

Through selected nursing interventions, the nurse will seek to

- Assist the person to recognize that he is bored and help him to work through and resolve his feelings about his current situation
- Help the person become aware of available activities and organizations to find new interests and favorite pastimes, and motivate him to seek out these activities
- Provide appropriate external stimuli to vary monotonous routines and stimulate thought (*e.g.*, music, games, visitors, volunteer services, relaxation therapy)

## Principles and Rationale for Nursing Care

1. All humans need stimulation. In the adult, lack of stimulation results in boredom and depression. In the infant or child, it causes "failure to thrive" and may stunt growth severely.
2. Boredom paralyzes an individual's productivity and causes a feeling of stagnation. It is often a major contributing factor to substance abuse (overeating, drug abuse, alcoholism, and smoking).
3. The bored person has introspective feelings of being oppressed and trapped, which give rise to conscious or unconscious anger or hostility.
4. Being aware that one is bored allows one to redirect activities to increase stimulation.
5. Nurses who understand the concept of boredom and are aware of their own patterns of reacting to and dealing with boredom are better able to deal with boredom in others.
6. Taking responsibility for doing something about a boring situation is a positive means of dispelling boredom.
7. Children in a strange environment need permission to be themselves and to play.
8. Immobilized children especially need play activity to make them feel less victimized.

# Diversional Activity Deficit
## Related to Monotony of Confinement

## Assessment

### Subjective data

The person states
"I'm bored; there's nothing to do"
"I feel trapped"
"I can't do anything"
"I'm tired of being here"
"I have no friends or family"
"I have no one to play with"
"I feel restless"

### Objective data

Inability to move
Confinement to room or building
Limited or no support system
Flat affect or facial expression
Lethargy or sleepiness
Restlessness/fidgeting
Hostility/anger

---

**Outcome Criteria**

The person will
- Recognize feelings of boredom and discuss methods of finding diversional activities
- Relate methods of coping with feelings of anger or depression caused by boredom
- Engage in a diversional activity

---

## Interventions

A. Assess causative factors
   Monotony
   Inability to make decisions concerning his own plan of care (see *Powerlessness*)
   Diminished socialization (see *Social Isolation*)
   Lack of motivation/depression

B. Reduce or eliminate causative factors
   1. Monotony
      a. Vary daily routine when possible (*e.g.*, give bath in the afternoon, so that the person can watch a special show or talk with a visitor who drops in to see him)

   b. Include the individual in planning schedule for daily routine
- Allow the person to make as many decisions as possible
- Make daily routine as normal as possible (*e.g.*, have the person wear street clothes during the day if feasible)

   c. Plan time for visitors
- Encourage person to make a schedule for visitors so everyone does not come at once or at an inconvenient time
- Spend quality time with the person (*i.e.*, not time that is task oriented; rather, sit down and talk)

   d. Be creative; vary the physical environment and daily routine when possible
- Update bulletin boards, change the pictures on the walls, move the furniture within the room
- Maintain a pleasant, cheerful environment (*i.e.*, plenty of light, flowers, conversation pieces)
- Place the person near a window if possible
- Provide reading material, radio, TV, "books on tape" (if person is visually impaired)
- Plan an activity daily to give person something to look forward to and always keep your promises
- Discourage the use of television as the primary source of recreation unless it is highly desired
- Consider using a volunteer to spend time reading to the person or helping with an activity
- Encourage suggestions and new ideas (*e.g.*, "Can you think of things you might like to do?")

2. Lack of motivation

   a. Stimulate motivation by showing interest and encouraging sharing of feelings and experiences
- Discuss the person's likes and dislikes
- Encourage sharing of feelings of present and past experiences
- Spend time with the person purposefully talking about other topics (*e.g.*, "I just got back from the shore. Have you ever gone there?")
- Create a climate of appreciation, expressing enjoyment in having spent time with the person (*e.g.*, "I enjoyed this")

   b. Help the person to work through feelings of anger and grief
- Allow him to ventilate
- Take the time to be a good listener
- See *Anxiety* for additional interventions

   c. Plan appropriate activities for children
- Set an environment with accessible playthings that suit the child's developmental age and see that they are well within reach
- Keep toys in all waiting areas
- Encourage family to bring in child's favorite playthings, including items from nature that will help to keep the real world alive (*e.g.*, goldfish, leaves in fall)

# Diversional Activity Deficit
## Related to Post-Retirement Inactivity (Change in Life-Style)

### Assessment

Subjective data

The person reports
    "There's nothing to do"
    "I'm too old"
    "I feel useless"
    "No one needs me any more"
Recent retirement
Empty nest (children gone from home)
Career terminated
Loss of significant others

Objective data

Flat affect
Lethargy
Anger

---

**Outcome Criteria**

The person will
  • Relate feelings of improved self-esteem and productivity
  • Relate available community services and agencies that can be used for
    hobbies or recreational activities
  • Use his strengths to contribute to himself and others
  • Redirect energy toward interests that are personally fulfilling

---

### Interventions

A. Assess causative factors

    Lack of significant others (loneliness, "empty nest")
    Loss of independence (*e.g.,* inability to drive, climb stairs)
    Fear of being unwanted or not needed
    Retirement
    Career termination or changes

B. Identify factors that promote activity and socialization

  1. Encourage socialization with peers and all age groups (frequently the very young
     and the very old mutually benefit from interaction with each other)
  2. Acquire assistance to increase the person's ability to travel
     • Arrange transportation to activities if necessary

- Acquire aids for safety (*e.g.*, wheelchair for going to shopping center, a walker for ambulating in hallways)

3. Increase the person's feelings of productivity and self-worth
   - Encourage person to use his strengths to help others and himself (*e.g.*, give him tasks to perform in a general project)
   - Acknowledge efforts made by the person (*e.g.*, "You look nice tonight" or "Thank you for helping Mr. Jones with his dinner")
   - Encourage open communication; value the person's opinion ("Mr. Jones, what do you think about———?")
   - Encourage the person to challenge himself with learning a new skill or pursuing a new interest
   - Refer to *Social Isolation* for additional interventions

## C. Initiate referrals if indicated

1. Suggest joining AARP (American Association of Retired Persons)
2. Write the local Health and Welfare Council
3. Provide a list of associations with senior citizen activities

    YMCA
    Churches
    Golden Age Club
    Encore Club
    MORA (Men of Retirement Age)
    Gray Panthers
    Sixty Plus Club
    XYZ Group (Extra Years of Zest)
    Young at Heart Club
    SOS (Senior Outreach Services)
    Leisure Hour Group

## Bibliography

### Books

Burnside I: Psychosocial Nursing Care of the Aged. New York, McGraw-Hill, 1973
Carlson C: Behavioral Concepts in Nursing. Philadelphia, JB Lippincott, 1979
Carneveli D, Patrick M: Nursing Management of the Elderly. Philadelphia, JB Lippincott, 1980
Travelbee M: Interpersonal Aspects of Nursing. Philadelphia, FA Davis, 1971
Weiner M: Working with the Aged. Englewood Cliffs, NJ, Prentice-Hall, 1978

### Articles

Ames B: Art and the dying patient. Am J Nurs 80:1094–1096, 1980
Billings C: Emotional first aid. Am J Nurs 80:2005–2009, 1980
Brooten D: Career guide: To change what needs changing . . . doesn't take Wonder Woman. Nursing 11(3):81–83, 1981
Clark C: Burnout: Assessment and intervention. J Nurs Adm 10(9):39–43, 1980
Kauffman M: Sharing the patient experience. Am J Nurs 78:860–862, 1978
Koch K: Teaching poetry writing to the old and the ill. Milbank Memorial Fund Quarterly/ Health and Society 56(1):113–125, 1978
Kovecses J: Burnout doesn't have to happen. Nursing 10(10):105–110, 1980
Lore A: Supporting the hospitalized elderly person. Am J Nurs 79:496–499, 1979

Martin D: Enjoyable activity for everyone. Geriatric Nursing 2:210–213, 1981
McGoran S: On developing empathy: Teaching students self-awareness. Am J Nurs 78:859–860, 1978
Piche J: Tell a story. Am J Nurs 78:1189–1193, 1978

## Pertinent Organization for the Consumer

American Association of Retired Persons, 1909 K Street NW, Washington, DC

# Family Processes, Alterations In

*Related to* **an Ill Family Member**

## Definition
Alterations in family processes: The state in which a normally supportive family experiences a stressor that challenges its previously effective functioning ability.*

## Etiological and Contributing Factors
Any factor can contribute to an alteration in family processes. Some common factors are listed below.

### Pathophysiological
Illness of family member

|  |  |
|---|---|
| Discomforts related to the illness's symptoms | Time-consuming treatments |
| Change in the family member's ability to function | Disabling treatments |
|  | Expensive treatments |

Trauma

|  |  |
|---|---|
| Surgery | Loss of body part or function |

### Situational
Loss of family member

|  |  |
|---|---|
| Death | Incarceration |
| Going away to school | Desertion |
| Separation | Hospitalization |
| Divorce |  |

Gain of new family member

|  |  |
|---|---|
| Birth | Marriage |
| Adoption | Elderly relative |

Poverty
Disaster
Relocation
Economic crisis

|  |  |
|---|---|
| Unemployment | Financial loss |

Change in family roles

|  |  |
|---|---|
| Working mother | Retirement |

Birth of child with defect
Conflict

|  |  |
|---|---|
| Goal conflicts | Cultural conflict with reality |
| Moral conflict with reality | Personality conflict in family |

*The nursing diagnosis *Alterations in Family Processes* describes a family that usually functions optimally but is challenged by a stressor which has altered or may alter the family's function. This diagnosis differs from *Ineffective Family Coping*, which describes a family that has a pattern of destructive behavior responses.

Breach of trust between members

|                | |            |
|----------------|-|------------|
| Dishonesty     | | Adultery   |

History of psychiatric illness in family
Social deviance by family member (including crime)

## Defining Characteristics

Family system cannot or does not
    Meet physical needs of all its members
    Meet emotional needs of all its members
    Meet spiritual needs of all its members
    Express or accept a wide range of feelings from other family members
    Seek or accept help appropriately
    Adapt constructively to crisis
    Communicate openly and effectively between family members

## Focus Assessment Criteria

1. Character of family
    Age and sex of members
    Ethnic background
    Religious background
        What is the religious affiliation?
        Does the family participate in religious activity?
        How often?
2. Health status
    What is the current health status of each member?
    Are children within the appropriate range for growth and development?
    What is the health history of each family member?

|            |          |
|------------|----------|
| Illness    | Accidents |
| Surgery    | Allergies |

What preventive measures are practiced?
    Immunizations
    Health exams

|          |                |
|----------|----------------|
| Dental   | Eye            |
| General  | Gynecological  |

    Health practices

| | |
|---|---|
| Family planning | Abstention from or moderate use |
| Regular exercise (2–3 times | of alcohol |
| a week for 30 minutes) | Daily dental care |
| Weight control | Self-breast exam (for women) |
| Abstention from smoking | Testes exam (for men) |

Are the parents knowledgeable about

| | |
|---|---|
| First aid? | Adequate exercise? |
| Growth and developmental stages? | Adequate signs of cancer and |
| Sex education? | heart attack? |
| Accident prevention? | Safety (automobile, home, |
| Adequate nutrition? | consumer)? |

Are the children knowledgeable about

| | |
|---|---|
| Safety (street, home, fire)? | Physical fitness? |
| Sexual development? | Dental care? |
| Nutritious foods? | Facts about drugs and alcohol? |

3. Nutritional status
>  Request a diet recall for past 24 hours.
>> What are the family's eating patterns?
>> Which meals are eaten at home?
>  Are members well-nourished?
>  Are meals nutritionally balanced (four food groups)?
>  Is food purchased economically? (In quantity? During seasonal savings?)

4. Sleeping patterns
>  Where do family members sleep?
>  What are their usual sleep hours?

5. Economic status
>  What is the current and past occupational history of each working member?
>  Does the income adequately meet the needs of the members?

6. Activity patterns
>  What are the usual activities of members (adults, children)?
>  What are the leisure activities (individual, group)?
>  Does the family have joint activities? How often?

7. Relationship patterns
>  How well do members relate to each other (adult to adult, adult to children, children to children)?
>  How well do members help each other?
>  How does the family reach decisions?
>  How does the family communicate?
>  Who does each family member interact with socially (peers, clubs, churches)?

8. Role responsibilities
>  What tasks are assigned to each member?
>  Does the family have rules?
>  How are children disciplined? By whom?
>  Are parents consistent in child-rearing practices?

9. Values
>  What are the values of the family? Examples are

| | |
|---|---|
| Frugality | Materialism |
| Productivity | Future orientation |
| Education | Orderliness |
| Health | |

>  Do all family members hold similar values?
>  Are there any value conflicts?

10. Coping patterns
>  Has there been a change in the family recently?
>  How does the family respond to stress or crisis?
>> Constructive responses

| | |
|---|---|
| Relies on each other | Seeks knowledge and resources |
| Shares feelings, thoughts | Utilizes support systems |
| Appraises problem accurately | |

>> Destructive responses

| | |
|---|---|
| Denial | Abandonment |
| Exploitation of members (threats, violence, neglect, scapegoating) | Authoritarianism |

>  Do any adults have a history of ineffective coping patterns (depression, violence, substance abuse)?

What are the strengths of the family?
What are the limitations of the family?

## Principles and Rationale for Nursing Care

### The nature of the human family

1. Each family has a personality to which each member contributes.
2. The family unit may be viewed as a system with
     Interdependency between members
     Interactional patterns that provide structure and support for members
     Boundaries between the family and the environment and between members
       with varying degrees of permeability
3. Families change with time. They must accomplish specific tasks that originate
   from the needs of their members. Table II-2 illustrates the tasks of the family.
4. Each family responds to life challenges in ways that reflect experiences in the
   past and goals for the future.
5. Within a family, members interact in a variety of roles, which result from
   individual and group needs: parent, spouse, child, sibling, friend, teacher, and so
   on.
6. Communication patterns of the family determine the quality of the family life.
7. Each family member influences the family unit. Thus, the health of an
   individual will influence the health of the family.

### Crisis and family coping

1. Stress is defined as the body's response to any demand made on it. Stress has the
   potential for becoming a crisis when the person or family cannot cope constructively.
2. A crisis is an event that occurs when the person's usual problem-solving methods
   are inadequate to resolve the situation.
3. The family in response to crisis will do one of the following: return to pre-crisis
   functioning, develop a more optimal level of functioning (higher level), or develop
   a destructive form of functioning (lower level).
4. The goal of crisis management is to assist the family to return to its pre-crisis
   functioning. If the pre-crisis functioning was destructive (*e.g.*, alcoholism), the
   goal would be to develop a more optimal level of functioning. (See Appendix VI
   for guidelines for crisis management.)
5. Common sources of family stress are (Minuchin)
     External sources of stress that one member is experiencing (*e.g.*, job- or
       school-related)
     External sources of stress that influence the family unit (*e.g.*, finances, relo-
       cation)
     Developmental stressors (*e.g.*, child-bearing, new baby, child-rearing,
       adolescence, new member or members—arrival of older grandparent,
       marriage of single parents—or loss of spouse)
     Situational stressors (*e.g.*, illness, hospitalization, separation)
6. Constructive or functional coping mechanisms of families faced with a stress
   crisis are (Friedman)
     Greater reliance on each other
     Maintenance of a sense of humor
     Increased sharing of feelings and thoughts
     Promotion of each member's individuality

Table II-2.    **Stage-Critical Family Developmental Tasks
Through the Family Life Cycle**

| Stage of the family life cycle | Positions in the family | Stage-critical family developmental tasks |
|---|---|---|
| 1. Married couple | Wife<br>Husband | Establishing a mutually satisfying marriage<br>Adjusting to pregnancy and the promise of parenthood<br>Fitting into the kin network |
| 2. Childbearing | Wife-mother<br>Husband-father<br>Infant daughter or son or both | Having, adjusting to, and encouraging the development of infants<br>Establishing a satisfying home for both parents and infant(s) |
| 3. Preschool-age | Wife-mother<br>Husband-father<br>Daughter-sister<br>Son-brother | Adapting to the critical needs and interests of preschool children in stimulating, growth-promoting ways<br>Coping with energy depletion and lack of privacy as parents |
| 4. School-age | Wife-mother<br>Husband-father<br>Daughter-sister<br>Son-brother | Fitting into the community of school-age families in constructive ways<br>Encouraging children's educational achievement |
| 5. Teenage | Wife-mother<br>Husband-father<br>Daughter-sister<br>Son-brother | Balancing freedom with responsibility as teenagers mature and emancipate themselves<br>Establishing postparental interests and careers as growing parents |
| 6. Launching center | Wife-mother-grandmother<br>Husband-father-grandfather<br>Daughter-sister-aunt<br>Son-brother-uncle | Releasing young adults into work, military service, college, marriage, etc., with appropriate rituals and assistance<br>Maintaining a supportive home base |
| 7. Middle-aged parents | Wife-mother-grandmother<br>Husband-father-grandfather | Rebuilding the marriage relationship<br>Maintaining kin ties with older and younger generations |
| 8. Aging family members | Widow/widower<br>Wife-mother-grandmother<br>Husband-father-grandfather | Coping with bereavement and living alone<br>Closing the family home or adapting it to aging<br>Adjusting to retirement |

(Duvall EM: Marriage and Family Development, 5th ed. Philadelphia, JB Lippincott, 1977; reproduced with permission)

Accurate appraisal of the meaning of the problem

Search for knowledge and resources about the problem

Utilization of support systems

7. Destructive or dysfunctional coping mechanisms of families faced with a stress or crisis are (Friedman)

Denial of the problem

Exploitation of one or more of the family members (threats, violence, neglect, scapegoating)

Separation (hospitalization, institutionalization, divorce, abandonment)

- Authoritarianism (no negotiation)
- Preoccupation of family or members (who lack affection) to appear close

8. Parenthood is a crisis. Some common problems are

Increase in mate arguments

Fatigue resulting from schedule

Disrupted social life

Diminished sexual life

Multiple losses—actual or perceived (*e.g.*, independence, career, beauty, attention)

9. Characteristics of families prone to crisis include

Apathy (resigned to state in life)

Poor self-concept

Low income

Inability to manage money

Unrealistic preferences (materialistic)

Lack of skills and education

Unstable work history

Frequent relocations

History of repeated inadequate problem-solving

Lack of adequate role model

Lack of participation in religious or community activities

Environmental isolation (no telephone, inadequate public transportation)

## Illness in the family

1. Successful coping with illness requires the family to complete the following tasks: acknowledge the problem and seek help, accept the problem and its implications, and adjust as the member begins reconstruction.
2. The family acknowledges the problem by identifying the symptoms and accepting their legitimacy, interpretating symptoms as serious enough to warrant investigation, and gaining knowledge of accessible resources.
3. There exists a time lag between identification of symptoms and help-seeking behavior, which may vary between families, depending upon previous experience with the health care system, cultural interpretations of health and illness, and financial concerns.
4. The family must face the diagnosis and its implications. This task is multidimensional, including

Experiencing the initial shock

Engaging in open communication between members

Minimizing anxiety and its disabling consequences

Preventing prolonged despair, guilt, blame, hostility

Accepting a valid diagnosis

5. The family must adjust, as the member begins to recover, by

Adapting to new ways of living and making appropriate changes as recovery ensues

Fostering independence of recovering member

Accepting residual disability and making any necessary accommodations

Recognizing depression and anxiety in family member during change from "sick role" to "well role"

6. The family must return to normalcy by returning to previous activities as much as is possible and incorporating the recovered member back into the flow of family activities and responsibilities.

# Alterations in Family Processes
## Related to an Ill Family Member*

## Assessment

### Subjective data

Family members verbalize fear, anxiety, and anger

Family members engage in destructive bickering

Individual family members make direct or subtle appeal for help, such as

"I can't cry but feel like I need to" (asking for permission to cry)

"I don't want her to know how worried I am" (asking for help with communication)

"I haven't eaten anything since this morning" (asking for permission to leave the bedside of ill family member)

"I don't know where I went wrong" (requesting reassurance that illness is not his fault)

Family members are unable to make a decision together

One or more family members refuse to assist with ill member's care

### Objective data

Absence of family interaction (both verbally and nonverbally)

Tendency of family members to interfere with necessary nursing and medical interventions

Sudden outburst of emotions without apparent cause and/or emotional liability of family members

*This specific diagnosis applies to most illnesses, but not to terminal illness. See *Grieving Related to Anticipated Loss* for specific interventions.

**Outcome Criteria**

The person (family members) will
• Frequently verbalize feelings to professional nurse and each other
• Participate in care of ill family member
• Facilitate return of ill family member from sick role to well role
• Maintain functional system of mutual support for each member
• Seek appropriate external resources when needed

## Interventions

A. Assess causative and contributing factors
 1. Illness-related factors
   Sudden, unexpected nature of illness
   Burdensome problems of a chronic nature
   Potentially disabling nature of illness
   Symptoms creating disfiguring change in physical appearance
   Social stigma associated with illness
   Financial burden
 2. Factors related to behavior of ill family member
   Refuses to cooperate with necessary interventions
   Engages in socially deviant behavior associated with illness: suicide attempts, violence, substance abuse
   Isolates self from family
   Acts out or is verbally abusive to health professionals and family members
 3. Factors related to the family as a whole
   Presence of unresolved guilt, blame, hostility, jealousy
   Inability to problem-solve adequately
   Ineffective patterns of communication among members
 4. Factors related to illness in family
   Absence of caring
   Lack of family members available for support
 5. Factors related to health care environment
   Intervening professionals lack expertise in crisis intervention, counseling, or basic communication skills
   Not enough health professionals can spend time with the family
   Lack of continuity of care
   Lack of physical facilities in institution to ensure privacy or individualized care

B. Acknowledge your feelings about the family and their situation
 • Attempt to resolve these feelings
   Pity
   Identifying with own family
   Blaming ill person and/or family for circumstances
   Judgmental attitude toward family
   Practicing punishing behavior (*e.g.*, ignoring people involved)
 • Gain experience in crisis intervention and communication skills
 • Approach the family with warmth, respect, and support

- Avoid vague and confusing advice and clichés such as "Take it easy, everything will be OK"
- Reflect family emotions to confirm these feelings ("This is very painful for you"; "You are very frightened")
- Keep family members abreast of changes in ill member's condition when appropriate

C. Create a private and supportive hospital environment for family
- Keep client's door closed if possible
- Provide family members with a meeting place alternative to client's room
- Make sure family members are oriented to visiting hours, bathrooms, vending machines, cafeteria, etc.
- If possible, provide pillows/blankets for family members spending the night

D. Facilitate family strengths
- Acknowledge these strengths to family when appropriate
  "I can tell you are a very close family"
  "You know just how to get your mother to eat"
  "Your brother means a great deal to you"
- Involve family members in care of ill member when possible (feeding, bathing, dressing, ambulating)
- Include family members in patient care conferences when appropriate
- Encourage family to acquire substitutes to care for the ill person, to provide the family with time away

E. Intervene when family weaknesses dominate
- Facilitate communication
- Encourage verbalization of guilt, anger, blame, and hostility and subsequent recognition of own feelings in family members
- Enlist help of other professionals when problems extend beyond realm of nursing (*e.g.*, social worker, clinical psychologist, nurse therapist, clinical specialist, psychiatrist, child care specialist)

F. Facilitate understanding, in other family members, of how ill member feels
- Discuss stresses of hospitalization
- Describe implications of "sick role" and how it will return to "well role"
- Aid family members to change their expectations of the ill member in a realistic manner

G. Assist family with appraisal of the situation
- What is at stake? Encourage family to have a realistic perspective by providing accurate information and answers to questions
- What are the choices? Assist family to reorganize roles at home and set priorities to maintain family integrity and reduce stress
- Where is there help? Direct family to community agencies, home health care organizations, and sources of financial assistance as needed (see *Impaired Home Maintenance Management* for additional interventions)

H. Provide the family with anticipatory guidance as illness continues
- Inform parents of the effects of prolonged hospitalization on children (appropriate to developmental age)

- Prepare family members for signs of depression, anxiety, and dependency, which are a natural part of the illness experience
- If the ill family member is an elderly parent undergoing surgery, inform the children that the patient may be confused or disoriented for a limited period of time following surgery

## I. Initiate health teaching and referrals as necessary

- Include family members in group education sessions
- Refer families to lay support and self-help groups.
  Al-Anon
  Syn-Anon
  Alcoholics Anonymous
  Sharing and Caring (American Hospital Association)
  Ostomy Association
  Reach for Recovery
  Lupus Foundation of America
  Arthritis Foundation
  National Multiple Sclerosis Society
  American Cancer Society
  American Heart Association
  American Diabetes Association
  American Lung Association

## Bibliography

Burr B, Good BJ, Good MD: The impact of illness on the family. In Taylor RB (ed): Family Medicine: Principles and Practice, pp 221–232. New York, Springer-Verlag, 1978

Christensen KE: Family epidemiology: An approach to assessment and intervention. In Hymovich DP, Barnard MV (eds): Family Health Care, 2nd ed, vol 1, pp 17–30. New York, McGraw-Hill, 1979

Duvall EM: Marriage and Family Development, 5th ed. Philadelphia, JB Lippincott, 1977

Friedman M: Family Nursing: Theory and Assessment. New York, Appleton-Century-Crofts, 1981

Geary MC: Supporting family coping. Supervisor Nurse 10(3):57–59, 1979

Giacquinta B: Helping families face the crisis of cancer. Am J Nurs 77:1585–1588, 1977

Hymovich DP, Barnard MV (eds): Family Health Care, 2nd ed. New York, McGraw-Hill, 1979

Johnson SH: High-Risk Parenting. Philadelphia, JB Lippincott, 1979

Miller S, Winstead-Fry P: Family Systems Theory in Nursing Practice, Reston Publishing, 1982

Minuchin A: Families and Family Therapy. Cambridge, MA, Harvard University Press, 1974

# Fear

## Definition

Fear: The state in which the individual experiences a painfully uneasy feeling that is related to an identifiable source (stimulus) which the person perceives as dangerous. The responses to the perceived threat may be adaptive or maladaptive.*

## Etiological and Contributing Factors

Fear can occur as a response to a variety of health problems, situations, or conflicts. Some common sources are indicated below.

### Pathophysiological

Loss of body part
Loss of body function
Disabling illness

Long-term disability
Terminal disease

### Situational

Hospitalization
Influences of others
Surgery and its outcome
Anesthesia
Treatments
Invasive procedures
Pain

New environment
New people
Lack of knowledge
Change or loss of significant
 other
Divorce
Success
Failure

### Maturational

Children: Age-related fears (dark, strangers), influence of others
Adolescent: school adjustments, social and intellectual competitiveness, independence, authorities
Adult: marriage, pregnancy, parenthood
Elderly: Retirement, relinquishing roles, functional losses

## Defining Characteristics

Feeling of physiological or emotional disruption related to an identifiable source
Feeling of loss of control (actual or perceived)

### Associated defining characteristics

Increased pulse and respiratory rate
Increased blood pressure

*Fear differs from anxiety in that the person can identify the threat, while in anxiety the threat cannot be accurately identified.

Diaphoresis
Voice tremors/voice pitch changes
Increased questioning/verbalization

## Focus Assessment Criteria

### Subjective data

Onset
   Have the person tell you his "story" about his fearfulness
Manner of communication
   How does the person organize his ideas?
   Are his thoughts clear, coherent, logical, confused, or forgetful?
   Can he concentrate, or is he preoccupied with one thought?
Control behaviors
   Does fear interfere with life-style?
   Are control behaviors expressed outwardly or are they expressed inwardly
      through bodily symptoms?
   Can the person use several control behaviors or only one persistent behavior?
Perception and judgment
   Is fear still present after stressor is eliminated?
   Do only major events lead to fearfulness, or do minor events trigger fears?
   Can the person comprehend the present and focus on his actions, or is he
      overwhelmed by future anticipations?
   Is the fear a response to a present stimulus, or is it distorted by influences in the
      past?
Emotional state
   Is emotional feeling tone appropriate or inappropriate to the situation?
   Do facial expressions, voice tone, and body posture correspond to the intensity of
      the person's verbal expression of fear?
Thought content
   What understanding does the person have about his fear?
   Do the coping mechanisms help him solve problems (functional) or do they con-
      tribute to further problems (maladaptive)?
   Do misperceptions interfere with reality testing?
Relatedness to others
   Does the person's intensity of fear cause movement away from others?
   What or who are his support systems?
   Can he accept support from the nurse or others?
Children
   Is the child's fear normal and expected for his age group?
   What actions of the parents contribute to the fear?
   What actions of the parents reduce the fear?

### Objective data

Body posture
   Relaxed
   Tense
Verbal expression
   Does verbal expression consist of constructive talking or destructive arguing?
   Does the person have rapid speech? Speechlessness? Excessively loud or quiet
      tone of voice?

Physical manifestations
Assess for the presence of

*Musculoskeletal*

Muscle tightness
Fatigue

*Cardiovascular*

Palpitations
Rapid pulse
Increased blood pressure

*Respiratory*

Shortness of breath
Increase rate

*Gastrointestinal*

Anorexia
Nausea/vomiting
Diarrhea

*Genitournary*

Urinary frequency

*Skin*

Flush/Pallor
Sweating
Paresthesia

*CNS/perceptual*

Syncope
Insomnia
Lack of concentration
Irritability
Absentmindedness
Nightmares

## Nursing Goals

Through selected interventions the nurse will seek to assist the individual to
 • Identify effective and ineffective coping behaviors
 • Promote adaptive coping styles
 • Maintain psychological equilibrium

## Principles and Rationale for Nursing Care

### General

1. Psychological defense mechanisms are distinctly individual and can be adaptive or maladaptive.
2. Fear differs from anxiety in that fear is the feeling aroused when there is an accurate perception of an external threat; anxiety is a feeling aroused when the perception is of an imagined danger in response to internal beliefs.
3. Both fear and anxiety lead to disequilibrium.
4. Activity uses energy and dissipates the physical reaction to fear.
5. Anger may be an adaptive response to certain fears.
6. Safety feelings increase when a person identifies with another person who has successfully dealt with a similar fearful situation.
7. A sense of adequacy in confronting danger reduces fear. Fear disguises itself. The expressed fear may be a substitute for other fears that are not socially acceptable. Awareness of factors that cause intensification of fears enhances controls and prevents heightened feelings. Fear is reduced when the safe reality of a situation is confronted.
8. Fear can become anxiety, *e.g.*, fear becomes internalized and serves to disorganize instead of becoming adaptive.
9. Chronic physical reactions to stressors lead to susceptibility and chronic disease.
10. Physiological responses are manifested throughout the body primarily from the hypothalmus's stimulation of the autonomic and endocrine systems.

11. Individuals interpret the degree of danger from a threatening stimulus. The physiological and psychological systems react with equal intensity to the perceived threat ($\uparrow$ BP, $\uparrow$ heart rate, $\uparrow$ respiratory rate).
12. Fear is adaptive and is a healthy response to danger.

## Children

1. A child learns fear from unpleasant direct experiences with people and things or from adults or other children who communicate their fears to him.
2. Adults increase fears in children when they utilize fear to encourage obedience (*e.g.,* "If you don't wear your boots you'll get sick and have to get a needle at the hospital"; "If you are bad that policeman will get you and put you in jail")
3. Preschool children (2 to 5 years) with their egocentric thinking and their limited ability for conceptual thinking experience distress when they witness another person hurting. For example, a 3-year-old child who witnesses another child receive an injection may cry as violently as the child who actually received the injection.
4. Fears throughout childhood follow a developmental sequence.

*Birth–2 years*

Fears evolve from physical stimuli, *e.g.*
    Loud noises (thunder)
    Strange people
    Strange places
    Sudden movements
    Flashes of light

*2–5 years*

Fears evolve from real and imagined situations, *e.g.*
    Injury or mutilation
    Ghosts, devils, monsters
    Dark
    Bathtub and toilet drains

*6 years*

Fears are numerous, *e.g.*
    Loud noises
    Ghosts, devils, monsters
    Large animals
    Imagined unseen persons (outside window, under bed)
    Fire, thunder, lightning, water
    Being lost
    Being hurt
    Something will happen to parents

*7 years*

Fears are still numerous, *e.g.*
    Dark, cellar, attic
    Burglars
    Imagined unseen persons (outside window, under bed)
    Failure (with friends; in school, sports)

Not being liked
Various subjects presented by radio or on TV

*8–9 years*

Fears and worries are fewer, *e.g.*
Things that cannot be explained or proved nonexistent (death, pain)
Poor achievement (grades, being late)

*10 years*

Fears are many but child worries less, *e.g.*
Animals (snakes, wild animals)
High places
Fires, ghosts
Dark, blood
Poor achievement (grades, sports)

*11 years*

This is the most worried and fearful stage, *e.g.*
Strong fear of being alone
Worry about school, money, parent's welfare, illness
Rejection by opposite sex
Strange animals
Pain, disease, and loss of mother (by girls)

*12 years*

This is a less fearful time, *e.g.*
The dark
Noises at night
Intruders

---

**Outcome Criteria**

The adult will
- Experience increase in psychological and physiological comfort
- Differentiate real from imagined situations
- Recognize effective and ineffective coping patterns
- Identify his own coping responses

The child will
- Discuss his fears
- Experience an increase in psychological comfort

---

## Interventions

The nursing interventions for the diagnosis *Fear* represent interventions for any individual with fear regardless of the etiological or contributing factors.

### A. Assess possible contributing factors

1. Perception of threatening stimulus (realistic)
   Unfamiliar environment (new home, admission, new people)
   Intrusion on personal space

Life-style change (promotion, marriage, retirement)
Biological change (dysfunction, pregnancy)
Self-esteem threat (abandonment, rejection)
2. Distorted perceptions of dangerous stimulus
3. Age-related fears

B. Reduce or eliminate contributing factors
1. Unfamiliar environment
   - Orient to environment using simple explanations
   - Speak slowly and calmly
   - Avoid surprises and painful stimulus
   - Use soft lights and music
   - Remove threatening stimulus
   - Plan one-day-at-a-time familiar routine
   - Encourage gradual mastery of a situation
   - Provide transitional object with symbolic safeness (security blanket, religious medals)
2. Intrusion on personal space
   - Allow personal space
   - Move person away from stimulus
   - Remain with him until fear subsides (listen, use silence)
   - Later, establish frequent and consistent contacts; utilize family members and significant others to stay with him
   - Use touch as tolerated (sometimes holding person firmly will help him maintain control)
3. Threat to self-esteem
   - Support preferred coping style when adaptive mechanisms are used (some prefer details; others, general explanations)
   - Initially, decrease the person's number of choices
   - Use simple direct statements (avoid detail)
   - Give direct suggestion to manage everyday events
   - Encourage expression of feelings (helplessness, anger)
   - Give feedback about his expressed feelings (support realistic assessments)
   - Refocus interaction on areas of capability rather than dysfunction
   - Encourage normal coping mechanisms
   - Encourage sharing common problems with others
   - Give feedback of effect his behavior has on others
   - Encourage him to face the fear
4. Distorted perceptions
   - Encourage responses that reflect reality
   - Ask straightforward questions ("Do you feel pain?" "Does my asking you about your feelings make you uncomfortable?")
   - Provide information to reduce distortions ("No, I will not harm you!" "That was only a shadow and not the boogey man")
   - Encourage specifics and discourage generalizations; have him give details, not vague general assumptions ("Who are you referring to when you say 'they' are trying to kill you?")
   - Explore superficial interactions
     a. Examine the person's reason for avoiding feelings
     b. Allow him to know that it is OK to feel
     c. Share your reaction to the event ("I can see why you're upset; if that happened to me I would have felt like screaming")

- Provide an emotionally nonthreatening atmosphere
  a. Provide situations that are predictable
  b. Allow for consistency in personnel to enhance comfort and familiarity
  c. Announce changes in the environment
5. Age-related fears (Refer to Principles and Rationale for Nursing Care)
  - Provide child with opportunities to express his fears and to learn healthy outlets for anger or sadness, *e.g.*, play therapy (see Appendix III for Guidelines for Play Therapy)
  - Acknowledge illness, death, pain as real and refrain from protecting children from the reality of its existence; encourage open, honest sharing
  - Accept the child's fear and provide him with an explanation, if possible, or some form of control; share with child that these fears are okay
    a. Fear of imaginary animals, intruders ("I don't see a lion in your room, but I will leave the light on for you, and if you need me again, please call")
    b. Fear of parent being late (establish a contingency plan, *e.g.*, "If you come home from school and Mommy is not here, go to Mrs. S. next door")
    c. Fear of vanishing down a toilet or bathtub drain
       Wait until child is out of tub before releasing drain
       Wait until child is off the toilet before flushing
       Leave toys in bathtub and demonstrate how they don't go down the drain
    d. Fear of dogs, cats
       Allow child to watch a child and a dog playing from a distance
       Don't force child to touch the animal
    e. Fear of death
       See Principles and Rationale of Nursing Care for *Grieving*
    f. Fear of pain
       See *Alterations in Comfort: Pain in Children*
  - Discuss with parents the normalcy of fears in children; explain the necessity of acceptance and the negative outcomes of punishment or of forcing the child to overcome the fear

## C. Initiate health teaching and referrals as indicated

1. When intensity of feelings has decreased, bring behavioral cues into the person's awareness
   - Teach signs that indicate increased fear ("Your face flushes and you clench your fists when we discuss your discharge")
   - Indicate adaptiveness of behavior
2. Explain how expressed fear of one thing may be hidden fear of something else
3. Teach how to problem-solve
   What is the problem?
   Who or what is responsible for the problem?
   What are the options?
   What are advantages and disadvantages of each option?
4. Teach ways for enhancing control
   - Include the person in the treatment process ("Please raise your hand if the procedure causes pain")
   - Share test results when appropriate
     a. Inform ahead of time about tests (time interval depends on ability to cope)

   b. Identify activities that rechannel emotional energy to diffuse intensity
   c. Use nightlight or flashlight to diffuse fear (child with fear of dark can be given a flashlight to use ad lib)
   d. Before tests or surgery, prepare patient as to what to expect, especially sensations, and define this role and how to participate in the role (*e.g.*, breathing exercises postoperatively may take mind off of fears and dissipate physical reaction)

5. Recommend or instruct concerning methods that increase comfort or relaxation (see Appendix IV for Guidelines)·
   Progressive relaxation technique
   Reading, music, breathing exercises
   Desensitization, self-coaching
   Thought stopping, guided fantasy
   Yoga, hypnosis, assertiveness training

6. Participate in community functions to teach parents age-related fears and constructive interventions, *e.g.*, parent-school organizations, newsletters, civic groups

## Bibliography

Clark C: Assertive Skills For Nurses, pp. 195–214. Wakefield, MA, Contemporary Publications, 1978

Fann W, Karacan I, Porkosny A et al: Phenomenology and Treatment of Anxiety. New York, Jamaica, NY, Spectrum Publications, 1979

"How one hospital allays children's fears of surgery. JAMA 242(23):2526, 1979

Knowles R: Control your thoughts. Am J Nurs 81:353, 1981

Lincoln L: Effects of illness and procedures on body image in adolescents. Matern Child Nurs 7:55–60, 1978

Olsen L: Intervention in pathological cycle of anxiety. Journal of Psychosocial Nursing and Mental Health Service 12(2):21–25, 1974

Rearick T, Hecht J, Schmidt E et al: Gaining insight into fear. Nursing 8(4):46–51, 1978

Smitherman C: Nursing Actions For Health Promotion, pp. 108–259. Philadelphia, FA Davis, 1981

Sutterly Doris: Stress and health: A survey of self-regulation modalities. Topics in Clinical Nursing, 1(2):1–20, 1979

Weil H: The Nightmares of Childhood. American Baby 42(1):60–61, 1980

Whaley L, Wong D: Nursing Care of Infants and Children, pp. 952–955, 429–777. St Louis, CV Mosby, 1979

# Fluid Volume Deficit

*Related to* **Decreased Fluid Intake**

*Related to* **Abnormal Fluid Loss**

## Definition

Fluid volume deficit: The state in which the individual experiences or is at risk of experiencing vascular, cellular, or intracellular dehydration.

## Etiological and Contributing Factors

### Pathophysiological

Excessive urinary output
    Uncontrolled diabetes
    Diabetes insipidus (inappropriate antidiuretic hormone)
Burns
Fever or increased metabolic rate
Overzealous dialysis (peritoneal dialysis, hemodialysis)
Shock

        Neurogenic        Hypovolemic
        Cardiogenic     Anaphylactic
        Septic

Fluid shift to extravascular space
    Ascites
    Pleural effusion
Infection
Abnormal drainage
    Wound
    Excessive menses
    Other
Serum electrolyte imbalance
Acid–base imbalance (acidosis–alkalosis)
Eclampsia (albumin loss)
Peritonitis
Diarrhea

### Situational

Vomiting or nasogastric suctioning
Excessive use of
    Laxatives or enemas
    Diuretics or alcohol
Imposed fluid restrictions
    Preoperative period
    Intra-operative period
    Postoperative period

Decreased motivation to drink liquids
    Depression
    Fatigue
Blood loss
    Overt (visible)
    Occult (hidden)
Dietary problems
    Fad diets/fasting
    Anorexia
    High solute tube feedings
Difficulty swallowing or feeding self
    Oral pain
    Fatigue
Climate exposure
    Extreme heat/sun
    Excessive dryness
Hyperpnea
Extreme exercise effort/diaphoresis

### Maturational

Infant/child: Decreased fluid reserve, decreased ability to concentrate urine
Elderly: Decreased fluid reserve, decreased sensation of thirst

## Defining Characteristics

Decreased urine output or excessive urine output
Concentrated urine or urinary frequency
Decreased fluid intake
Output greater than intake
Weight loss (rapid)
Decreased venous filling
Hemoconcentration
Increased serum sodium
Increased pulse rate
Decreased pulse volume/pressure
Increased body temperature
Decreased skin turgor
Dry skin/mucous membranes
Thirst/nausea/anorexia
Weakness/lethargy/confusion

## Focus Assessment Criteria

### Subjective data

1. History of symptoms
    The person complains of

        Nausea/vomiting/anorexia        Thirst
        Weight loss        Polyuria/dysuria
        Diarrhea/loose stools/black        Fever/diaphoresis
            stools/bloody stools
      Onset/duration
      Location

Description
Frequency
Precipitated by what?
Relieved by what?
Aggravated by what?
2. History of contributing and causative factors
Diabetes mellitus (diagnosed, family history)
Cardiac disease
Renal disease
Blood loss
Gastrointestinal disorders or surgery
Alcohol use
Medications
    Laxatives/enemas               Side-effects that are GI irritants
    Diuretics                       (antibiotics)
Allergies (food, milk)
Extreme heat/humidity
Extreme exercise effort accompanied by sweating
Depression
Pain
3. Current drug therapy
    Type, dosage               Frequency (last dose taken
                             when?)

## Objective data

1. Assess for presence of contributing factors
Abnormal or excessive fluid loss
    Liquid stools             Abnormal or excessive drainage
    Vomiting or gastric suction   (e.g., fistulas, drains)
    Diuresis or polyuria       Loss of skin surfaces (e.g., burns)
    Diaphoresis              Fever
Decreased fluid intake related to
    Order of NPO            Depression/disorientation
    Fatigue                 Nausea or anorexia
    Decreased level of consciousness   Physical limitations (e.g., unable
                           to hold glass)

2. Assess for signs of dehydration
Vital signs
    Pulse (increased)
    Respirations (increased)
    Blood pressure (decreased)
Skin
    Mucosa (lips, gums) (dry)
    Tongue (furrowed/dry)
    Turgor (decreased)
    Color (pale or flushed)
    Moisture (dry or diaphoretic)
    Fontanelles of infants (depressed)
    Eyeballs (sunken)
Urine output
    Amount (varied; very large or minimal amount)

Color (amber; very dark or very light)
Specific gravity (increased or decreased)
Intake vs. output (less intake than output)
Weight (loss)
Neck veins (collapsed when lying flat)
3. Diagnostic studies
Hemoglobin/hematocrit
Electrolytes
Blood urea nitrogen (BUN)
Urinalysis
Central venous pressure (CVP)
Pulmonary artery pressure (PAP)
Creatinine
Pulmonary wedge pressure (PWP)

## Nursing Goals

Through selected nursing interventions, the nurse will seek to
 • Prevent abnormal fluid loss
 • Promote adequate fluid replacement (intake)
 • Maintain fluid and electrolyte balance

## Principles and Rationale for Nursing Care

General
1. Fluid intake is primarily regulated by the sensation of thirst. Fluid output is primarily regulated by the kidneys' ability to concentrate urine.
2. The average daily fluid loss for the normal individual is urine, 1500 ml; stool, 200 ml; and perspiration/respiration ("insensible water loss"), 300 ml.
3. The body gains water in two ways: from food and drink absorbed through the gastrointestinal tract (this is the major source) and from the cellular oxidation of nutrients.
4. Excreted body fluids pull electrolytes with them, resulting in electrolyte loss:
Urine ($K^+Na^+$)
Gastric juices ($K^+$, $H^+$)
Perspiration ($Na^+$ $Cl^-$)
Stool ($K^+$)
5. Normal serum electrolytes are

| Cations | Sodium (137–148 mEq/liter) |
|---|---|
| (Positive ions) | Potassium (3.5–5 mEq/liter) |
| | Calcium (8.5–10.5 mg/dl) |
| | Magnesium (1.5–2.5 mEq/liter) |
| Anions | Chloride (95–106 mEq/liter) |
| (Negative ions) | Bicarbonate (21–28 mEq/liter) |
| | Protein (6.0–8.5 gm/dl) |
| | Organic acids (2.4–4.5 mg/dl) |
| | Phosphate (2.5–4.8 mg/dl) |
| | Sulfate (minuscule) |

6. A balance of water and sodium is necessary for normal body fluid levels. Water provides 90% to 93% of the volume of body fluids, while sodium provides 90% to 95% of the solute of extracellular fluid.
7. Excessive fluid loss can be expected during
Fever or increased metabolic rate

Extreme exercise or diaphoresis
Climate extremes (heat/dryness)
Excessive vomiting or diarrhea
Burns, tissue insult, fistulas

8. Blood is the cooling fluid of the body. Dehydration (and resulting decrease in blood volume) causes an increased body temperature, pulse, respirations.

9. Water can normally be found in three spaces of the body: within the blood vessels and within the interstitial spaces (extracellular) and within the cell itself (intracellular).

10. Dehydration may occur within the vascular tree, while water within the interstitial spaces may be excessive (edema). Abnormal shifts between body compartments may cause fluid excess or deficit.

11. The specific gravity of the urine reflects the kidney's ability to concentrate urine; the range of urine specific gravity varies with the state of hydration and the solids to be excreted. (Specific gravity is elevated when dehydration is present, signifying concentrated urine.) Values are

Normal: 1.010–1.025
Concentrated: >1.025
Diluted: <1.010

12. Serum electrolytes serve four major functions

Assisting in regulating fluid balance
Assisting in enzyme reactions
Participating in acid-base regulation to maintain normal pH
Playing an essential role in nervous and muscular activity

13. A normal balance of cations (positive ions), anions (negative ions), and buffers are necessary for normal blood pH. (Normal arterial pH is 7.37–7.45.) *A very slight variation in these normals can cause death.*

14. Potassium is the major cation of the intracellular fluid-influencing acid–base balance and cellular hydration. High or low potassium interferes with the conduction of nerve impulses through skeletal, smooth, and cardiac muscle. *This may be manifested by cardiac and muscular irritability or flaccidity, which can cause life-threatening arrhythmias.*

15. Conditions that increase the incidence of hypokalemia (low potassium) are

Diuretic therapy ($K^+$ loss in urine)
Ascites ($K^+$ loss to accumulation of fluid in the abdomen)
Poor dietary habits (poor $K^+$ intake)
Extreme diaphoresis ($Na^+$ and $K^+$ loss)
Prolonged diarrhea/malabsorption syndrome ($K^+$ loss via stool)
Prolonged gastric suction ($K^+$ loss from gastric contents)
Surgery/tissue trauma (Cellular loss of $K^+$)

16. Persons undergoing lengthy abdominal or chest surgery lose large amounts of fluid through direct evaporation from the open surgical cavity to the air in the operating room. (This additional insensible loss may account for immediate postoperative fluid deficit.)

## Nutrition

1. The average adult requires 2,000 ml–3,000 ml of fluid intake per day.

2. To correctly assess a person's potential for fluid imbalance, close examination of the previous 24 to 72 hours' intake and output is necessary. (In renal or cardiac disease, it may be necessary to consider intake and output for the previous 5 to 7 days, as well as body weight.)

3. People at high risk for fluid imbalance include

People on medication for fluid retention, high blood pressure, seizures, or "anxiety" (tranquilizers)

People who suffer from diabetes, cardiac disease, excessive alcohol intake, malnourishment, obesity, or GI distress

Adults over 60, and children under 6

People who are confused, depressed, comatose, or lethargic (no sensation of thirst)

4. In determining the 24-hour intake requirement for an infant or child, both caloric and fluid intake should be measured. The following calculations can be utilized:

*Caloric Intake*

For a child up to 10 kg of body weight: 100 cal/kg
For a child between 11 kg and 20 kg: 1000 cal plus 50 cal/kg for each kg above 20

*Fluid Intake (for maintenance)*

Approximately 120 ml per 100 cal of metabolism
*Abnormal fluid loss must be replaced in addition to the above.*

5. With inadequate caloric intake, metabolism of the body's stores of fat and muscle may provide significant increase in total body water, resulting in weight gain that may hide malnutrition (*e.g.*, the "bloating" of terminal malnutrition).

6. Adequate protein intake is necessary to maintain normal osmotic pressures. Foods that have a high protein content are meats, fish, fowl, soybeans, eggs, legumes, and cheese.

7. Large amounts of sugar, alcohol, and caffeine act as diuretics that increase urine production and may cause dehydration.

8. People receiving tube feedings are at high risk for dehydration, because the high solute concentration of the tube feeding may cause diarrhea and diuresis. *Tube feedings must be supplemented with specified amounts of water to maintain adequate hydration.*

9. A high intake of sodium causes increased retention of water.

Foods with high sodium content include salted snacks, bacon, cheddar cheese, pickles, soy sauce, processed luncheon meats, MSG (monosodium glutamate), canned vegetables, catsup, and mustard. Some over-the-counter drugs such as bicarbonate of soda, antacids, cough suppressants, and many oral hygiene products also have a high sodium content.

Foods with moderate sodium content include eggs, milk, hamburger, canned corn, and canned tomato juice.

Foods with low sodium content include fruits, chicken, liver, fresh vegetables, unsalted bread, and unsalted crackers.

10. Foods with a high potassium content include bananas, dates, raisins, oranges, tomatoes, puffed wheat cereal, potatoes, liver, Pepsi, and Gatorade.

## Edema

1. People with cardiac pump failure are at high risk for both vascular and tissue fluid excess (*i.e.*, pulmonary and peripheral edema). Acute pulmonary edema should be considered a medical emergency.

2. The most frequent vascular cause of tissue edema is increased venous pressure, which causes increased capillary blood pressure.

3. Edema inhibits blood flow to the tissue, resulting in poor cellular nutrition and increased susceptibility to injury.
4. Edema is often seen as a result of

Venous obstruction (pressure point, such as sitting with legs crossed) and resulting venous pooling

Heart failure (decreased cardiac output) resulting in backup of blood in the heart, lungs, and vessels

Lymphatic obstruction (*e.g.*, after a lymph node disection)

Trauma (tissue injury that releases histamines, causing vasodilation and increased permeability and movement of fluid); examples are burns, sprains, fractures

Hypoxia of the cell

Vitamin C deficiency or extreme malnutrition

Prolonged steroid therapy

# Fluid Volume Deficit
## Related to Decreased Fluid Intake

### Assessment

### Subjective data

The person reports

Nausea and vomiting

Altered ability to drink or swallow (sore throat, dysphagia)

Upper limb limitations

Decreased motivation to obtain fluids (weakness, depression, fatigue)

### Objective data

Decreased urine output

Increased specific gravity of urine

Dry skin or dry mucous membranes

Decreased lacrimal secretions and decreased saliva

Poor skin turgor

Furrowed tongue

---

**Outcome Criteria**

The person will

- Increase intake of fluids to a minimum of 2,000 ml (unless contraindicated)
- Relate the need for increased fluid intake during stress or heat
- Maintain a urine specific gravity within a normal range

---

**Interventions**

A. Assess causative factors

Inability to feed self
Dislike of available liquids
Sore throat
Extreme fatigue or weakness
Lack of knowledge (of the need for increased fluid intake)

B. Reduce or eliminate causative factors

1. Inability to feed self
See *Self-Care Deficit Related to Inability to Feed Self*
2. Dislike of available liquids
   - Assess likes and dislikes; provide favorite fluids within dietary restrictions
   - Plan an intake goal for each shift (*e.g.*, 1000 ml during day; 800 ml during evening; 300 ml at night)
   - For children offer
        a. Appealing forms of fluids (popsicles, frozen juice bars, snow cones, water, milk, Jell-O with vegetable coloring added; let child help make it)
        b. Unusual containers (colorful cups, straws, syringe to squirt liquid into child's mouth)
        c. A game or activity
   - Read a book to child and have him drink a sip when a page is turned
   - Tea party
   - Have child take a drink when it is his turn in a game
   - Make a set schedule for supplementary liquids to promote the habit of in-between meal fluids (*e.g.*, juice or Kool-Aid at 10 a.m. and 2 p.m. each day).
3. Sore throat
   - Offer warm or cold fluids; consider frozen ices
   - Consider warm saline gargle or anesthetic lozenges before fluids
4. Extreme fatigue or weakness
   - Give smaller amounts more frequently
   - Provide for periods of rest prior to meals
5. Lack of knowledge
   - Assess the person's understanding of the reasons for maintaining adequate hydration, and methods for reaching goal of fluid intake
   - Include significant others
   - See Principles and Rationale for Nursing Care under *Knowledge Deficit*

C. Proceed with health teaching
   - Give verbal and written directions for desired fluids and amounts
   - Include the person/family in keeping a written record of fluid intake
   - Provide a list of alternative fluids (*e.g.*, ice cream, pudding).
   - Explain the need to increase fluids during exercise, fever, infection, and hot weather
   - Teach the person how to observe for dehydration (especially in infants) and to intervene by increasing fluid intake (see objective and subjective data for signs of dehydration)
   - Seek medical consultation for continued dehydration

# Fluid Volume Deficit
## Related to Abnormal Fluid Loss

Abnormal fluid loss describes fluid loss by vomiting, diarrhea, excessive diaphoresis, or drains.

### Assessment

#### Subjective data
The person reports
"I keep going to the bathroom all the time"
"I have to get up several times a night to urinate"
"I have loose bowels [diarrhea]"
"I've been vomiting a lot"
"I break out in a cold sweat"
"I'm thirsty all the time"

#### Objective data
Extreme diaphoresis
Increased body drainage
  Vomitus/nasogastric suction
  Chest tubes/thoracentesis
  Sump drains/paracentesis
  T-tubes
  Liquid or loose stools
  Polyuria
  Wound drainage (pus, serous, etc.)
Weight loss
Output exceeds intake

---

**Outcome Criteria**
The person will
- Maintain adequate intake of fluid and electrolytes
- Identify his abnormal fluid loss and relate methods of decreasing this loss if possible
- Relate relief of symptoms of dehydration

---

### Interventions

A. Assess causative factors
  Vomiting
  Fever
  Gastric suction
  Diarrhea/loose stools

## B. Remove or reduce causative factors

1. Vomiting
   - Encourage small, frequent amounts of ice chips or clear liquids such as weak tea or flat cola or ginger ale* (adults 30 ml, children 15 ml; see *Alterations in Nutrition: Less Than Body Requirements)*
2. Fever
   a. Maintain temperature lower than 101° F (38.4° C) through tepid water sponging and medication (*e.g.*, A.S.A. or acetaminophen)*
      - Eliminate excessive clothing and bed covers
      - Keep the room temperature cool
      - Encourage cool, clear liquids when medication is at peak effectiveness and temperature is lowest
      - Substitute frozen ices or popsicles if necessary (be resourceful)
      - If the temperature is extremely high, >103° F (39.5° C), apply ice packs to pulse points (groin, axilla)*
   b. Specifically for children under 5 with a sudden rise in temperature ("spiking fever"):
      - Work to attain a temperature <101° F (38.4° C) as soon as possible with medication* (A.S.A., acetaminophen) and sponging
      - Use tepid water (85°–90° F/29.4°–37.7° C) for sponging or bathing the child
      - Caution parents not to cover the child with blankets, and to be aware of the increased risk of febrile seizures
      - Give the child small amounts of *clear liquids only* (15 ml)
      - Teach the parents how to protect the child, should a seizure occur, and *instruct them to seek immediate medical consultation*
3. Gastric suction (nasogastric or other)
   - Use only normal saline for irrigation of gastric tubes to minimize electrolyte imbalance
   - Do not allow swallowing of water or ice chips; a "few small sips" can readily add up over a period of time
   - For the thirsty individual with gastric suction, *unless contraindicated by surgery or renal failure*, consult with the physician concerning ingestion of measured sips of Gatorade (1 oz/hr)
   - Always subtract all fluid ingested (via either tube or mouth) from any total gastric drainage to attain net drainage
   - Keep a careful, clear record of intake and output: amount, character, color
   - Offer frequent mouth care
4. Diarrhea/loose stools, see *Alterations in Bowel Elimination: Diarrhea*
5. Wound drainage
   - Keep careful records of the amount and type of drainage
   - Weigh dressings, if necessary, to estimate fluid loss (weigh the wet dressing; weigh a dry dressing of the same type; compare the difference)
   - Weigh the person daily if the drainage is excessive and difficult to measure (*e.g.*, soaked sheets)
   - Replace fluid loss (may be contraindicated in cardiac failure, renal failure, or head trauma)

*May require a physician's order.

C. Initiate health teaching as indicated

1. Assess the person's understanding of the type of fluid loss he is experiencing (what electrolytes are lost) and the fluids that provide replacement (see Principles and Rationale for Nursing Care)
2. Give verbal and written instructions for fluid replacement (*e.g.*, "Drink at least 3 quarts of liquid a day, including 1 quart of Gatorade")
3. Teach the person to
    * Avoid sudden and overexposure to heat/sun/and exercise
    * Gradually increase exposure and activity in hot weather
    * Eat three balanced meals a day
    * Increase fluid intake during hot days
    * Decrease activity during extreme weather

## Bibliography

See *Fluid Volume Excess*

# Fluid Volume Excess:

### Edema

## Definition

Fluid volume excess: The state in which the individual experiences or is at risk of experiencing vascular, cellular, or extracellular fluid overload.

## Etiological and Contributing Factors

### Pathophysiological
Renal failure, acute or chronic
Decreased cardiac output
          Myocardial infarction           Valvular disease
          Congestive heart failure     Tachycardia/arrhythmias
          Left ventricular failure
Varicosities of the legs
Liver disease
          Cirrhosis               Cancer
          Ascites
Tissue insult
          Injury to the cell wall       Hypoxia of the cell
Inflammatory process
Hormonal disturbances
          Pituitary             Estrogen
          Adrenal
Steroid therapy
Effusion (abnormal fluid accumulation)
          Pleural             Pericardial

### Situational
Excessive fluid intake (IV therapy)
Overtransfusion
          Blood/packed cells       Plasma expanders
Excessive sodium intake
Low protein intake
          Fad diets            Malnutrition
Dependent venous pooling/venostasis
          Immobility          Standing or sitting for long periods of time

Venous pressure point
          Tight cast or bandage
Pregnancy
Inadequate lymphatic drainage

## Defining Characteristics

Edema
Weight gain
Taut, shiny skin
Increased pulse volume or blood pressure
Tachycardia or arrhythmia
Jugular vein distention
Increased respiratory rate
Cough
Rales or rhonchi
Increased venous filling
Change in mental state (lethargy or confusion)
Hemodilution
Intake greater than output
Orthopnea/dyspnea on exertion
Weakness/fatigue

## Focus Assessment Criteria

### Subjective data

1. History of symptoms
   Complaints of
   Shortness of breath          Weakness/fatigue
   Weight gain                  Edema
   Onset/duration
   Location
   Description
   Aggravated by?
   Precipitated by?
   Relieved by?
2. History of contributing and causative factors
   Family or personal history of diabetes
   Pregnancy
   Pre-menses period
   Cardiac or renal disease
   Liver disease
   Alcoholism
   Hyper- or hypothyroidism
   Hypertension
   Steroid therapy
   Malnutrition
   Excessive salt intake
   Excessive use of tap-water enemas
   Lymphatic obstruction (*e.g.*, post lymph node dissection)
   Excessive parenteral fluid replacement
3. Current drug therapy
   Type, dosage
   Frequency
   Last dose taken when?
4. Dietary intake
   Estimated protein intake (adequate/inadequate)
   Estimated caloric intake (adequate/inadequate/excess)

Estimated fluid intake (adequate/inadequate/excess)

Daily alcohol consumption       Type _____ Amount _____

## Objective data

1. Assess vital signs for signs of fluid overload
   Pulse (bounding or arrhythmic)
   Respirations
      Rate (tachypnea)
      Quality (labored or shallow)
      Lung sounds (rales or rhonchi)
   Blood pressure (elevated)
2. Palpate for edema
   Press thumb for at least 5 seconds into the skin and note any remaining
      indentations
   Note degree and location (feet, ankles, legs, arms, sacral, generalized)
3. Assess for weight gain (weigh daily on the same scale, at the same time)
4. Assess for neck vein distention (distended neck veins at 45° elevation of the head
   may indicate fluid overload or decreased cardiac output)
5. Diagnostic studies
   Electrolytes
   Hemoglobin and hematocrit
   Blood urea nitrogen (BUN)
   Creatinine
   Urinalysis
   Central venous pressure (CVP)
   Pulmonary artery pressure (PAP)
   Pulmonary wedge pressure (PWP)

## Nursing Goals

Through selected nursing interventions, the nurse will seek to

- Prevent fluid overload
- Promote optimum cellular nutrition and oxygenation in cases of fluid overload
- Maintain normal fluid balance within the intracellular and extracellular spaces
- Promote the return of sequestered fluid to the vascular compartment, unless
  contraindicated

## Principles and Rationale for Nursing Care

See *Fluid Volume Deficit.*

# Fluid Volume Excess: Edema
Related to (specify)

## Assessment

### Subjective data

The person reports
   "I'm not supposed to eat salt"

"I feel bloated (tired, weak)"
Sudden or abnormal weight gain
History of
 Fingers, feet, or ankles swelling
 "Bad heart"
 "Bad kidneys"
 Hypertension
 Cancer or lymph node dissection
 Liver disease or alcoholism
 Immobility or neurological deficit (*e.g.*, stroke or spinal cord injury)
 Recent trauma or burn

## Objective data

Pedal or sacral puffiness
Puffing of face and extremities
Shiny, taut skin
Pitting edema (skin, when depressed by thumb, remains indented)
Increased blood pressure (especially diastolic)
Distended neck and leg veins
Weight gain
Fluid intake greater than fluid output
Decreased urinary output

---

**Outcome Criteria**

The person will
- Relate causative factors and methods of preventing edema
- Exhibit decreased peripheral edema

---

## Interventions

### A. Identify contributing and causative factors

Improper diet (excessive sodium intake; inadequate protein intake)
Dependent venous pooling/venostasis
Venous pressure point (*e.g.*, tight cast or bandage)
Inadequate lymphatic drainage
Immobility/neurologic deficit
Lack of knowledge of or compliance with medical regimen

### B. Reduce or eliminate causative contributing factors

1. Improper diet
   - Assess dietary intake and habits that may contribute to fluid retention
       a. Be specific; record daily and weekly intake of food and fluids
       b. Assess weekly diet for adequate protein or excessive sodium intake
           Discuss likes and dislikes of foods that provide protein
           Teach to plan weekly menu that provides protein at a price that is affordable
   - Encourage the person to decrease salt intake
       a. Teach the person to
           Read labels for sodium content

Avoid convenience foods, canned foods, and frozen foods

Cook without salt and to use spices to add flavor (lemon, basil, tarragon, mint)

Use vinegar in place of salt to flavor soups, stews, etc., *e.g.*, 2–3 teaspoons of vinegar to 4–6 quarts, according to taste

   b. Ascertain with physician whether salt substitute may be used (caution individual that he must use exactly the substitute that is prescribed)

2. Dependent venous pooling
   - Assess for evidence of dependent venous pooling or venostasis
   - Encourage alternating periods of horizontal rest (legs elevated) with vertical activity (standing) (this may be contraindicated in congestive heart failure)
   - Keep edematous extremity elevated above the level of the heart whenever possible (unless contraindicated by heart failure)
     a. Keep edematous arms elevated on two pillows or with IV pole sling
     b. Elevate legs whenever possible, using pillows under legs (avoid pressure points, especially behind knees)
     c. Discourage leg and ankle crossing
   - Reduce constriction of vessels
     a. Assess wearing apparel for proper fit and constrictive areas
     b. Instruct person to avoid panty girdles/garters, knee highs, leg crossing and to practice keeping legs elevated when possible
   - Consider using antiembolism stockings or Ace bandages; measure legs carefully for stockings/support hose*
     a. Measure from back of heel to back of knee, or top of thigh, depending on desired stocking length
     b. Measure circumference of calf and thigh
     c. Consider both measurements in choosing a stocking, matching measurements with size requirement chart that accompanies the stockings
     d. Apply stockings while lying down (*e.g.*, in the morning before arising)
     e. Check extremities frequently for adequate circulation and evidence of constrictive areas

3. Venous pressure points
   - Assess for venous pressure point associated with casts, bandages, tight stockings
     a. Observe circulation at edges of casts, bandages, stockings
     b. For casts, insert soft material to cushion pressure points at edges
     c. Check circulation frequently
   - Shift body weight in cast to redistribute weight within the cast (unless contraindicated)
     a. Encourage person to do this himself every 15 to 30 minutes during waking hours to prevent venostasis
     b. Encourage wiggling of fingers or toes, and isometric exercise of unaffected muscles within the cast*
     c. If the person is unable to do this himself, assist him at least hourly to shift body weight
     d. See *Impaired Physical Mobility*

4. Inadequate lymphatic drainage
   - Keep extremity elevated on pillows

*May require a physician's order.

      a. If edema is marked, the arm should be elevated, *but not in adduction* (this position may constrict the axilla)

      b. The elbow should be higher than the shoulder

      c. The hand should be higher than the elbow

- Take blood pressures in unaffected arm
- Do not give injections or start intravenous fluids in affected arm
- Protect the affected arm from injury

      a. Teach the person to avoid strong detergents, carrying heavy bags, holding a cigarette, injuring cuticles or hangnails, reaching into a hot oven, wearing jewelry or a wristwatch, or using Ace bandages

      b. Advise the person to apply lanolin cream several times a day to prevent dry, flaky skin

      c. Encourage the person to wear a "Medic Alert" tag engraved with *Caution: lymphedema arm — no tests — no needle injections*

      d. Caution the person to see a physician if the arm becomes red, swollen or unusually hard

- After a mastectomy, encourage range-of-motion exercises and use of affected arm to facilitate development of a collateral lymphatic drainage system (explain to the person that lymphedema is often decreased within a month, but that she should continue massaging, exercising, and elevating the arm for 3 or 4 months following surgery)

5. Immobility/neurologic deficit
   - Plan passive or active range-of-motion exercises for all extremities every 4 hours, including dorsiflexion of the foot to massage veins
   - Change the individual's position at least every 2 hours, utilizing the four positions (left side, right side, back, abdomen), if not contraindicated (see *Impairment of Skin Integrity*)
   - If the person must be maintained in high Fowler's position, assess for edema of the buttocks and sacral area and help the person to shift body weight every 2 hours to prevent pressure on edematous tissue

6. Lack of knowledge
   - Assess the person's knowledge of
     Medical diagnosis (*e.g.,* congestive heart failure, renal failure)
     Diet
     Medications (*e.g.,* diuretics, cardiotonics)
     Activity
     Use of Ace bandages, antiembolus stockings

## C. Protect edematous skin from injury

- Inspect skin for redness and blanching
- Reduce pressure on skin areas; pad chairs and footstools
- Prevent dry skin
  Use soap sparingly
  Rinse off soap completely
  Use a lotion to moisten skin
- See *Impairment of Skin Integrity* for additional information to prevent injury

## D. Initiate health teaching and referrals as indicated

- Give clear instructions verbally and in writing for all medications: what, when, how often, why, side-effects; pay special attention to drugs directly influencing fluid balance (*e.g.,* diuretics, steroids)

- Write down instructions for diet, activity, use of Ace bandages, stockings, etc. Have the person demonstrate his understanding of the instructions
- With severe fluctuations in edema, have the person weigh himself every morning and before bedtime daily, instructing the person to keep a written record of weights
- For less severe illness, the person may need to weigh himself daily only and record
- Caution the person to call physician for excessive edema/weight gain (>2 lbs/day) or increased shortness of breath at night or on exertion
- Explain that the above may be indicative of early heart problems and may require medication to prevent them from getting worse
- Consider home care or visiting nurses referral to follow at home
- Provide literature concerning low-salt diets; consult with dietician if necessary

## Bibliography

### Books

Aspinall MJ, and Tanner C: Decision Making and the Nursing Process. New York, Appleton-Century-Crofts, 1981

Brunner LS, Suddarth DS: Textbook of Medical-Surgical Nursing, 4th ed. Philadelphia, JB Lippincott, 1980

Fischbach F: A Manual of Laboratory Diagnostic Tests for Nurses. Philadelphia, JB Lippincott, 1980

Kintzel KC: Advanced Concepts in Clinical Nursing, 2nd ed. Philadelphia, JB Lippincott, 1977

Metheny NM, Snively WD Jr: Nurses' Handbook of Fluid Balance, 3rd ed. Philadelphia, JB Lippincott, 1979

Wieczorek RR, Natapoff JN: A Conceptual Approach to the Nursing Care of Children. Philadelphia, JB Lippincott, 1981

### Articles

Bindler RN, Howry RN: Nursing care of children with febrile seizures. Am J Nurs 78:270–273, 1978

Boh D: The water load test. Am J Nurs 82:112–113, 1982

Boyd Shurett PH, Coburn C: Heat and heat related illness. Am J Nurs 81:1298–1301, 1981

Boylan A, Marbach B: Dehydration: Subtle, sinister . . . preventable. RN 42(8):37–41, 1979

Castle M, Watkins J: Fever: Understanding the sinister sign. Nursing 9(2):26–33, 1979

Chambers J: Assessing the dialysis patient at home. Am J Nurs 81:750–754, 1981

Dale R: Symposium on fluid, electrolyte, and acid–base balance. Nurs Clin North Am 15, NC. 3:535–536, 1980

Felver L: Understanding the electrolyte maze. Am J Nurs 80:1591–1599, 1980

Guthrie D, Guthrie R: DKA (diabetic ketoacidosis): Breaking the vicious cycle. Nursing 11(6):54–61, 1981

Lane G: When persistence pays off: Resolving the mystery of unexplained electrolyte imbalance. Nursing 12(1):44–47, 1982

McConnell E: Urinalysis: A common test, but never routine. Nursing 12(2):108–111, 1982

Twombly M: The shift into third space. Nursing 8(1):38–46, 1978

Urrows ST: Physiology of body fluids. Nurs Clin North Am 15:603–615, 1980

# Grieving

*Related to* **an Actual or Perceived Loss**

*Related to* **Anticipated Loss**

## Definition

Grieving: A state in which an individual or family experiences an actual or a perceived loss (person, object, function, status, relationship) or the state in which an individual or family responds to the realization of a future loss (anticipatory grieving).

## Etiological and Contributing Factors

### Pathophysiological

Loss of function (actual or potential) related to a body-system alteration

| | |
|---|---|
| Neurological | Digestive |
| Cardiovascular | Respiratory |
| Sensory | Renal |
| Musculoskeletal | |

Loss of function or body part related to

Trauma

Surgery (mastectomy, colostomy, hysterectomy)

### Situational

Chronic pain

Terminal illness

Changes in life-style

| | |
|---|---|
| Childbirth | Child leaving home (*e.g.*, college |
| Marriage | or marriage) |
| Separation | Loss of career |
| Divorce | |

Type of relationship (with the person who is leaving or is gone)

Multiple losses or crises

Lack of social support system

### Maturational

Loss associated with aging

| | |
|---|---|
| Friends | Function |
| Occupation | Home |

## Defining Characteristics

The person

Reports an actual or perceived loss (person, object, function, status relationship)

Anticipates a loss

Associated defining characteristics

| | |
|---|---|
| Denial | Crying |
| Guilt | Sorrow |
| Anger | |

## Focus Assessment Criteria

Subjective data

1. Family

    Previous coping patterns to crisis

    Quality of the relationship of the ill or deceased person to each family member

    Position or role responsibilities of the ill or deceased person

    Sociocultural expectations for bereavement

    Religious expectations for bereavement

2. Individual family members

    Previous experiences with loss or death (as child, adolescent, or adult)

    Did family talk out their grief?

    Did they practice any particular religious rituals associated with bereavement?

    Present interactions between or among family members

    Adults

    Children

    Maturational level

    Understanding of crisis

    Degree of participation

    Knowledge of expected grief reactions

    Relationship to ill or deceased person

3. Expressions of

    | | |
    |---|---|
    | Ambivalence | Anger |
    | Denial | Depression |
    | Fear | Guilt |
    | Concerns | |

4. Report of

    Gastrointestinal disturbances

    | | |
    |---|---|
    | Indigestion | Weight gain or loss |
    | Nausea or vomiting | Constipation or diarrhea |
    | Anorexia | |

    Insomnia

    Preoccupation with sleep

    Fatigue (decreased or increased activity level)

Objective data

1. Normative (simple bereavement)

    | | |
    |---|---|
    | Shock | Sorrow |
    | Disbelief | Withdrawal |
    | Anger | Preoccupation with lost object |
    | Crying | Hopelessness |

2. Pathological pattern (profound; increases in intensity; continuous over 6 months)

    | | |
    |---|---|
    | Anger | Denial |
    | Depression | Regression |
    | Isolation | Obsession |

Despair                     Hallucinations
Worthlessness               Delusions
Guilt                       Phobias
Suicidal thoughts

## Nursing Goals

Through selected nursing interventions the nurse will seek to
- Provide for the concept of hope but not false hope
- Provide for person/family to have autonomy of their situation
- Provide for anticipatory grieving for losses
- Provide for person/family to engage in a life review
- Identify delayed reactions to grief

## Principles and Rationale for Nursing Care

### General

1. American culture is devoted to youth and life. Even though death surrounds each person, it is viewed as pertaining to someone else, not oneself.
2. Loss can be viewed as consisting of four components: dying, death, grief, and mourning.
3. Loss can occur without death; when a person experiences any loss (object, relationship), grief and mourning ensue.
4. Grief is the emotional response to loss; grief work is the adaptive process of mourning. It can be identified as
   Emancipation from bondage to the deceased
   Readjustment to the environment
   Formation of new relationships
5. An individual's grief is affected by many factors, such as personality, previous losses, intimacy of relationship, and personal resources.
6. Staging (of grieving process) can create problems if the nurse applies the stages universally to all persons, disregarding individual differences. Staging also may encourage the nurse to focus on the symptoms as opposed to the strength of the person/family.
7. The following stages (Engle) are specific enough to assist the nurse to intervene and broad enough to prevent labeling.

---

I. Shock and disbelief
    Initial denial            Decreased activity
    Numbed feelings       Sporadic periods of despair
II. Developing awareness of loss
    Sadness                Guilt
    Anger                 Crying
III. Restitution (usually requires at least a year)
    The work of mourning     Preoccupation with thoughts
    Painful void in life         of loss
IV. In the months to follow
    Beginning to put the lost rela-
    tionship in perspective (its
    positive and negative qualities)

---

8. Unresolved grief is a pathological response of prolonged denial of the loss or a profound psychotic response. Examples of such responses are

Progressively deeper regression, depression

Progressively deeper isolation

Somatic manifestations (prolonged)

Obsessions, phobias

Delusions, hallucinations

Attempted suicide

9. Factors that contribute to unresolved grief are

Quality of the individual's attachment to the loved object

Presence of ambivalence toward the loved object

Presence of lowered self-esteem

Inability to grieve

10. Grief work cannot begin until the loss is acknowledged. Nurses can encourage this acknowledgment by open honest dialogue and by providing the family with an opportunity to view the dead person.

11. Life review is a process whereby a dying person reminisces about the past, especially unresolved conflicts, in an attempt to resolve them. Life review also provides the person with an opportunity to evaluate his successes and failures.

12. Terminal illness with its concurrent treatments and its progression produces a multitude of losses

Loss of function (all systems)

Loss of financial independence

Change in appearance

Loss of friends

Loss of self-esteem

Loss of self

## Children

1. The child responds to death depending on his developmental age (see table) and the response of significant others.

**Developmental Understanding of Death**

| Age | Degree of Understanding |
| --- | --- |
| < 3 years | Cannot comprehend death, fears separation |
| 3 to 5 | Views illness as a punishment for real or imagined wrong-doing |
| | Has little concept of death as final because of immature concept of time |
| | May view death as a kind of sleep |
| | May feel he caused the event to happen (magical thinking), *e.g.*, by bad thoughts about person |
| 6 to 10 | Begins to fear death |
| | Attempts to put meaning to the event, *e.g.*, devil, ghost, God |
| | Associates death with mutilation and punishment |
| | Can feel responsibility for the event |
| 10 to 12 | Usually has an adult concept of death (inevitable, irreversible, universal) |
| | Attitudes greatly influenced by reactions of parents and others |
| | Very interested in postdeath services and rituals |
| Adolescence | Has priorities for group acceptance and independence |
| | Illness threatens both sets of priorities |

2. Children may learn early that discussions about death are taboo.

3. Children may utilize symbolic or nonverbal language to communicate their awareness of death and dying.

4. Children can be encouraged to communicate symbolically through writing or telling stories or by drawing pictures (see Appendix III for play therapy guidelines).
5. Children need to feel the joys and sorrows of life in order to begin to incorporate both in their lives appropriately.

# Grieving
## Related to an Actual or Perceived Loss

### Assessment

Subjective data

The person expresses

| | |
|---|---|
| Sadness | Fear |
| Depression | Denial |
| Shock | Guilt |

Objective data
Crying
Inability to cry
Withdrawn behavior
Apathetic behavior

---

**Outcome Criteria**

The individual will
- Express his grief
- Describe the meaning of the death or loss to him
- Share his grief with significant others (children, spouses)

---

### Interventions

A. Assess for causative and contributing factors that may delay the grief work

| | |
|---|---|
| Lack of support system | Inability to grieve (cultural, |
| Denial | social, age-related) |
| Shock | History of previous emotional |
| Anger | illness |
| Depression | Personality structure |
| Guilt | Early object loss |
| Fear | Nature of the relationship with |
| Dependency | the lost person or object |

B. Reduce or eliminate causative or contributing factors if possible
1. Promote a trust relationship
   - Promote feelings of self-worth through one-on-one and/or group sessions

- Allow for established time to meet and discuss feelings
- Communicate clearly, simply, and to the point
- Assess what the person and the family are learning by the use of feedback
- Offer support and reassurance
- Create a therapeutic milieu
- Establish a safe, secure, and private environment
- Demonstrate respect for the person's culture, religion, race, and values

2. Support the person and the family's grief reactions
- Explain grief reactions
   Shock and disbelief
   Developing awareness
   Restitution
- Describe varied acceptable expressions
   Elated or manic behavior as a defense against depression
   Elation and hyperactivity as a reaction of love and protection from depression
   Various states of depression
   Various somatic manifestations (weight loss or gain, indigestion, dizziness)
- Assess for past experiences with loss
   Loss of significant other in childhood
   Losses in later life

3. Promote family cohesiveness
- Support the family at its level of functioning
- Encourage self-exploration of feelings with family members
- Explain the need to discuss behaviors that interfere with relationships
- Recognize and reinforce the strengths of each family member
- Encourage the family to evaluate their feelings and support one another

4. Promote grief work with each response
   a. Denial
      - Recognize that this is a useful and necessary response
      - Explain the use of denial by one family member to the other members
   b. Isolation
      - Convey a feeling of acceptance by allowing grief
      - Create open, honest communications to promote sharing
      - Reinforce the person's self-worth by allowing privacy
   c. Depression
      - Reinforce the person's self-esteem
      - Identify the level of depression and develop the approach accordingly
      - Use empathetic sharing; acknowledge grief ("It must be very difficult")
      - Identify any indications of suicidal behavior (frequent statements of intent, revealed plan)
      - See *Potential for Violence* for additional information
   d. Anger
      - Understand that this feeling usually replaces denial
      - Explain to family that anger serves to try to control one's environment more closely because of inability to control loss
      - Encourage verbalization of the anger
      - See *Anxiety* for additional interventions for anger
   e. Guilt
      - Acknowledge the person's expressed self-view

- Avoid arguing and participating in the person's system of shoulds and should nots
- Discuss the person's preoccupation with him and attempt to move verbally beyond the present

f. Fear
- Focus on the present and maintain a safe and secure environment
- Help the person to explore reasons for a meaning of the behavior
- Consider alternative ways of expressing his feelings

g. Rejection
- Reassure the person by explaining what is happening
- Explain this response to family members

h. Hysteria
- Reduce environmental stresses, *e.g.*, limit personnel
- Provide person with a safe, private area to display grief

5. Promote grief work in children
- Encourage parents and staff to be truthful and offer explanations that can be understood
- Explore with child his concept of death in the context of his maturational level

  "What does death mean to you?"

  "Have you ever known a person or a pet that died?"

  "What happens when someone dies?"
- Correct misconceptions about death, illness, and rituals (funerals)

  Person was not bad

  Person is not asleep

  Body doesn't go to God but soul does
- Prepare the child for grief responses of others

  Explain that people are sad and cry when someone dies

  Explain the need to cry and how helpful it is

  Discuss with the family the inclusion of the child in postdeath services
- If the child plans to attend the funeral or visit the funeral home, a thorough explanation of the setting, rituals, and expected behaviors of mourners is necessary before (the family can plan the visit of the child to be short and also before the other mourners arrive)
- Reduce the fear of separation and feelings of guilt

  Allow child to share fears

  Allow child to remain with significant others while they grieve at home

  Reinforce to child that they are not responsible for the sadness

  Provide child with close contact and holding
- Provide accurate explanations for sibling illness or death

  Prepare child if sibling is terminal

  Explain the illness to the child in terms he can understand

  Stress that the illness or death did not result from being bad or because the well child wished it

6. Identify persons who are at high risk for potential pathological grieving reactions

   Absence of any emotion

   Previous conflict with deceased person

   History of ineffective coping patterns

7. Teach individual/family signs of pathological grieving, especially persons who are at risk

   Hallucinations

Delusions
Isolation
Egocentricity
Overt hostility (usually toward a family member)

C. Provide health teaching and referrals as indicated
  · Teach the person and the family signs of resolution
    Griever no longer lives in past but is future oriented and establishing new goals
    Griever breaks ties with lost object/person after approximately 6 to 12 months of grieving
  · Identify agencies that may be helpful
    Community agencies
    Religious groups

# Grieving
## Related to Anticipated Loss

### Assessment

Subjective data

The person expresses

| | |
|---|---|
| Sadness | Fear |
| Depression | Denial |
| Shock | Guilt |
| Anger | |

Objective data

Crying
Inability to cry
Withdrawn behavior
Apathetic behavior

---

**Outcome Criteria**

The person will
  · Express his grief
  · Participate in decision-making for the future
  · Share his concerns with significant others

---

### Interventions

A. Assess for causative and contributing factors of anticipated or potential loss

| | |
|---|---|
| Terminal illness | Socioeconomic status |
| Separation, (divorce, hospitalization, marriage, relocation, job) | Alteration in body image |
| | Alteration in self-esteem |
| | Aging |

## B. Assess individual response

| | |
|---|---|
| Denial | Shock |
| Rejection | Anger |
| Bargaining | Depression |
| Isolation | Guilt |
| Helplessness | Fear |

1. Encourage the person to share concerns
   - Utilize communication techniques of open-ended questions and reflection ("What are your thoughts today?" "Are you depressed?")
   - Acknowledge the value of the person and his grief by using touch and by sitting with him and verbalizing your concern ("This must be a very difficult time for you")
   - Recognize that some individuals may choose not to share their concerns but convey that you are available if they desire to do so later
2. Assist the person and the family to identify strengths
   "What do you do well?"
   "What are you willing to do to improve your life?"
   "Is religion a source of strength for you?"
   "Do you have close friends?"
   "Who do you turn to in times of need?"
   "What does this person do for you?"
3. Promote the integrity of the person and the family by acknowledging strengths
   "Your brother looks forward to your visit"
   "Your family is so concerned for you"
4. Support person and family with grief reactions
   - Prepare person and family for grief reactions
   - Explain grief reactions to person and family
   - Focus on the present life situation until the person or family indicates the desire to discuss future
5. Promote family cohesiveness
   - Identify availability of a support system
     a. Meet consistently with family members
     b. Identify family member roles, strengths, weaknesses
   - Assess communication patterns
     a. Listen and clarify the messages being sent
     b. Identify the patterns of communication within the family unit by assessing positive and negative feedback, verbal and nonverbal communications, and body language
   - Provide for the concept of hope by
     Supplying accurate information
     Resisting the temptation to give false hope
     Discussing concerns willingly
   - Promote group decision-making to enhance group autonomy
     a. Establish consistent times to meet with person and family
     b. Encourage members to talk directly with each other and to listen to each other
6. Promote grief work with each response
   a. Denial
      - Initially support and then strive to increase the development of awareness (when individual indicates readiness for awareness)
   b. Isolation
      - Listen and spend designated time consistently with person and family

- Offer the person and the family opportunity to explore their emotions
- Reflect back on past losses and acknowledge loss behavior (past and present)

  c.  Depression
- Begin with simple problem solving and move toward acceptance
- Enhance self-worth through positive reinforcement
- Identify the level of depression and indications of suicidal behavior or ideas
- Be consistent and establish times daily to speak with person and family

  d.  Anger
- Allow for crying to release this energy
- Listen to and communicate concern
- Encourage concerned support from significant others as well as professional support

  e.  Guilt
- Listen and communicate concern
- Allow for crying
- Promote more direct expression of feelings
- Explore methods to resolve guilt

  f.  Fear
- Help person and family recognize the feeling
- Explain that this will help cope with life
- Explore person and family's attitudes about loss, death, etc.
- Explore person and family's methods of coping

  g. Rejection
- Allow for verbal expression of this feeling state in order to diminish the emotional strain
- Recognize that expression of anger may create a rejection of self to significant others

7. Provide for expression of grief
- Encourage emotional expressions of grieving
- Caution the use of sedatives and tranquilizers which may prevent and/or delay emotional expressions of loss
- Encourage verbalization of clients and families of all age groups
  - a.  Support family cohesiveness
  - b.  Promote and verbalize strengths of the family group
- Encourage person and family to engage in life review
  - a.  Focus and support the social network relationships
  - b.  Reevaluate past life experiences and integrate them into a new meaning
  - c.  Convey empathetic understanding

8. Identify potential pathological grieving reactions

| | |
|---|---|
| Delusions | Difficulty crying or controlling |
| Hallucinations | crying |
| Phobias | Loss of control of environment |
| Obsessions | leading to hopelessness, |
| Isolations | helplessness |
| Conversion hysteria | Intense reactions lasting longer |
| Agitated depression | than 6 months with few signs |
| Delay in grief work | of relief |
| Suicidal indications | Restrictions of pleasure |

9. Refer individual with potential for pathological grieving responses for counseling (psychiatrist, nurse therapist, counselor, psychologist)

## C. Provide health teaching and referrals as indicated

- Explain what to expect

  | | |
  |---|---|
  | Sadness | Fear |
  | Feelings of aloneness | Rejection |
  | Guilt | Anger |

- Teach person and family signs of resolution
    a. Griever no longer lives in past but is future oriented, establishing new goals
    b. Griever breaks ties with lost object/person after approximately 6 to 12 months of grieving
- Teach signs of pathological responses and referrals needed
    a. Defenses used in uncomplicated grief work that become exaggerated or maladaptive responses
    b. Persistent absence of any emotion
    c. Abnormal intense reactions of anxiety, anger, fear, guilt, helplessness
- Identify agencies that may enhance grief work

  Self-help groups
  Widow-to-widow groups
  Parents of deceased children
  Single parent groups
  Bereavement groups

## Bibliography

### Books

Battin D, Aakin A, Gerber I et al: Coping and vulnerability among the aged bereaved. In Schroenber B, Gerber I, Wiener A et al (eds): Bereavement: Its Psychosocial Aspects. New York, Columbia University Press, 1975

Barton D (ed): Dying and Death: A Clinical Guide for Caregivers. Baltimore, Williams & Wilkins, 1977

Beitler R: 1968. The life review: An interpretation of reminiscence in the aged. In Neugarten BL (ed): Middle Life and Aging. Chicago, University of Chicago Press, 1968

Caughill R (ed): The Dying Patient: A Supportive Approach. Boston, Little, Brown, 1976

Fulton R (ed): Death and Identity. Bowie, MD, Charles Press, 1976

Hamilton M, Reid H (eds): A Hospice Handbook: A New Way to Care for the Dying. Grand Rapids, Wm B Eerdmans, 1980

Kastenbaum R: Death, Society, and Human Experience. St. Louis, CV Mosby, 1977

Kastenbaum R: Psychological death. In Pearson L (ed): Death and Dying. Cleveland, Case Western Reserve University Press, 1969

Kyes JJ, Hofling CK: Basic Psychiatric Concepts in Nursing, 4th ed. Philadelphia, JB Lippincott, 1980

Kübler-Ross, E: Death: The Final Stage of Growth. Englewood Cliffs, NJ, Prentice-Hall, 1975

Packes C: Bereavement: Studies of Grief in Adult Life. New York, International Universities Press, 1972

Werner-Beland, JA: Grief Responses to Long-Term Illness and Disability. Virginia, Reston Publishing, 1980

### Periodicals

Butler RN: The life review. Psychiatry 26:65–76, 1963

Domming J, Stackman J, O'Neill P et al: Experiences with dying patients. Am J Nurs 73:1058–1064, 1973

Engle G: Grief and grieving. Am J Nurs 64:93–97, 1964

Hutton L: Annie is alone: The bereaved child. Matern Child Nurs J 6:274–277, 1981

Kowalski K, Osborn MR: Helping mothers of stillborn infants to grieve. Matern Child Nurs J 2:29–32, 1977

Philpot T: St. Joseph's Hospice: Death—a part of life. Nursing Mirror 151(16):20–23, 1980

Oehler J: The frog family books: Color pictures sad or glad. Matern Child Nurs J 6:281, 1981

Radford C: Nursing care to the end. Nursing Mirror 150(2):30–31, 1980

Schultz CA: The dynamics of grief. Journal of Emergency Nursing 15(5):26–30, 1979

Sheer BL: Help for parents in a difficult job: Broaching the subject of death. Matern Child Nurs J 5:320–324, 1977

Willans JH: Appetite in the terminally ill patient. Nursing Times 76(10):875–876, 1980

Williams H, Rivara FP, Rothenberg, MB: The child is dying: Who helps the family? Matern Child Nurs J 6:261–265, 1981

Wong D: Bereavement: The empty mother syndrome. Matern Child Nurs J 5:384–389, 1980

Wooten B: Death of an infant. Matern Child Nurs J 6:257–260, 1981

# Health Maintenance, Alterations in

## Definition

Alterations in health maintenance: States in which the individual experiences or is at risk of experiencing a disruption in his present state of wellness because of inadequate preventive measures or an unhealthy life-style.

**Note:** This diagnostic category should be used to describe an asymptomatic person. However, it can be used for a person with a chronic disease to help that person attain a higher level of wellness. For example, a woman with lupus erythematosus can have a diagnosis: *Potential Alterations in Health Maintenance Related to Lack of a Regular Exercise Program.*

This diagnostic category can also be used for persons with acute conditions to describe other dimensions of their health. For example, a child with acute otitis media may have a diagnosis: *Alterations in Health Maintenance Related to Lack of Immunizations for Age.*

## Etiological and Contributing Factors

### Pathophysiological

Not directly related to alterations in health maintenance

### Situational

Loss of independence
Changing support systems
Change in finances
Lack of knowledge
Poor learning skills (illiteracy)
Crisis situation
Lack of accessibility to adequate health care services
Substance abuse (alcohol, tobacco)
Inadequate health practice
Lack of supervision for dependents (children, elderly)
Health beliefs (lack of perceived threat to health)
Religious beliefs
External locus of control
Cultural or folk beliefs
Alterations in self-image (poor self-esteem, distorted body image)

### Maturational

See Table II-3 for age-related conditions.

## Defining Characteristics (in the absence of disease)

Skin and nails

| | |
|---|---|
| Malodorous | Sunburn |
| Unclean | Unusual color, pallor |
| Lesion (pustule, rash, dry, scaly) | Unexplained scars |

(*text continues on page 221*)

Table II-3. **Primary and Secondary Prevention for Age-Related Conditions**

| Developmental Level | Primary Prevention | Secondary Prevention |
|---|---|---|
| Infancy (0–1 year) | Parent education | Complete physical exam every 2–3 months |
| | Infant safety | Screening at birth |
| | Nutrition | Congenital hip |
| | Breast feeding | PKU |
| | Sensory stimulation | Sickle cell |
| | Infant massage and touch | Cystic fibrosis |
| | Visual stimulation | Vision (startle reflex) |
| |   Activity | Hearing (response to and localization of |
| |   Colors |   sounds) |
| | Auditory stimulation | TB test at 12 months |
| |   Verbal | Developmental assessments |
| |   Music | Screen and intervene for high risk |
| | Immunizations | Low birth weight |
| |   DPT ⎫ at 2, 4, and 6 months | Maternal substance abuse during pregnancy |
| |   TOPV ⎭ |   Alcohol: fetal alcohol syndrome |
| | Oral hygiene |   Cigarettes: SIDS |
| | Teething biscuits |   Drugs: addicted neonate |
| | Fluoride | Maternal infections during pregnancy |
| | Avoid sugared food and drink | |
| Preschool (1–5 years) | Parent education | Complete physical exam between 2 and 3 years |
| | Teething |   and preschool (U/A, CBC) |
| | Discipline | TB test at 3 years |
| | Nutrition | Developmental assessments (annual) |
| | Accident prevention | Speech development |
| | Normal growth and development | Hearing |
| | | Vision |

Table II-3 (continued)

| Developmental Level | Primary Prevention | Secondary Prevention |
|---|---|---|
| Preschool (continued) (1–5 years) | Child education<br>  Dental self-care<br>  Dressing<br>  Bathing with assistance<br>  Feeding self-care<br>Immunizations<br>  DPT<br>  TOPV } at 18 months<br>  MMR at 15 months<br>Dental/oral hygiene<br>  Fluoride treatments<br>  Fluoridated water<br>  Dietary counsel | Screen and intervene<br>  Lead poisoning<br>  Developmental lag<br>  Neglect or abuse<br>  Strabismus<br>  Hearing deficit<br>  Vision deficit |
| School age (6–11 years) | Health education of child<br>  "Basic 4" nutrition<br>  Accident prevention<br>  Outdoor safety<br>  Substance abuse counsel<br>  Anticipatory guidance for physical changes at<br>    puberty<br>Immunizations<br>  Tetanus age 10<br>  DPT<br>  TOPV } boosters between 4 and 6 years<br>Dental hygiene every 6–12 months<br>Continue fluoridation<br>Complete physical exam | Complete physical exam<br>TB test every 3 years (at ages 6 and 9)<br>Developmental assessments<br>  Language<br>  Vision: Snellen charts at school<br>    6–8 years, use "E" chart<br>    Over 8 years, use alphabet chart<br>  Hearing: audiogram |

(continued)

Table II-3 *(continued)*

| Developmental Level | Primary Prevention | Secondary Prevention |
|---|---|---|
| Adolescence (12–19 years) | Health education<br>Proper nutrition and healthful diets<br>Sex education with family planning, male/female<br>Safe driving skills<br>Adult challenges<br>Seeking employment and career choices<br>Dating and marriage<br>Confrontation with substance abuse<br>Safety in athletics<br>Skin care<br>Dental hygiene every 6–12 months<br>Immunizations<br>Tetanus without trauma<br>TOPV booster at 12–14 years | Complete physical exam (prepuberty or age 13)<br>Blood pressure<br>Cholesterol<br>TB test at 12 years<br>VDRL, CBC, U/A<br>Female: breast self-exam<br>Male: testicular self-exam<br>Female, if sexually active: Pap and pelvic exam twice, one year apart (cervical gonorrhea culture with pelvic); then every 3 years if both are negative<br>Screening and interventions if high risk<br>Depression<br>Suicide<br>Substance abuse<br>Pregnancy (more than 18 years old)<br>Family history of alcoholism or domestic violence |
| Young adult (20–39 years) | Health education<br>Weight management with good nutrition as BMR changes<br>Lifestyle counseling<br>Stress management skills<br>Safe driving<br>Family planning<br>Parenting skills<br>Regular exercise<br>Environmental health choices | Complete physical exam at about 20 years, then every 5–6 years<br>Cancer checkup every 3 years<br>Female: BSE monthly<br>Male: TSE monthly<br>All females: baseline mammography between ages 35 and 40<br>Parents-to-be: high-risk screening for Downs syndrome, Tay-Sachs<br>Female pregnant: screen for VD, rubella titer, Rh factor |

Table II-3 (continued)

| Developmental Level | Primary Prevention | Secondary Prevention |
|---|---|---|
| Young adult (continued ) (20–39 years) | Dental hygiene every 6–12 months<br><br>Immunizations<br>  Tetanus at 20 years and every 10 years<br>  Female: rubella, if serum negative for antibodies | Screening and interventions if high risk<br>  Female with previous breast cancer: annual mammography at 35 years and after<br>  Female with mother or sister who has had breast cancer, same as above<br>  Family history colorectal cancer or high risk: annual stool guaiac, digital rectal, and sigmoidoscopy<br>  PPD if exposed to TB |
| Middle-aged adult (40–59 years) | Health education: continue with young adult<br>Midlife changes, male and female counseling<br>  "Empty-nest syndrome"<br>Anticipatory guidance for retirement<br>Grandparenting<br>Dental hygiene every 6–12 months<br><br>Immunizations<br>  Tetanus every 10 years<br>  Pneumococcal } annual if high risk, i.e.,<br>  Influenza } major chronic disease (COPD, CAD) | Complete physical exam every 5–6 years with complete laboratory evaluation (serum/urine tests, x-ray, EKG)<br>Cancer checkup every year<br>  Female: BSE monthly<br>  Male: TSE monthly<br>  All females: annual mammography 50 years and over<br>  Schiotz's tonometry (glaucoma) every 3–5 years<br>  Female pregnant: perinatal screening by amniocentesis if desired<br>  Sigmoidoscopy at 50 and 51, then every 4 years if negative<br>  Stool guaiac annually at 50 and thereafter<br>  Screening and intervention if high risk<br>  Endometrial cancer: have endometrial sampling at menopause<br>  Oral cancer: screen more often if substance abuser<br>                    (continued) |

Table II-3 *(continued)*

| Developmental Level | Primary Prevention | Secondary Prevention |
|---|---|---|
| Elderly adult (60–74 years) | Health education: continue with previous counseling<br>Home safety<br>Retirement<br>Loss of spouse<br>Special health needs<br>Nutritional changes<br>Changes in hearing or vision<br>Alterations in bowel or bladder habits<br>Dental/oral hygiene every 6–12 months<br>Immunizations<br>Tetanus every 10 years<br>Pneumococcal ⎰⎱ annual if high risk<br>Influenza | Complete physical exam every 2 years with laboratory assessments<br>Annual cancer checkup<br>Blood pressure annually<br>Female: BSE monthly<br>Male: TSE monthly<br>Female: annual mammogram<br>Annual stool guaiac<br>Sigmoidoscopy every 4 years<br>Schiotz's tonometry every 3–5 years<br>Podiatric evaluation with foot care PRN<br>Screen for high risk<br>Depression<br>Suicide |
| Old-age adult (75 years and over) | Complete physical exam annually<br>Laboratory assessments<br>Cancer checkup<br>Blood pressure<br>Stool guaiac<br>Female: mammogram, sigmoidoscopy every 4 years<br>Schiotz's tonometry every 3–5 years<br>Podiatrist PRN | Health education: continue counsel<br>Anticipatory guidance<br>Dying and death<br>Loss of spouse<br>Increasing dependency upon others<br>Dental/oral hygiene every 6–12 months<br>Immunizations<br>Tetanus every 10 years<br>Pneumococcal ⎰⎱ annual<br>Influenza |

Respiratory system

Frequent infections          Dyspnea with exertion

Chronic cough

Oral cavity

Frequent sores (on tongue, buc-     Lesions associated with lack of

cal mucosa)                           oral care or substance abuse

Loss of teeth at early age        (leukoplakia, fistulas)

Gastrointestinal system and nutrition

Obesity                       Chronic anemia

Anorexia                    Chronic bowel irregularity

Cachexia                   Chronic dyspepsia

Musculoskeletal system

Frequent muscle strain, backaches, neck pain

Diminished flexibility and muscle strength

Genitourinary system

Frequent venereal lesions and infections

Frequent use of potentially unhealthful over-the-counter products (chemical douches, vaginal perfumed products)

Constitutional

Chronic fatigue, malaise, apathy

Neurosensory

Presence of facial tics (nonconvulsant)

Headaches

Psychoemotional

Emotional fragility

Behavior disorders (compulsiveness, belligerence)

Frequent feelings of being overwhelmed

## Nursing Goals

Through selected interventions the nurse will seek to

- Establish a therapeutic nursing relationship with person and family that facilitates their sharing of personal information and readiness to learn
- Educate person and family about health maintenance behaviors that are appropriate to developmental level and chronological age
- Act as a resource person for the person and the family by answering their questions and thereby facilitate understanding of developmental needs
- Perform some screening procedures within the context of the work setting
- Identify those persons at high risk and make appropriate referrals

## Principles and Rationale for Nursing Care

### Screening

1. Screening is the administration of a specific procedure to an asymptomatic person for the purpose of early detection of disease.
2. Assumptions concerning screening are

The procedure is acceptable to the at-risk population, is relatively simple and not time-consuming, and is available at a reasonable cost

The disease would not ordinarily be suspected due to lack of symptoms

Detection of the disease during this period will improve morbidity/mortality from that condition

The disease is significantly prevalent

Adequate treatment for the disease is available

Treatment for the disease will improve the quality of life, and this outcome outweighs any adverse effects of the screening procedure

3. The tasks of screening are to

Identify major disabling conditions

Investigate the personal and social benefits of early detection and intervention for asymptomatic persons with the condition (*e.g.*, facilitate family coping, minimize disability and cost, prevent premature death, improve productivity of affected persons, decrease overall morbidity and mortality)

Identify persons at high risk for specific conditions, through *personal medical history* (*e.g.*, concurrent diseases such as diabetes mellitus involves greater risk for hypertension), *family medical history* (*e.g.*, breast cancer, diabetes, hypertension), and *social history* (*e.g.*, substance abuse—cancer, heart disease; sexual patterns—venereal disease; domestic violence—person abuse)

Identify tests and procedures that accurately detect the condition (who will do them? how often are they done? who bears the cost?)

Plan a strategy for disseminating screening information to health care professionals and the public

Plan evaluation of screening effectiveness

4. Screening must be individualized based upon personal health risk profile, developmental level and age, and the right to self-determination and protection of dignity.

5. Screening is directed toward two populations: those identified as high risk, and the general population.

6. Types of screening measures include

Physical findings (periodic exams by health care professionals and self-exams of breast, testicles, and skin)

Survey of risk factors (smoking, alcohol abuse)

Laboratory tests (serum—*e.g.*, sickle-cell in blacks, PKU in newborns; urine—*e.g.*, renal disease in the elderly; x-ray—*e.g.*, dental caries, chest TB)

7. Nurses are in an especially effective position to screen because they

Permeate every segment of society

Are knowledgeable about health and physical examination

Believe in a holistic philosophy of care

Consider client teaching a vital aspect of the nursing role

Interface with multiple health professions

## Prevention

1. The goals of prevention are
   - Avoidance of disease by choosing a healthy life-style
   - Decrease in mortality due to disease by early detection and intervention
   - Improvement of quality of life and limitation of disability
2. The three levels of prevention are primary, secondary, and tertiary.
3. The primary level of prevention involves actions that prevent disease and accidents and promote well-being. Key concepts are as follows:

| Concept | Examples |
|---------|----------|
| **Wellness**<br>A life-style that incorporates the principles of health promotion and is directed by self-responsibility | Diet low in salt, sugar, and fat<br>Regular exercise and stress management<br>Elimination of smoking<br>Minimal alcohol intake |
| **Self-help**<br>Mutual sharing with others who have similar needs | La Leche League<br>Childbirth Education<br>Assertiveness training<br>Specific written resources (books, pamphlets, magazines)<br>Public media (radio, TV) |
| **Safety** | Adherence to speed limits<br>Use of seat belts and car seats<br>Proper storage of household poisons |
| **Immunizations** | Children: DPT<br>Pregnant women: rubella<br>Elderly: influenza, pneumonia |

4. The secondary level of prevention concerns actions that promote early detection of disease and subsequent intervention (see screening principles), both routine physical examination by a health professional at regular intervals and self-examination. Self-examination is a two-fold process.

   (1) A general awareness of changes in body parts, functions, sensations, and the possible implications of these changes.

   *Cancer warning signs*

   Change in bowel or bladder habits
   Sore that does not heal
   Unusual bleeding or discharge
   Thickening or lump in breast or elsewhere
   Indigestion or difficulty in swallowing
   Obvious change in wart or mole
   Nagging cough or hoarseness

   *Arthritis warning signs*

   Stiffness on arising
   Persistent pain
   Pain or tenderness in one or more joints
   Swelling in one or more joints
   Recurrence of these symptoms, especially when they involve one or more joint

   *Heart attack signals*

   Chest pain, usually behind sternum
   Pain in jaw, neck, or arm
   Pressure or tight sensation in chest, possibly associated with sweating, nausea, shortness of breath, and feeling weak

   (2) Specific and purposeful examination of one's own body parts for abnormality (*e.g.*, breast, testicles, skin)

5. The tertiary level of screening involves actions that restore and rehabilitate in the presence of illness. For example, for a person with coronary artery disease, these would be

Restorative (surgery, such as coronary bypass, and medications)

Rehabilitative (stress management, exercise program, stop smoking, "zipper club" [self-help group])

6. Potential barriers to prevention are found in both the health care system and in the individual. The system may be

Disease-oriented rather than health-oriented

Composed of health care professionals who are taught to focus on fragment systems of the human body rather than take a holistic approach

Functioning on a financial systems that rewards treatment of illness, not prevention

Difficult to reach or has previously proved unsatisfactory

The client may

Believe that the health/illness state is determined by forces (fate, luck) outside himself (external locus of control)

Perceive the behavior needed as unacceptable or uncomfortable

Practice sociocultural behaviors that are not healthful (*e.g.*, obesity is considered desirable, salt is prevalent in diet)

Experience psychological disturbances that impede incentive to practice healthy behaviors

Lack financial resources

## Nutrition

See Principles and Rationale for Nursing Care for *Alterations in Nutrition*

## Exercise

1. A regular exercise program should

Be enjoyable

Utilize a minimum of 400 calories in each session

Sustain a heart rate of approximately 120 to 150 beats per minute

Involve rhythmical alternately contracting and relaxing of muscles

Be integrated into the person's life-style 4 to 5 days per week (at least 30 to 60 minutes)

2. Regular exercise can provide the person with increased

Cardiovascular-respiratory endurance

Muscle strength

Muscle endurance

Flexibility

Ability to deliver nutrients to tissue

Ability to tolerate psychological stress

Ability to reduce body fat content

3. An exercise program should include

A warm-up session (10 minutes of stretching exercises)

Endurance exercises

A cool-down session (5 to 10 minutes)

4. Before beginning an exercise program, the person must consider

Physical limitations (consult nurse or physician)

Personal preferences

Life-style

Community resources

5. The person must know

When to stop exercising (pain, muscle strain)

What clothing is needed (shoes)

How to monitor pulse before, during, and after exercise

6. The person is taught to monitor his pulse before, during, and after exercise to assist him to achieve his target heart rate and not to exceed his maximum advisable heart rate for his age (Kuntzelman).

| Age | Maximum Heart Rate | Target Heart Rate |
|-----|--------------------|--------------------|
| 30 | 190 | 133–162 |
| 40 | 180 | 126–153 |
| 50 | 170 | 119–145 |
| 60 | 160 | 112–136 |

---

**Outcome Criteria**

The person will
- Identify factors that increase the potential for injury
- Utilize safety measures to prevent injury (*e.g.*, remove throw rugs or anchor them)
- Practice selected prevention measures (*e.g.*, wear sunglasses to reduce glare)
- Increase his daily activity, if feasible

---

## Interventions

A. Assess for factors that contribute to the promotion and the maintenance of health

Knowledge of disease and preventive behavior

Appropriate screening practices for age and risk

Good nutrition and weight control

Regular exercise program

Constructive stress management

Supportive social networks

B. Promote health behaviors in the person and the family

1. Determine the person or family's knowledge or perception of
   a. Specific diseases (*e.g.*, heart disease, cancer, respiratory disease, childhood diseases, infections, dental disease)
   b. Susceptibility (*e.g.*, presence of risk factors, family history)
   c. Seriousness
   d. Value of early detection
2. Determine the person or family's past patterns of health care
   a. Expectations
   b. Interactions with health care system or providers
   c. Influences of family, cultural group, peer group, mass media
3. Provide specific information concerning screening for age-related conditions (refer to Table II–3)
4. Discuss the role of nutrition in health maintenance and the prevention of illness (see Principles and Rationale for Nursing Care for *Alterations in Nutrition* for specific explanations)

   a.  Basic four food groups

   b.  Nutrient needs relate to age, level of physical activity, pregnancy and lactation

   c.  The prudent use of
> Salt (see *Fluid Volume Excess* for foods high in sodium)
> Canned vegetables
> Fried foods
> Red meats
> Fats (butter, margarines)
> High-calorie desserts
> Snack foods (potato chips, candy, soda)
> Refined sugar

   d.  See *Alterations in Nutrition* for specific information concerning weight control

5. Discuss the benefits of a regular exercise program
   - See Principles and Rationale for Nursing Care for the positive effects of a regular exercise program
   - Determine the optimal exercise for the individual, considering physical limitations preferences, and life-style
     > Walking briskly
     > Jogging
     > Running
     > Aerobic exercises
     > Aerobic dancing
     > Swimming
     > Bicycling
     > Skipping rope
   - Stress the importance of beginning any physical activity slowly
   - See *Alterations in Nutrition: More Than Body Requirements* related to intake for walking program

6. Discuss the elements of constructive stress management
   > Assertiveness training
   > Problem-solving
   > Relaxation techniques
   > See Appendix III for relaxation techniques and Appendix VI for guidelines for problem-solving
   > See Pertinent Literature for the Consumer on assertiveness and problem-solving self-help books

7. Discuss strategies for developing positive social networks

   a.  Relate the functions of a support system
   - Provide love and affection
   - Share common social concerns
   - Serve as buffers for life's stressors
   - Prevent isolation
   - Respect mutual pursuits of members
   - Cooperate for the purpose
   - Provide dependable assistance (emotional and economic, if appropriate)

   b.  Suggest methods for strengthening this system
   - Be supportive of others
   - Practice active listening by allowing yourself to listen attentively to the other person

- Don't interrupt the person
- Allow a few seconds to lapse between dialogue to provide time to gather thoughts and to reduce the "rush to speak"

c. Provide others with opportunities to share their concerns without judgment. Refrain from giving solutions to problems of others; rather, a discussion of options may be indicated (e.g., "You have several options: You can quit your job, request a transfer, discuss the problem with your boss, or do nothing)

d. When confronted with a relationship problem, review the situation
   What is the problem?
   Who/what is responsible for the problem?
   What are the options?
   What are the advantages and disadvantages of each option?
   (See Appendix VI guidelines for problem solving)

e. Provide warmth and affection to significant others
   - Praise a child's accomplishments
   - Praise all attempts at accomplishments
   - Practice open shows of affection, *e.g.*, with children (boys and girls), with spouse, and with others

f. Practice mutual goal setting to direct common efforts and reevaluate them periodically

g. Offer sincere assistance to individuals to promote trust

h. Build relationships with individuals and families who share common interests and values

i. Recognize when additional assistance is needed
   Marital counseling
   Self-help groups
   Health professional
   Religious affiliation

j. Allow oneself and each member of the family —children, spouse, parents—to enhance personal identity by pursuing individual interests (refer to Appendix VII for age-related needs of children)

## C. Initiate health teaching and referrals as indicated

1. Review the daily health practices of the individual (adults, children)
   Dental care
   Food intake
   Fluid intake
   Exercise regime
   Leisure activities
   Responsibility in the family
   Use of
   Tobacco
   Salt, sugar, fat products
   Alcohol
   Drugs (over-the-counter, prescribed)
   Knowledge of safety practices
   Fire prevention
   Water safety
   Automobile (maintenance, seat belts)
   Bicycle
   Poison control

2. Refer to selected nursing diagnoses for additional information on and assessment of

> Safety needs: see *Potential for Injury*
> Activity needs: see *Diversional Activity Deficit*
> Affiliative needs: see *Social Isolation*
> Parenting needs: see *Alterations in Parenting*
> Family needs: see *Alterations in Family Processes*
> Spiritual needs: see *Spiritual Distress*
> Sexual needs: see *Sexual Dysfunction*
> Self-care needs: see *Impaired Home Maintenance Management; Knowledge Deficit*
> Emotional needs: see *Ineffective Individual Coping; Anxiety; Fear; Grieving; Disturbance in Self-Concept;* and *Powerlessness*

## Bibliography

American Cancer Society: The Cancer-Related Health Checkup. New York, American Cancer Society, 1980

Breslow L, Somers A: The lifetime health-monitoring program. N Engl J Med 296:601–608, 1977

Carlson CE, Blackwell B: Behavioral Concepts and Nursing Intervention, 2nd ed. Philadelphia, JB Lippincott, 1978

Chow MP, Durand BA, Feldman MN et al: Handbook of Primary Care. New York, John Wiley & Sons, 1979

Duvall EM: Marriage and Family Development, 5th ed. Philadelphia, JB Lippincott, 1977

Hymovich DP, Barnard MV: Family Health Care, 2nd ed. New York, McGraw-Hill, 1979

Kandzari J, Howard J: The Well Family: A Developmental Approach to Assessment. Boston, Little, Brown & Co, 1981

Lieberman MA, Borman LD: Self-Help Groups for Coping with Crisis. San Francisco, Jossey-Bass, 1979

Periodic health exam: A guide for designing individualized preventive health care in the asymptomatic adult. Ann Intern Med 95:729–732, 1981

Smitherman C: Nursing Actions for Health Promotion. Philadelphia, FA Davis, 1981

Spitzer WO: Report of the task force on the periodic health examination. Can Med Assoc J 121:193–254, 1979

## Pertinent Literature and Organizations for the Consumer

National Self-Health Clearinghouse, Graduate School and University Center of the City University of New York (CUNY), 33 West 42nd Street, Room 1227, New York, NY 10036, (212) 840-7606. Publishers of *Self-Help Reporter.*

### General

Eisenberg A, Eisenberg H: Alive and Well: Decision in Health. New York, Mc-Graw-Hill, 1979

### Stress Management

Alberti RE, Emmons ML: Your Perfect Right: A Guide to Assertive Behavior. San Luis Obispo, CA, Impact Publishers, 1974

Bloom L, Coburn K; Pearlman J: The New Assertive Woman. New York, Dell Publishers, 1976

Girdano DD, Everly GS: Controlling Stress and Tension. Englewood Cliffs, NJ, Prentice-Hall.

Girdano DD, Everly GS: The Stress-Mess Solution. Bowie, MD, Robert J. Brady, 1980

Martin RA, Poland EY: Learning to Change: A Self-Management Approach to Adjustment. New York, McGraw-Hill, 1980

## Exercise

Cantu RC: Toward Fitness: Guided Exercise for Those with Health Problems. New York, Human Sciences Press, 1980

Ellfeldt L, Lowman CL: Exercises for the Mature Adult. Springfield, IL, Charles C Thomas, 1973

Getchell L: Physical Fitness: A Way of Life, 2nd ed. New York, John Wiley & Sons, 1979 1973

Kuntzleman CT: The Complete Book of Walking. New York, Simon and Schuster, 1979

## Nutrition/Dental

Beal VA: Nutrition in the Life Span. New York, John Wiley & Sons, 1980

Diet and Dental Health. Chicago, IL, American Dental Association, 1975

A Healthier Mouth: It's Up to You. Jersey City, NJ, Block Drug Company, 1975

McGill M, Pye O: The No-Nonsense Guide to Food and Nutrition. New York, Butterick Publishing, 1978

## Community Wellness Resource Centers

The Center for Health Promotion, 601 Brookdale Towers, 2810 Fifty-seventh Avenue N, Minneapolis, MN 55430

Good Health Program, Skokie Valley Community Hospital, 9600 Gross Point Road, Skokie, Illinois 60076

## Organizations

American Cancer Society
American Dental Association
American Heart Association

# Home Maintenance Management, Impaired

## Definition

Impaired home maintenance management: The state in which an individual or family experiences or is at risk to experience a difficulty in maintaining self or family in a safe home environment

## Etiological and Contributing Factors

Pathophysiological

Chronic debilitating disease

|  |  |
|---|---|
| Diabetes mellitus | Cancer |
| Chronic obstructive pulmonary | Arthritis |
| disease | Multiple sclerosis |
| Congestive heart failure | Muscular dystrophy |

Situational

Injury to individual or family member (fractured limb, spinal cord injury)
  Surgery (amputation, ostomy)
  Impaired mental status (memory lapses, depression, anxiety—severe, panic)
  Substance abuse (alcohol, drugs)
  Unavailable support system
  Loss of family member
  Addition of family member (newborn, aged parent)
  Lack of knowledge
  Insufficient finances

Maturational

Infant: Newborn care, high risk for sudden infant death syndrome
Elderly: Family member with deficits (cognitive, motor, sensory)

## Defining Characteristics

Outward expressions of difficulty by individual or family
  In maintaining the home (cleaning, repairs, financial needs)
  In caring for self or family member at home
Poor hygienic practices

|  |  |
|---|---|
| Infections | Unwashed cooking and eating |
| Infestations | equipment |
| Accumulated wastes | Offensive odors |

Impaired caregiver

|  |  |
|---|---|
| Overtaxed | Lack of knowledge |
| Anxious | Negative response to ill member |

Unavailable support system

## Focus Assessment Criteria

Owing to the variability and complexity of this diagnostic category, the nurse must determine whether the entire assessment must be performed or just selected areas. For example, if an elderly man lives alone, delete the assessment of the family. If a family is in crisis (financial or emotional), delete assessment of the functional status of the individual.

If a member is ill or disabled, the entire assessment may be indicated.

### Subjective data

### Assessment of individual function

Vision
    Adequate
    Corrected (date of last prescription)
    Complaints of
            Blurriness                Difficulty in focusing
            Loss of side vision       Inability to adjust to darkness
Hearing
    Adequate
    Use of hearing aid (condition, batteries)
    Need to lip-read
Thermal/tactile
    Adequate
    Altered sense of cold/hot
Mental status
    Alert
    Drowsy
    Confused
    Oriented to time, place, events
    Complaints of
            Vertigo                  Orthostatic hypotension
            Altered sense of balance
Mobility
    Ability to ambulate
            Around room           Around house
            Up and down stairs     Outside house
    Ability to travel
            Drive car (date of last     Use public transportation
              reevaluation)         Get in and out of vehicles
    Devices
            Cane                   Prosthesis
            Wheelchair          Condition of devices
            Walker              Competence in their use
    Shoes/slippers
            Proper fit             Nonskid soles
            Condition
Self-care activities: ability to
            Dress and undress     Use the toilet
            Groom self           Eat
            Bathe

Housekeeping activities: ability to

| | |
|---|---|
| Clean | Shop |
| Launder clothes | Prepare food |

Miscellaneous

Drug therapy

| | |
|---|---|
| Type, dosage | Storage |
| Labeling | Ability to self-medicate safely |

Communication: ability to

| | |
|---|---|
| Write | Contact emergency assistance |
| Use phone | |

Support system

| | |
|---|---|
| Help available from relatives, friends, neighbors | Club or religious contacts |
| | Emergency help available |

Community resources (*e.g.,* public health nurses, homemaker service, Meals on Wheels)

## Objective data

### Assessment of individual function

Physical appearance (groomed, unkempt)
Gait (steady, unsteady, use of aids)
Cognitive processes
Ability to communicate needs
Ability to interact
History of wandering (witnessed, reported by others)
Assess for presence of

| | |
|---|---|
| Anger | Withdrawal |
| Depression | Faulty judgment |

Treatment-related activities
Presence of barriers to performance

| | |
|---|---|
| Lack of knowledge | Sensory deficits (visual, tactile) |
| Lack of resources (support system, equipment, financial) | Cognitive deficits |
| | Emotional deficits |
| Motor deficits (weakness, paralysis, amputation) | Environmental (bathroom/water not accessible) |

### Assessment of family function

(The following focuses on the assessment of the ability of the family to care for family member at home. For an assessment of the family unit, refer to assessment criteria for *Alterations in Family Processes.*)
Knowledge and skills
Assess the family or caretaker for ability to perform the following safely and correctly

| | |
|---|---|
| Treatments | Emergency treatment if appropriate (*e.g.,* cardiac arrest, seizures) |
| Bathing | |
| Medication administration | |

Emotional response
Assess the family or caretaker for the presence of

| | |
|---|---|
| Overprotecting the person | Inability to ask for or accept relief from responsibilities |
| Neglect of other family members | |
| Neglect of other responsibilities | Unrealistic expectations of future recovery |
| Resentment of responsibilities | |

Assess the disabled or ill individual for the presence of

| Impossible demands upon time of caretaker | Lack of diversional activities |
| Resentment when caretaker is away | Lack of vocational or educational pursuits |

Resources

Assess knowledge of family or caretaker of resources available for

| Emergency care | Relief from caretaking |
| Equipment | responsibilities |
|   Purchase |   Close relative or neighbor |
|   Maintenance |   Church group |
|   Repair |   Community agency |
|   Financial support | Medical follow-up care |

## Assessment of housing

Type (rent, own)

    Apartment        Duplex        Single family house

Appearance: presence of

| Insects (flies, roaches) | Unwashed cooking equipment |
| Rodents/vermin | Accumulation of dirt, food |
| Offensive odors |   wastes, or hygiene wastes |

Physical facilities

| Number of rooms for family members | Lighting |
| | Water supply |
| Toilet facilities (accessibility) | Sewage |
| Heating | Garbage disposal |
| Ventilation | |

Safety

Are there any adaptations that need to be made in the home for the individual?

    Better communication (telephone)

    Access (in and out of home, to rooms)

    Bathroom (*e.g.*, grab bar, bath bench, nonskid floors).

Refer to Focus Assessment Criteria for *Potential for Injury* for an assessment of hazards in the home.

## Nursing Goals

Through selected interventions the nurse will

- Identify potential home maintenance problems before discharge
- Assist the person or the family to acquire the needed assistance at home
- Educate the person and the family when additional assistance is indicated

## Principles and Rationale for Nursing Care

1. Home care by professionals should be preventive, supportive, and therapeutic.

   *Preventive* measures include health education, home safety, and stress management.

   *Supportive* care can be legal, financial, nutritional, social, religious, and homemaking.

   *Therapeutic* care involves nursing care, therapists (occupational, speech), dental, and medical.

2. Discharge planning begins at admission, with the nurse determining the anticipated needs of the person and family after discharge: the individual's self-care

ability, the availability of support, homemaker services, equipment needs, community nursing services, and therapy (physical, speech, occupational).

3. The home environment must be assessed for safety prior to discharge: location of bathroom, access to water, cooking facilities, and environmental barriers (stairs, narrow doorways).

4. Community agencies can provide the opportunity for home care and allow for the person to remain at home.

5. In determining an individual's ability to care for himself at home, assess his ability to function and protect self. Consider such things as: motor deficits, sensory deficits, and mental status.

6. To assess, teach, and evaluate the individual or the family's ability to perform learned skills after discharge, use on-unit situations, whereby the person(s) takes responsibility for care, and day, overnight, or weekend leave to home. A home visit may be indicated by a nurse or a community health nurse.

7. Some families are unable to meet the home needs of ill members and require assistance. Families who are able to meet the needs of ill members should also be provided with periodic assistance or relief.

8. The effects on the life of a caretaker of a chronically ill person depend on (Goldstein):

   The ill person's level of disability and dependence

   The health and functional mobility of the caretaker

   The availability of assistance (type and frequency)

   The other responsibilities the caretaker has

9. The time and energy demands of caretaking may compete with other role responsibilities, e.g., spouse, mothering, occupational.

10. Role fatigue describes the situation when the caregiver must devote the majority of time to caregiving, thus requiring that all other roles and responsibilities be subordinated to the demands of caretaking.

11. Persons and families with cancer have certain ongoing needs that may necessitate interventions at home:

    Teaching needs (disease, treatment, diagnostic studies)

    Surgery (recovery, wound care)

    Coping with the diagnosis

    Fear of the future

    Treatment effects and side-effects (radiotherapy, chemotherapy)

    Inability to perform role responsibilities

    Biologic needs (disease- or treatment-related), *e.g.*, nutrition, elimination, comfort

# Impaired Home Maintenance Management
Related to (specify etiological or contributing factors)

*Example:* **Impaired Home Maintenance Management**
       *related to*  **Inability to Perform Household Activities**
       *related to*  **Post Myocardial Infarction**

**Assessment**

Refer to Defining Characteristics

---

**Outcome Criteria**

The person or caretaker will
- Identify factors that restrict self-care and home management
- Demonstrate the ability to perform skills necessary for the care of the individual or home
- Express satisfaction with home situation

---

**Interventions**

The following interventions apply to most individuals with impaired home management, regardless of etiology.

A. Assess for causative or contributing factors

Lack of knowledge
Insufficient funds
Lack of necessary equipment or aids
Inability to perform household activities (illness, sensory deficits, motor deficits)
Impaired cognitive functioning
Impaired emotional functioning

B. Reduce or eliminate causative or contributing factors if possible

1. Lack of knowledge for home care
   - Determine with the person and family the information needed to be taught and learned
   - Initiate the teaching
   - Refer to a community nursing agency for follow-up
   - Refer to *Knowledge Deficit* for additional interventions on teaching
2. Lack of necessary equipment or aids
   - Determine the type of equipment needed, considering availability, cost, and durability
   - Seek assistance from agencies that rent or loan supplies
     a. Teach the care and maintenance of supplies to increase length of use
     b. Consider adapting equipment to reduce cost
3. Insufficient funds
   - Consult with social service department for assistance

- Consult with service organizations for assistance
    - American Heart Association
    - The Lung Association
    - American Cancer Society
4. Inability to perform household activities
    Determine the type of assistance needed (*e.g.*, meals, housework, transportation) and assist the individual to obtain them
    a. Meals
        - Discuss with relatives the possibility of freezing complete meals that require only heating (*e.g.*, small containers of soup, stew, casseroles)
        - Determine the availability of meal services for ill persons (Meals on Wheels, church groups)
        - Teach persons about foods that are easily prepared and nutritious (*e.g.*, hard-boiled eggs)
    b. Housework
        - Contract with an adolescent for light housekeeping
        - Refer to community agency for assistance
    c. Transportation
        - Determine the availability of transportation for shopping and health care
        - Request rides with neighbors to places they drive routinely
5. Impaired mental processes
    - Assess the ability of the individual to safely maintain a household
    - Refer to *Potential for Injury* related to lack of awareness of hazards
6. Impaired emotional functioning
    - Assess the severity of the dysfunction
    - Refer to *Ineffective Individual Coping* for additional assessment and interventions

## C. Initiate health teaching and referrals as indicated

1. Discuss the implications of caring for a chronically ill family member
    Amount of time
    Effects on other role responsibilities (spouse, children, job)
    Physical requirements (lifting)
2. Share alternatives to reduce strain and fatigue of caretaking responsibilities
    - Acquire relief from responsibilities at least twice a week for at least 3 hours (sitter, neighbors, relatives)
    - Enlist the aid of others to meet some of the needs of the ill person (hairdresser, transporting to physician's office)
    - Plan to utilize at least one hour each day as leisure time (*e.g.*, after ill person is asleep)
    - Maintain contacts with friends and relatives even if only by phone; let friends know that you do use sitters so they can include you in some social activities
    - Allow the caretaker opportunities to share problems and feelings
    - Commend caregivers for their concern, diligence, and perseverance in caring for the loved one at home

## Bibliography

Craven R: The effects of illness on family function. Nurs Forum 2:191–193, 1972
Davis AJ: Disability, home care, and the caretaking role in family life. J Adv Nurs 5:475–484, 1980

Edstrom S, Miller MW: Preparing the family to care for the cancer patient at home: A home care course. Cancer Nursing 4:49–52, 1981

Eggert GM, Granger CV, Morris R et al: Caring for the patient with long-term disability. Geriatrics 32(6):102–106, 1977

Ellmyer P, Thomas N: A guide to your patient's safe home use of oxygen. Nursing 12(1):55–57, 1982

Ford M, Wasilewicz C: Bridging the gap between hospital and home. Canadian Nurse 77(1):44–47, 1981

Fortinsky R, Granger CV, Seltzer GB: The use of functional assessment in understanding home care needs. Med Care 19:489–497, 1981

Goldstein V: Caretaker Role Fatigue. Nurs Outlook 29:23–30, 1981

Googe M, Varricchio C: A pilot investigation of home health care needs of cancer patients and their families. Oncology Nursing Forum 8(3):24–28, 1981

Harvey BL: Your patient's discharge plan: Does it include home care referral? Nursing 11(7):48–51, 1981

Heller BR, Walsh FJ, Wilson KM: Seniors helping seniors: Training older adults as new personnel resources in home health care. Journal of Gerontological Nursing 7:552–555, 1981

Hunter G, Johnson SH: Physical support systems for the homebound oncology patient. Oncology Nursing Forum 7(3):21–23, 1980

Jelneck LJ: The special needs of the adolescent with chronic illness. Matern Child Nurs J 2: 57–61, 1977

Klopovich P, Suenram D, Cairns N: A common sense approach to caring for children with cancer: The community health nurse. Cancer Nursing 3:201–208, 1980

MacVicar M, Archoid PA: A framework for family assessment in chronic illness. Nurs Forum 15:180–194, 1976

Pigg J: Fifty helpful hints for active arthritis patients. Nursing 4(4):39–41, 1974

Rathlev M, McNamara M: Teaching families to give trach care at home. Nursing 12(6):70–71, 1982

Symposium on community health/home care. Nurs Clin North Am 15:321–428, 1980

White HA, Briggs AM: Home care of persons with respiratory problems. Topics in Clinical Nursing 2(4):69–77, 1980

# Injury, Potential for

*Related to* **Sensory or Motor Deficits**

*Related to* **Lack of Awareness of Environmental Hazards**

## Definition

Potential for injury: The state in which an individual is at risk for injury because of a perceptual or physiological deficit, a lack of awareness, or maturational age.

## Etiological and Contributing Factors

Pathophysiological

Altered cerebral function

| | |
|---|---|
| Tissue hypoxia | Syncope |
| Post trauma | Confusion |
| Vertigo | |

Altered mobility

| | |
|---|---|
| Unsteady gait | Loss of limb |

Impaired sensory function

| | |
|---|---|
| Vision | Thermal/touch |
| Hearing | Smell |

Pain

Fatigue

Situational

Faulty judgment

Drugs

Alcohol

Poisons (plants, toxic chemicals)

Household hazards

| | |
|---|---|
| Unsafe walkways | Faulty electric wires |
| Unsafe toys | Improperly stored poisons |

Automotive hazards

| | |
|---|---|
| Lack of use of seat belts or child seats | Mechanically unsafe vehicle |

Fire hazards

| | |
|---|---|
| Smoking in bed | Improperly stored petroleum products |
| Gas leaks | |

Unfamiliar setting (hospital, nursing home)

Improper footwear

Inattentive caretaker

Improper use of aids (crutches, canes, walkers, wheelchairs)

## Maturational

Infant/child
> Suffocation hazards (improper crib, pillow in crib, plastic bags, unattended in water—bath, pool)
> Improper use of bicycles, kitchen utensils/appliances, sports equipment, lawn equipment
> Poison (plants, cleaning agents, medications)
> Fire (matches, fireplace, stove)

Adolescent: Automobile, bicycle, alcohol, drugs
Adult: Automobile, alcohol
Elderly: Motor and sensory deficits, medication (accidental overdose)

## Defining Characteristics

> Evidence of environmental hazards*
> Lack of knowledge of environmental hazards
> Lack of knowledge of safety precautions
> History of accidents
> Impaired mobility
> Sensory deficits

## Focus Assessment Criteria

This entire assessment is only indicated when the individual is at high risk for injury because of personal deficits or alterations (*e.g.*, mobility problems). In households without such a family member, the functional assessment of the individual can be deleted.

### Subjective data

### Physical capabilities of the individual

1. Vision
   Adequate
   Corrected (date of last prescription)
   Complaints of

|  |  |
|---|---|
| Blurriness | Difficulty in focusing |
| Loss of side vision | Inability to adjust to darkness |

2. Hearing

|  |  |
|---|---|
| Adequate | Need to read lips |
| Use of hearing aid (condition, batteries) | Inadequate |

3. Thermal/tactile

|  |  |
|---|---|
| Adequate | Altered sense of hot/cold |

4. Mental status

|  |  |
|---|---|
| Alert | Complaints of |
| Drowsy | Vertigo |
| Confused | Altered sense of balance |
| Oriented to time, place, events | Orthostatic hypotension |

*(See Etiological and Contributing Factors and Focus Assessment Criteria for specific hazards)

5. Mobility
Ability to ambulate

| | |
|---|---|
| Around room | Around house |
| Up and down stairs | Outside house |

Ability to travel

| | |
|---|---|
| Drive car (date of last reevaluation) | Use public transportation |

Devices

| | |
|---|---|
| Cane | Prosthesis |
| Wheelchair | Condition of devices |
| Walker | Competence in their use |

Shoes/slippers

| | |
|---|---|
| Condition | Nonskid soles |
| Fit | |

6. Self-care activities: ability to

| | |
|---|---|
| Dress and undress | Bathe self |
| Groom self | Eat |
| Reach the toilet | |

7. Housekeeping activities: ability to

| | |
|---|---|
| Clean | Shop |
| Launder clothes | Prepare food |

8. Miscellaneous
Drug therapy

| | |
|---|---|
| Type, dosage | Storage |
| Labeling | Ability to self-medicate safely |

Communication

| | |
|---|---|
| Can write | Contact emergency assistance |
| Use phone | |

Support system

| | |
|---|---|
| Help available from relatives, friends, neighbor | Club and church contacts |

## Objective data

## Physical capabilities of the individual

Gait

| | | |
|---|---|---|
| Steady | Unsteady | Requires aids |

Cognitive processes
Ability to communicate needs
Ability to interact
History of wandering (witnessed and reported by others)
Assess for presence of

| | |
|---|---|
| Anger | Withdrawal |
| Depression | Faulty judgment |

Self-care activities: ability to

| | |
|---|---|
| Dress and undress | Bathe |
| Groom self | Eat |
| Reach toilet | |

## Housing assessment

Rent or own
Type (apartment, duplex, single family house)
Physical amenities

| | |
|---|---|
| Number of rooms for family members | Lighting |
| | Water supply |
| Toilet facilities | Sewage |
| Heating | Garbage disposal |
| Ventilation | |

Safety
    Adaptations that may need to be made
        Better communication facilities (telephone)
        Easier passage from room to room and into and out of house
        Bathroom safety (grab bar, bath bench, nonskid floors)
    Walkways (inside and outside)
        Sidewalks (uneven, broken)
        Stairs (inside and outside)

| | |
|---|---|
| Broken steps | Lighting |
| No hand rails | Protection for children |

        Halls

| | |
|---|---|
| Cluttered | Poor lighting |

    Electrical considerations
        Cords frayed and unanchored
        Outlets overloaded; accessible to children; near water
        Switches too far from bedside
    Lighting
        Adequate or inadequate
        At night; and outdoors
        To bathroom at night
    Floors
        Even or uneven
        Highly polished
        Rugs not anchored
    Kitchen
        Stove (grease or flammable objects on stove)
        Refrigerator (improperly stored food; inadequate temperatures)
    Toxic substances
        Stored in food containers and not properly labeled
        Medications kept beyond date of expiration
    Fire protection
        No fire extinguishers
        Improper storage of corrosives, combustibles
        Lack of furnace maintenance
        No fire escape plan
        Emergency phone numbers not accessible (firehouse, police)
    Hazards for children in nursery
        Cribs with wide slat openings
        Plastic bags
        Pillows in crib
        Space between mattress and crib rails

        Unattended without crib rails up
        Unattended on changing table
        Pacifier hung around infant's neck
        A propped bottle placed in infant's crib
        Toys with pointed edges, removable parts
    Hazards for children in household
        Objects with lead paint
        Poisonous plants (see Table II–4 for specific plants)
        Open windows without screens
        Plastic bags
        Furniture with glass or sharp corners
        Open doorways, stairways
    Outdoor hazards for children
        Porches without rails
        Play area without fence
        Backyard pools

## Nursing Goals

Through selected interventions, the nurse will seek to
- Identify the accident-prone individual
- Assist the person and his family in identifying hazards and related safety measures
- Prevent injury to the individual

Table II-4.   **Poisonous Substances Around the House**

**Drugs**

| | | |
|---|---|---|
| Aspirin | Cough medicines | Laxatives |
| Tranquilizers | Vitamins | Oral contraceptives |
| Barbiturates | | |

**Petroleum products**

**Cleaning agents**

| | | |
|---|---|---|
| Soaps and polishes | Disinfectants | Drain cleaners |

**Poisonous plants**

| | | |
|---|---|---|
| Amaryllis | Holly | Oleander |
| Azalea | Iris | Poinsettia |
| Baneberry | Jack-in-the-pulpit | Poison hemlock |
| Belladonna | Jerusalem cherry | Poison ivy |
| Bittersweet | Jimsonweed | Pokeweed |
| Bloodroot | Lily of the valley | Potato leaves |
| Castor-bean plant | Marijuana | Rhododendron |
| Climbing nightshade | Mistletoe | Rhubarb leaves |
| Daffodil | Morning glory | Tomato leaves |
| Dieffenbachia | Mountain laurel | Wisteria |
| Foxglove | Mushrooms | Yew |

**Miscellaneous**

| | | |
|---|---|---|
| Baby powder | Cosmetics | Lead paint |

## Principles and Rationale for Nursing Care

### General

1. There is an increased incidence of injuries in the confused elderly. Confusion in the aged can result from
   Toxic effects of drugs
   Sensory overload (too many details in a new situation)
   Physiological states such as fatigue or elimination problems (*e.g.*, constipation or a full bladder) or pain
   Sensoriperceptual problems
   Hypoxia
2. Dangerous drugs and products that are accessible to children and confused persons can result in accidental poisoning.
3. Accidents occur more frequently
   During the initial period of hospitalization and between the hours of 6 and 9 P.M.
   During peak activity periods (mealtime, playtime)
   In unfamiliar surroundings
   With inadequate lighting
   At holidays
   On vacations
   During home repairs
4. Seventy percent of all fatal falls occur in people 65 years of age and over (National Safety Council).
5. The highest risk for falls occurs in people who are confused or agitated.
6. Persons over 60 usually need twice as much light to perform a task as a 20-year-old.
7. Visual difficulty because of glare is often responsible for falls in the aged, who have an increased susceptibility to glare. Incandescent (nonfluorescent) lighting produces less glare and therefore provides better illumination for the aged.
8. Color contrast between the object and the background increases visualization (*e.g.*, white against black).
9. Fasting for diagnostic tests causes dehydration and weakness that contribute to accidents.
10. Falls can result when urinary urgency and frequency cause a person to rush to the bathroom.
11. Some common drugs contributing to postural hypotension are:

| | |
|---|---|
| Diuretics | Antihistamines |
| Phenothiazides | Alcohol |
| Antidepressants | Levodopa |
| Barbiturates | Diazepam |

12. Table II-4 lists common sources of poisoning in the home.

### Children

1. Accidents rank number one as the cause of death and injury for children under the age of 19.
2. Mechanical suffocation is the most frequent accident for infants under 1 year of age.
3. Accidental poisoning is the major cause of death in children from 1 to 5 years old (see Table II-4).

4. In each stage of development, a child is prone to a specific type of accident.

| | |
|---|---|
| Under 1 | Mechanical suffocation |
| 1 to 3 | Burns and poisoning |
| 3 to 5 | Motor vehicles |
| School age | Fire, water, motor vehicles, bicycles, playground equipment, animal bites |

5. Traditional lap belts should only be worn by children over 40 or 50 pounds, and the shoulder belt should not be used for children weighing less than 55 pounds because the danger of strangulation.
6. Children should be taught early (when 2 years old) and constantly reminded about rules regarding streets, playground equipment, fires, water (pools, bathtubs), animals, strangers

# Potential for Injury
## Related to Sensory or Motor Deficits

## Assessment

### Subjective data

The person reports
Past history of falls and injuries

| | |
|---|---|
| Decreased or absent vision | Limited movement |
| Decreased or absent hearing | Pain |
| Decreased or absent thermal perception | Vertigo |

### Objective data

| | |
|---|---|
| Inflamed joints | Muscle spasm |
| Contractures | Crutches |
| Skeletal deformities | Walker, cane |
| Unsteady gait | Prosthesis |
| Paralysis | Evidence of past injuries |
| Weakness | (bruises, burn marks) |

---

### Outcome Criteria

The person will
- Identify factors that increase the potential for injury
- Utilize safety measures to prevent injury (*e.g.*, remove throw rugs or anchor them)
- Practice selected prevention measures (*e.g.*, wear sunglasses to reduce glare)
- Increase his daily activity, if feasible

---

**Interventions**

A. Assess for the presence of causative or contributing factors

Unfamiliar surroundings
Impaired vision
    Altered spatial judgment
    Blurred vision
    Diplopia
    Blind spots
    Cataracts
    Altered peripheral vision
    Hemianopia (loss of half the visual field)
    Increased susceptibility to visual glare
    Decreased ability to distinguish object from background
Decreased hearing acuity
Decreased tactile sensitivity (touch)
Orthostatic hypotension
Unstable gait
    Pain
    Fatigue
    Improper shoes or slippers
    Improper use of crutches, canes, walkers
    Joint immobility
Side-effects of medication (*e.g.*, tranquilizers, diuretics)
Hazardous environmental factors

B. Reduce or eliminate causative or contributing factors if possible

1. Unfamiliar surroundings
   - Orient each new admission to surroundings, explain the call system, and assess the person's ability to use it
   - Closely supervise the person during the first few nights to assess safety
   - Utilize night light
   - Encourage the person to request assistance during the night
   - Teach the person about side-effects of certain drugs (*e.g.*, dizziness, fatigue)
   - Keep bed at lowest level during the night
2. Impaired vision
   a. Provide safe illumination or teach person to
      - Provide adequate lighting in all rooms, with soft light at night
      - Have light switch easily accessible, next to bed
      - Provide background light that is soft
   b. Teach person to reduce glare
      - Avoid all glossy surfaces (*e.g.*, glass, highly polished floors)
      - Use diffuse light rather than direct light; use shades that darken the room
      - Turn head away when switching on a bright light
      - Wear sunglasses or hats with brims, or carry umbrellas, to reduce glare outside
      - Avoid looking directly at bright lights (*e.g.*, headlights)
   c. Teach person or family to provide sufficient color contrast for visual discrimination
      - Color-code edges of steps (*e.g.*, with colored tape)

- Avoid white walls, dishes, counters
- Avoid clear glasses (*i.e.,* use smoked glass)
- Choose objects colored black on white (*e.g.,* black phone)
- Avoid colors that merge (*e.g.,* beige switches on beige walls)
- Paint doorknobs bright colors

3. Decreased tactile sensitivity
   a. Teach preventive measures
      - Assess temperature of bath water and heating pads prior to use
      - Use bath thermometers
      - Assess extremities daily for undetected injuries
      - Keep feet warm and dry and skin softened with emollient lotion (lanolin, mineral oil)
   b. See *Alteration in Tissue Perfusion: Peripheral* for additional interventions

4. Decreased hearing acuity
   - Determine if the person has had his hearing evaluated professionally
   - Assist him in making a decision regarding the use or type of hearing aid if indicated
   - Teach him, when driving, to leave car window partially open to allow warning signals to be heard (*e.g.,* sirens) and set air conditioner, heater, or radio low so outside noises can be heard

5. Orthostatic hypotension
   a. Instruct individual to change positions slowly
      - Sit before standing
      - Stand still briefly before walking
      - Hold on to something
      - Avoid sudden movements (*e.g.,* sudden hyperextension of neck or back)
   b. See *Alteration in Tissue Perfusion: Cerebral: Orthostatic Hypotension* for additional interventions

6. Unstable gait
   a. Crutches
      - Teach exercises to strengthen arm and shoulder muscles to facilitate use of crutches; use weights and parallel bars
      - Measure and fit crutches to each person (2 to 3 inches between top of crutch and armpit); improper length of crutches may cause nerve damage or falls
      - Instruct person to wear shoes that fit properly and have nonskid soles
      - Assess ability to walk and climb up and down stairs
      - Consult with physical therapist for proper gait training
   b. Canes
      - Teach person to hold cane in hand opposite affected leg and move cane and impaired limb together
      - Cane should be proper length to allow person to extend elbow and bear weight on hand
      - Cane should be fitted with rubber tip
      - Consult with physical therapist for proper gait training
   c. Walkers
      - Teach person exercises to strengthen triceps muscles used in proper crutch walking
      - See that floors are clean and dry and free of obstacles and that rugs are anchored
      - Instruct person to wear properly fitted shoes with nonslip soles
      - Consult with physical therapist for proper gait training

  d.  Prosthesis
- Teach person to bathe and inspect stump daily
- Instruct to put on prosthesis soon after rising to minimize stump swelling
- Prepare person for crutch walking with triceps exercises using weights and parallel bars
- Consult with physical therapist for proper gait training
7. Side-effects of medications
- Assess for the presence of side-effects of drugs that may cause vertigo

| | |
|---|---|
| Hypotension | Vasodilation |
| Sedation | Vasoconstriction |
| Hypokalemia | |

8. Hazardous environmental factors
  a.  Teach person to
- Eliminate throw rugs, litter, and highly polished floors
- Provide nonslip surfaces in bathtub or shower by applying commercially available traction tapes
- Provide hand grips in bathroom
- Provide railings in hallways and on stairs
- Remove protruding objects (*e.g.*, coat hooks, shelves, light fixtures) from stairway walls
  b.  Instruct staff to
- Keep side rails on bed in place and bed at the lowest position when person is left unattended
- Keep bed at lowest position with wheels locked when stationary
- Teach person in wheelchair to lock and unlock wheels
- Ensure that person's shoes or slippers have nonskid soles

## C. Initiate health teaching and referrals as indicated

1. Teach measures to prevent auto accidents
- Frequently reevaluate ability to drive vehicles
- Wear good-quality sunglasses (gray or green) to reduce glare
- Keep windshields clean and wipers in good condition
- Place mirrors on both sides of car
- Stop periodically to stretch and rest eyes
- Know the effects of medications on driving ability
- Do not smoke while driving or drive after drinking

2. Teach measures to prevent pedestrian accidents
- Allow enough time to cross streets
- Wear garments that reflect light (beige, white) at night
- Wait to cross on the sidewalk, not the street
- Look both ways
- Do not rely solely on green traffic lights to provide safe crossing (right turn on red light may be legal, or driver may disobey traffic regulations)

3. Teach measures to prevent burns
- Equip home with smoke alarm system and check its function each month
- Have a hand fire extinguisher
- Set thermostats for water heater to provide warm but not scalding water
- Use baking soda or a lid cover to smother a kitchen grease fire
- Do not wear loose-fitting clothing (*e.g.*, robes, nightgowns) when cooking
- Do not smoke when sleepy

- Ensure that portable heaters are safely used
- See *Potential for Injury Related to Lack of Awareness of Environmental Hazards* for additional safety measures

4. Refer individuals with motor or sensory deficits for assistance in identifying environmental hazards
   - Local fire company
   - Community nursing agency
   - Accident-prevention information (see Bibliography)

5. Discuss the benefits of a walking program to increase circulation if permissible; instruct to
   - Rest 10 to 15 minutes before walking
   - Start slowly (10 minutes)
   - Increase time gradually
   - Refrain from drinking caffeine products (coffee, tea, chocolate, cola) 2 to 3 hours before walking
   - Wait 2 hours after meals to walk
   - Expect some muscle soreness; reduce activity if pain or breathlessness occur

6. Assist person and family to evaluate environmental hazards
7. Refer person to public health or visiting nurse for home visit
8. Refer person to physical therapist for evaluation of gait

# Potential for Injury
## Related to Lack of Awareness of Environmental Hazards

### Assessment

**Subjective data**

The person reports
    Past history of accidents

**Objective data**

Presence of hazards (see Focus Assessment Criteria)

---

**Outcome Criteria**

The person or family will
- Identify potentially hazardous factors in the environment
- Demonstrate safe practices in the home
- Teach children safety habits

## Interventions

A. Identify situations that contribute to accidents

Unfamiliar setting (homes of others, hotels)
Children
Peak activity periods (during meal preparation, holidays)
New equipment (bicycle, chain saw)
Lack of awareness of or disregard for environmental hazards

1. Unfamiliar setting
   * Instruct to leave a light on for access to bathroom during night
   * With small children, instruct parents to
     a. Inspect the area (inside and outside) for hazards before allowing child to play
     b. Expect the child to explore hidden areas
     c. Have infants sleep on floor on padding rather than in beds without rails

2. Children
   * Teach parents to expect frequent changes in infants' and children's ability and to take precautions (*e.g.*, infant who suddenly rolls over for the first time might be on a changing table unattended)
   * Discuss with parents the necessity of constant monitoring of small children
   * Provide parents with information to assist them in selecting a babysitter
     a. Determine previous experiences and knowledge of emergency measures
     b. Observe the interaction of the sitter with the child (*e.g.*, pick up the sitter one-half hour before you are ready to leave)
   * Teach parents to expect children to mimic them, and to teach children what they can do with or without supervision
     a. Tell the child to ask you before attempting a new task
     b. Don't take pills in front of children
   * Explain and expect compliance with certain rules (depending on age) regarding

     | | |
     |---|---|
     | Streets | Fire |
     | Playground equipment | Animals |
     | Water (pools, bathtubs) | Strangers |
     | Bicycles | |

   * Role-play with children to assess understanding of the problem
     "You are walking home from school and a strange man pulls up in a car near you. What do you do?"
     "While walking past a barbecue, your dress catches on fire. What do you do?"

3. Peak activity periods
   * Provide the child with a special distraction (*e.g.*, clay) while preparing the meal
   * Place the child in a playpen to provide a safe place that does not require close supervision
   * Assess the safety of holiday decorations prior to use
     Christmas trees

     | | |
     |---|---|
     | Fire or electrical hazard | Lighted candles |
     | Poorly anchored | Ceramic pieces |

4. New equipment
   - Teach to read directions completely before using a new appliance or a piece of equipment
   - Determine the limitations of the equipment
   - Unplug and turn off any appliance that is not functioning before examining (*e.g.*, lawnmower, snow blower, electric mixer)
   - Determine that a new bicycle is the correct size for the child before allowing unrestricted riding
   - Examine new toys for removable parts and chemical and electrical hazards before allowing child to play
5. Lack of awareness of or disregard for environmental hazards
   - Teach to avoid unsafe practices and prevent injury
     a. Automobiles
        Driving a mechanically unsafe vehicle
        Not using or misusing seat restraints
        Driving after partaking of alcohol or drugs
        Driving with unrestrained babies and children in the car
        Driving at excessive speeds
        Driving without necessary visual aids
        Driving with unsafe road or road crossing conditions
        Nonuse or misuse of necessary headgear for motorcyclist
        Children riding in front seat of car
        Backing up without checking location of small children
        Warming a car in a closed garage
     b. Bicycles, wagons, skateboards, and skates carrying passengers
        No reflectors or lights
        Not in single file
        Riding a too-large bicycle
        Lack of knowledge of rules of the road
        Use of skateboards or skates in heavily traveled areas
     c. Flammables
        Igniting gas leaks
        Delayed lighting of gas burner or oven
        Experimenting with chemicals or gasoline
        Unscreened fires, fireplaces, heaters
        Inadequately stored combustibles, matches, or oily rags
        Smoking in bed or near oxygen
        Highly flammable children's toys or clothing
        Playing with fireworks or gunpowder
        Playing with matches, candles, cigarettes
        Wearing of plastic aprons or flowing clothing around open flame
     d. Household
        Kitchen
              Grease waste collected on stoves
              Wearing of plastic aprons or flowing clothing around open flame
              Use of cracked glasses or dishware
              Use of improper canning, freezing, or preserving methods
              Knives stored in an uncovered fashion
              Pot handles facing front of stove
              Use of thin or worn potholders or oven mitts
              Stove controls on front

Bathroom
       Lack of grab rails in bathtub
       Lack of nonskid mats or emory strips in bathtub
       Poor lighting in bathroom and hallways
       Improper placement of electrical outlets
Chemicals and irritants
       Improperly labeled medication containers
       Medications kept in containers other than original ones
       Poor illumination at the medicine cabinet
       Improperly labeled containers of poisons and corrosive substances
       Expired medications that dangerously decompose
       Toxic substances stored in accessible areas (*e.g.*, under sink)
       Inadequately stored corrosives (*e.g.*, lye)
       Contact with intense cold
       Overexposure to sun, sunlamps, heating pads
Lighting and electrical
       Unanchored electrical wires
       Overloaded electrical outlets
       Overloaded fuse boxes
       Faulty electrical plugs, frayed wires, or defective electrical appliances
       Inadequate lighting over landings and stairs
       Inaccessible light switches (*e.g.*, bedside)
       Use of machinery or appliances without prior instruction
Miscellaneous
       Outdoor pools
       Obstructed passageways
       Unsafe window protection in home with young children
       Guns or ammunition stored in unlocked fashion
       Large icicles hanging from roof
       Icy walkways
       Glass sliding doors that look open when closed
       Low-strung clothesline
       Discarded or unused refrigerators or freezers without removed doors
e.  Infants and children
Household
       Pillows in crib
       Staircases without stair gates
       Crib mattresses that do not fit snugly
       Cribs with slat opening to allow child's body to fall through, catching the head
       Glass or sharp-edged tables
       Porches and decks without railings
       Poisonous plants (see Table II–4)
       Furniture painted with lead paint
       Unsupervised bathing
       Open windows
       Propped bottle in crib
Toys
       Sharp edges

Easily breakable parts
Removable small pieces
Balloons
Lollipops
Pacifier around neck
Miscellaneous
Unattended in shopping cart
Unattended in car
Cribs, walkers, high chairs with movable parts that trap child
(*e.g.*, springs)

## B. Initiate health teaching and referrals as indicated

- Instruct parents how to "child proof" the home
- Instruct parents to keep poisons and corrosive substances in tightly closed, carefully marked containers in locked closets
- Parents should discard unused supplies of medications and keep needed medications in locked, inaccessible medicine closet
- Parents should be taught how to administer antidotes for specific toxic substances
- Parents should also have the phone number of the Poison Control Center in a convenient place
- Refer individuals to local poison control center for "Mr. Yuk" poison warning stickers and advice on emergency procedures; teach the child what a Mr. Yuk sticker means
- Instruct parents on the use of ipecac and its availability
- Assist family to evaluate environmental hazards in home; consult public health agency
- Install specially designed locks to prevent children from opening closets where combustible, corrosive, or flammable materials or medications are stored
- Instruct parents to use socket covers to prevent accidental electric shocks to children
- Teach parents about hazards of lead paint ingestion and how to identify "pica" in a child
- Refer parents to public health department if lead paint screening is necessary
- Encourage use of child-proof caps
- Advise parents to avoid storing dangerous substances in containers ordinarily used for foods
- Refer parents to automobile club for information regarding safety car seats for children
- Refer parents to local fire department for assistance in staging home fire drills

## Bibliography

### Articles

Cooper S: Accidents and older adults. Geriatric Nursing 2:287–290, 1981

Kulikowski E: A study of accidents in a hospital. Supervisor Nurse 8(3):64–68, 1979

Lynn FH: Incidents—need they be accidents? Am J Nurs 80:1098–1101, 1980

McIntire M, Angle CR: Poison control: A model for childhood safety. Pediatrician 5:180–184, 1976

Rauckhorst LM: Community and home assessment. Journal of Gerontological Nursing 6:319–327, 1980

Riffle K: Falls: Kinds, causes, and prevention. Geriatric Nursing 3:165–169, 1982

Simons RS: The occupational health nurse: Safety's overlooked resource. Occupational Health Nurse 28(2):7–12, 1980

Wheatley G: Introduction: Childhood accidents. Pediatr Ann 6(11):12–26, 1977

Witte N: Why the elderly fall. Am J Nurs 79:1154–1160, 1979

## Pertinent Literature and Organizations for the Consumer

Making Products Safer (Pamphlet no. 524)

What Should Parents Expect from Children? (Pamphlet no. 357)

Request the above and a list of other publications from Public Affairs Pamphlets, 381 Park Avenue South, New York, NY 10016 (50 cents for each pamphlet).

Fontana VJ: A Parents' Guide to Child Safety. New York, TY Crowell, 1973

Poison Prevention Packaging available free from the Consumer Product Safety Commission, Washington, DC 20207

# Knowledge Deficit

## Definition

Knowledge deficit: The state in which the individual experiences a deficiency in cognitive knowledge or psychomotor skills that alters or may alter health maintenance.

## Etiological and Contributing Factors

A variety of factors can produce knowledge deficits. Some common causes are listed below.

### Pathophysiological

Any existing or new medical condition

### Situational

Language differences
Prescribed treatments (new, complex)
Diagnostic tests
Surgical procedures
Medications
Pregnancy
Personal characteristics

| | | |
|---|---|---|
| Lack of motivation | Ineffective coping patterns |
| Denial of situation | (*e.g.*, anxiety, depression) |

### Maturational

Children

| | | |
|---|---|---|
| Sexuality and sexual development | Substance abuse |
| | Nutrition |
| Safety hazards | |

Adolescents

| | |
|---|---|
| Same as children | Substance abuse (alcohol, drugs, |
| Automobile safety practices | tobacco) |
| | Health maintenance practices |

Adults

| | |
|---|---|
| Parenthood | Safety practices |
| Sexual function | Health maintenance practices |

Elderly

| | |
|---|---|
| Effects of aging | Sensory deficits |

## Defining Characteristics

Verbalizes a deficiency in knowledge or skill
Expresses "inaccurate" perception of health status
Does not perform correctly a desired or prescribed health behavior

Does not comply (noncompliance) with prescribed health behavior

Exhibits or expresses psychological alteration (*e.g.,* anxiety, depression) resulting from misinformation or lack of information.

## Focus Assessment Criteria

This assessment is structured primarily to collect data to determine the person's learning capabilities and limitations.

## Subjective data

1. Determine present knowledge of
   Illness

   | | |
   |---|---|
   | Severity | Susceptibility to complications |
   | Prognosis | Ability to cure it or control its progression |

   Treatment
   Preventive measures

2. What is the pattern of adhering to prescribed health behaviors?

   | | |
   |---|---|
   | Complete | Not adhering |
   | Modified | |

3. What is interfering with adherence to the prescribed health behavior?
4. History of disease
   Onset
   Symptoms
   Effects on life-style (relationships, work, leisure activities, finances)
5. Stage of adaptation to disease

   | | |
   |---|---|
   | Disbelief | Anger |
   | Denial | Awareness |
   | Depression | Acceptance |

6. Learning needs (perceived by client, family)
7. Learning ability (client, family)

   | | |
   |---|---|
   | Level of education | Language spoken |
   | Ability to read | Language understood |

8. Ethnic background

   | | |
   |---|---|
   | Traditions | Health care beliefs and practices |
   | Life-style | |

## Objective data

1. Ability to perform prescribed procedures

   | | |
   |---|---|
   | Competency | Accuracy |

2. Level of cognitive and psychomotor development

   | | |
   |---|---|
   | Age | Ability to read and write |

3. Presence of sensory deficits
   Vision

   | | |
   |---|---|
   | Problems in focusing | Partial or total blindness |
   | Inability to distinguish colors | |

   Hearing

   | | |
   |---|---|
   | Partial or total deafness | Tinnitus |

   Sense of smell (altered or lost)
   Sense of taste (altered or lost)
   Sense of touch

   | | |
   |---|---|
   | Anesthesia | Paresthesia |

4. Physical stability
   a.  Circulation/tissue perfusion
       General appearance
       Arterial blood pressure
       Pulse rate and regularity
       Pulse volume (weak, thready, full, bounding)
       Skin (color, temperature, moisture)
       Urine output
       Level of consciousness
   b.  Respiratory status
       Rate
       Pattern
       Presence of abnormal breath sounds
       Altered blood gases
       Restlessness
       Irritability
   c.  Nutritional/hydration status
       Fluid and electrolyte balance (Na, K, urine specific gravity, skin turgor)
       Intake and output
       Weight change
   d.  Activity tolerance (good, fair, poor; see *Activity Intolerance* for additional assessment criteria)

## Nursing Goals

Through selected interventions the nurse will seek to
  · Individualize the teaching approach of each person and family, following an assessment of the problem and any factors that will influence learning
  · Enable behavior changes that are required to prevent illness or allow a person to recover from or live with illness
  · Facilitate an increase in cognitive knowledge
  · Influence person/family attitudes and psychological responses
  · Guide the development of psychomotor skills
  · Evaluate the effectiveness of instruction by evaluating the presence of desired behavioral changes

## Principles and Rationale for Nursing Care

### Introduction

Patient/health education is the teaching-learning process of influencing client and family behavior through changes in knowledge, attitudes, and beliefs and through the acquisition of psychomotor skills. It should not be expected to accomplish more than behavior change. The teaching-learning process consists of "steps," which are actually the components of the nursing process: assessment, planning, implementing, and evaluating.

### Assessment of learning needs, readiness to learn, and factors that will influence learning

  1. An assessment prior to teaching will facilitate the meaningfulness, the efficiency, and the overall success of the teaching-learning process by defining *what* content should be presented, *how* the content should be given, *when* the client is ready to learn, and *who* should be included in the process.

2. Each person learns in his own unique way.
3. Learning is dependent on physical and emotional readiness. The client needs to be relatively free of pain and extreme anxiety to learn.
4. High anxiety decreases learning, while slight anxiety may increase learning.
5. Client motivation is one of the most important variables affecting the amount of learning that takes place.

## Planning for the attainment of realistic goals by client and family

1. Planning goals and teaching strategies must be started only after a thorough assessment.
2. Planning should include the involvement of the client and family in goal-setting.
3. Goals must be written in the format of behavioral objectives, which are specific and observable behaviors to be accomplished by client and family at the completion of the learning experience.
4. Planning should also include a determination of teaching strategies to be employed to enable the client and family to achieve the goals set.
5. The best combination of educational methods, content, and learning materials for some clients is not necessarily the best combination for others.

## Implementing the teaching plan

1. Teaching is planned, structured, and sequenced communication to produce learning.
2. Teaching can be formal with the use of audiovisual aids, or it can be informal, occurring in conjunction with other forms of nursing care.
3. Active participation on the part of the client and family enhances learning and retention and is essential if learning is to occur.
4. Learning is increased when roles are clearly defined, *i.e.*, who is the learner and who is the teacher.
5. Learning requires energy. More information is learned with the least amount of energy when the nurse presents the information at a level consistent with the client's ability, when there is an association between the content presented and something the client already knows or has experienced, and when information is given in response to an expressed need of the client and family.
6. Use of audiovisual aids enhances learning.
7. Retention of information is increased when the teaching-learning process involves a variety of senses.
8. Repetition strengthens learning. Retention is increased when facts or skills are repeated. Overlearning increases retention.
9. Retention is better when the information learned is put into immediate use than when its application is delayed.
10. No single educational input, by itself, should expect to have a lasting effect on behavior, unless it is reinforced by other educational efforts.
11. Teaching is most effective in changing behavior if it is in response to a newly diagnosed illness or new treatment for the client.
12. Learning is made easier when the learner is aware of his progress.
13. Reward is a stronger inducement to learning than punishment.
14. Learning is enhanced in an environment free of distractions and other obstacles.
15. Learning is increased when the nurse communicates the necessity of learning and her own enjoyment and expertise as a facilitator in the teaching-learning process.

## Evaluating the teaching-learning process

1. Evaluation involves determining whether or not the planned goals are able to be achieved by client and family.
2. Evaluation methods include observing client and family behaviors, skill performance, etc., and asking questions related to the behavioral objectives that were mutually planned with client and family.
3. If learning cannot be demonstrated, further assessments and revisions in the teaching plan are necessary.

## General

1. Each person should be assessed for the knowledge and skill needed to monitor health status (*e.g.*, urine testing in diabetes), control or cure disease or prevent disease (*e.g.*, diet, medication therapy, life-style changes), and prevent recurrence or complications (*e.g.*, postoperative leg exercises).
2. Inaccurate perceptions of health status usually involve misunderstanding of the nature and seriousness of the illness, susceptibility to complications, and the need for procedures for cure or control of illness.
3. Psychological manifestations of anxiety and denial may have resulted from misconceptions, not knowing what to do, or not knowing how to carry out prescribed behaviors.
4. Teaching should be routinely incorporated as an integral part of nursing care whenever a new diagnosis or change in regimen is made or when the client faces an unfamiliar situation.

## Factors affecting learning

## Factors affecting the learner

Physical factors that affect learning include
    Presence of acute illness
    Fluid and electrolyte imbalance
    Nutritional status
    Illness or treatments that interfere with mental alertness (pain, medications)
    Illness or treatments that interfere with motor abilities (fatigue, equipment)
    Activity tolerance (endurance)
Personal factors that affect learning include
    Age
    Intelligence
    Level of motivation
    Level of anxiety
    Denial of disease process
    Depression
    Stage of adaptation to illness
    Past experiences or knowledge
    Locus of control
    Perception of
        Seriousness of condition
        Susceptibility to complications
        Prognosis
        Ability to control progression or to cure condition
Socioeconomic factors that affect learning include
    Language

Life-style
Support system
Financial status
Past experiences with health care
Cultural background
Transportation
Health care facility
Drugstore

## Factors resulting in ineffective teaching

Inadequate or no assessment prior to teaching
Assessment data were not communicated or not considered when teaching (the
most influential assessment factors are psychological status, physical stabil-
ity, educational level, cultural background, socioeconomic status)
Teaching was not individualized
Information not presented at a level consistent with the client's ability
Tendency to talk down to client
Use of misunderstood terms
Fragmented presentation of information
Too much information given, with important information hidden or lost among
irrelevant information
No repetition of information
No feedback given in relation to process (or client is punished for not learning)
No evaluation of client learning made

## Factors reflecting ineffective interaction

Client and family not involved with planning learning goals—which may be
unrealistic
Cultural differences between nurse and client may create stereotyping, thus
interfering with teaching
Discouragement of questions, hindering learner involvement
No opportunity to practice psychomotor skills or put learned information into
practice
Distractions in environment

---

# Knowledge Deficit
## Related to (specify)

*Example:* **Knowledge Deficit Related to Dietary Management of
Diabetes Mellitus**

### Assessment

### Subjective data

The person states that he
Is aware of a knowledge deficit
Is anxious and fearful of unfamiliar situations
Needs instruction

## Objective data

The person

Does not participate in his care (when other reasons for noncompliance have been ruled out)

Exhibits anxious behavior, such as

| | |
|---|---|
| Increased verbalization | Restlessness |
| Inability to concentrate | Sweating palms |
| and retain information | Tremulousness |

Behaves in a way that indicates a knowledge deficit regarding

Preparation for diagnostic study, examination, surgical procedure

The need for diagnostic study, examination, surgical procedure, or treatment and follow-up medical supervision

What is involved with the diagnostic study, examination, surgery, or treatment prescribed

Delays seeking medical assistance when it is needed

Misuses health care system (seeks assistance when he himself could have solved the problem or used a more appropriate resource)

---

**Outcome Criteria**

The person will

- Actively participate in the health behaviors prescribed or desired (such as those behaviors required in preparation for a diagnostic test, surgery, or physical examination, or those behaviors related to recovery from illness and prevention of recurrence or complications)
- Experience less anxiety, related to fear of the unknown, fear of loss of control, misconceptions, or previously given misinformation
- Describe disease process, causes, and factors contributing to symptoms, and the procedure(s) for disease or symptom control

---

## Interventions

The following interventions represent the teaching/learning activities to deal with a new diagnosis or treatment or the anticipation of an unfamiliar test, procedure, or surgery.

A. Assess the causative and contributing factors (in situations requiring a planned teaching/learning intervention)

New diagnosis

Change in existing medical condition/health status

New or altered treatment regimen

Unfamiliar diagnostic study

Unfamiliar physical examination procedure

Surgery

Hospitalization

No previous instruction given

Instruction given was ineffective in producing learning

B. Reduce or eliminate barriers to learning
- Assist person in meeting basic physiological needs, if necessary
- Support person in progressing through stages of psychosocial adaptation to illness
  1. Stage of disbelief (denial)
     a. Orient person to hospital setting, routines affecting him
     b. Teach with a focus on the present
     c. Provide simple explanations of procedures as they are carried out
     d. Help person feel safe, secure
     e. Concentrate on one-to-one teaching, rather than group teaching
     f. Teach family about the denial that person is having
  2. Stage of developing awareness (guilt, anger)
     a. Listen carefully to person
     b. Continue teaching with a present-tense focus
     c. Allow hostility to be safely vented
     d. Avoid arguing with person
- Delay teaching until person is ready
- Adapt teaching to person's physical and psychological status
- Allow person to work through and express intense emotions prior to teaching
- Examine person's health beliefs and past experiences related to his illness and assess their impact on his desire to learn

C. Promote person/family learning
- Individualize the teaching approach after a thorough assessment
- Plan and share necessity of learning and learning outcomes with person/family
- Follow the principles of teaching/learning previously listed
- Evaluate person/family behaviors as evidence that learning outcomes have been achieved

D. Promote a positive attitude and active participation of the person and his family
- Solicit expressions of feelings, concerns, and questions from person and family
- Encourage person and family to seek information and become involved in making informed decisions
- Explain person/family responsibilities and how these can be assumed

E. Reduce anxiety
- Encourage verbalization
- Listen attentively
- Meet person's expressed needs prior to giving other information
- Develop trust with frequent, consistent interactions
- Give correct, relevant information
- Give nonthreatening information before more anxiety-producing information
- Explain reason(s) for and intended effect of regimen or surgery, emphasizing the positive
- Explore with person the effects of a new diagnosis, treatment, or surgery on his significant others
- Do not overwhelm person with too much information if anxiety is high or physical condition is unstable
- Allow person to maintain some control over himself and his routines by involving person in care

- Prepare person and family for what to expect concerning his environment, routines, the personnel giving care, sensations experienced, etc.
- Reorient as needed

## F. Proceed with health teaching and referrals as indicated; for example, for the person undergoing surgery

1. Before hospitalization, the person's physician should explain
   Nature of surgery needed
   Reason for and anticipated outcomes of surgery
   Risks involved
   Type of anesthesia
   Expectations regarding length of recovery and limitations imposed during the recovery period
2. The person's understanding and informed consent should be ascertained, preferably before hospitalization
3. Assess
   a. Past experiences related to surgery, and positive or negative effect on client
   b. Nature of concerns, fears
   c. Factors affecting learning (refer to Etiological and Contributing Factors and Focus Assessment Criteria)
4. Document and communicate these data to others involved with care to meet the client's needs and ensure continuity.
5. Plan
   a. Give bedside instruction concerning specific type of surgery and sensations and appearances (presence of machines, tubes, etc.) that client and family may be aware of, postoperatively
   b. Provide instruction (bedside or group) on general information pertaining to the need for active participation, routines, environment, personnel, postoperative exercises
6. Implement plan
   a. Proceed with group or bedside instruction, following principles of teaching and learning
   b. Utilize efficient and effective teaching methods
      - Give general information, pertaining to most people having surgery, in a group session for patients and families
      - Present information or reinforce learning with the use of written materials (booklets, posters for room on exercises, instruction sheets) or audiovisual aids (slides of surgical areas, personnel, films, videotapes)
      - Demonstrate and conduct practice session for postoperative exercises
      - Explain the rationale for routines, focusing on positive aspects. For example, "An enema may be ordered preoperatively, which will decrease your need to use the bedpan for a few days postoperatively"
      - Encourage participation by making person feel susceptible to complications if he does not participate, without scaring him
      - Defer postoperative teaching until after surgery so as not to overwhelm person
      - Give feedback on progress, rewarding person frequently
7. Evaluate
   a. Person/family ability to meet preset, mutually planned learning goals (behaviors)
   b. Need for further teaching and support

8. Assess, postoperatively
   a. Additional factors affecting learning (discomfort, sedation, mobility deficit, etc.)
   b. Complications, such as pneumonia, phlebitis, pulmonary emboli
9. Implement plan
   a. Review measures taught preoperatively to reduce discomfort and prevent complications; demonstrate and support person in his participation
   b. Encourage person to start resuming normal activities, as allowed
   c. Start teaching in preparation for discharge early; instruction may include an explanation or demonstration of incisional care, diet and medication instruction, and a discussion of physical activities permitted
   d. Incorporate the individual's participation and practice under supervision, as appropriate
   e. Use supplemental written materials and audiovisual aids to reinforce learning
10. Evaluate
    a. Performance of behaviors demonstrating client understanding; for example, "The client demonstrates proper care of his operative site"
    b. Need for further instruction and support from health care agencies, community support and self-help groups, etc., and make appropriate referrals

G. Refer to health care agencies and community agencies (commonly required for persons with learning barriers to ensure adequate nursing care following hospital discharge)

## Bibliography

Bille D (ed): Practical Approaches to Patient Teaching. Little, Brown, Boston, 1981

Cohen N: Three steps to better patient teaching. Nursing 10(2):72–74, 1980

Czerwinski B: Manual of Patient Education for Cardiopulmonary Dysfunctions. St Louis, CV Mosby, 1980

Implementing Patient Education in the Hospital. Chicago, American Hospital Association, 1979

Pritchett S: Patient, Family and Community Health Education. Atlanta, Pritchett and Hull Associates, 1977

Redman B: Curriculum in patient education. Am J Nurs 78:1363–1366, 1978

Redman B: The Process of Patient Teaching in Nursing. St Louis, CV Mosby, 1981

Storlie F: Patient Teaching in Critical Care. New York, Appleton-Century-Crofts, 1975

Zander K, Bower K, Foster S et al: Practical Manual for Patient Teaching. St Louis, CV Mosby, 1978

# Mobility, Impaired Physical

*Related to* **Alterations in Lower Limbs**

*Related to* **Alterations in Upper Limbs**

## Definition

Impaired physical mobility: A state in which the individual experiences or is at risk of experiencing limitation of physical movement.

## Etiological and Contributing Factors

Pathophysiological

Neuromuscular impairment
  Autoimmune alterations (multiple sclerosis, arthritis)
  Nervous system diseases (Parkinsonism, myasthenia gravis)
  Muscular dystrophy
  Partial or total paralysis (spinal cord injury, stroke)
  Central nervous system (CNS) tumor
  Increased intracranial pressure
  Sensory deficits
Musculoskeletal impairment
  Spasms
  Flaccidity, atrophy, weakness
  Connective tissue disease (systemic lupus erythematosus)
  Edema (increased synovial fluid)

Situational
  Trauma or surgical procedures
  Nonfunctioning or missing limbs (fractures, amputations)
  External devices (casts or splints, braces, IV tubing)
  Pain
  Bedrest

Maturational

Elderly: Decreased motor agility, muscle weakness

## Defining Characteristics

  Inability to move purposefully within the environment, including bed mobility, transfers, ambulation
  Inability to move because of imposed restrictions (*e.g.*, bed rest, mechanical and medical protocols)
  Range-of-motion limitations
  Limited muscle strength or control
  Impaired coordination
  Impaired perception of position or presence of body parts

### Focus Assessment Criteria

Subjective data

1. History of systemic disorders
   Neurologic
         CVA, head trauma, increased intracranial pressure
         Multiple sclerosis, polio, Guillain-Barré, myasthenia gravis
         Spinal cord injury, tumor, birth defect
   Cardiovascular

| Myocardial infarction | Congenital heart anomaly |
|---|---|
| Congestive heart failure | |

   Musculoskeletal

| Osteoporosis | Fractures |
|---|---|
| Arthritis | |

   Respiratory

| Chronic obstructive pulmonary | Orthopnea |
|---|---|
|   disease (COPD) | Pneumonia |
| Dyspnea on exertion | |

   Debilitating diseases

| Cancer | Endocrine disease |
|---|---|
| Renal disease | |

2. History of symptoms that interfere with mobility

| Onset | Frequency |
|---|---|
| Duration | Precipitated by what? |
| Location | Relieved by what? |
| Description | Aggravated by what? |

3. History of symptoms (complaints of)
   Pain
   Muscle weakness
   Fatigue

| Attributed to? | Amount of time out of bed |
|---|---|
| Induced by? | Amount of time sleeping or resting |

4. History of recent trauma or surgery
   Fractures
   Head injury
   Abdominal surgery or injury
5. Current drug therapy
   Sedatives, hypnotics, CNS depressants
   Laxatives
   Other

Objective data

1. Dominant hand

| Right | Left | Ambidextrous |
|---|---|---|

2. Motor function

| | | | |
|---|---|---|---|
| Right arm | Strong | Weak | Absent | Spastic |
| Left arm | Strong | Weak | Absent | Spastic |
| Right leg | Strong | Weak | Absent | Spastic |
| Left leg | Strong | Weak | Absent | Spastic |

3. Mobility

| | | | |
|---|---|---|---|
| Ability to turn self | Yes | No | Assistance needed (specify) |
| Ability to sit | Yes | No | Assistance needed (specify) |
| Ability to stand | Yes | No | Assistance needed (specify) |
| Ability to transfer | Yes | No | Assistance needed (specify) |
| Ability to ambulate | Yes | No | Assistance needed (specify) |

Weight-bearing (assess both right and left sides)

| | |
|---|---|
| Full | As tolerated |
| Partial | Non-weight bearing |

Gait

| | |
|---|---|
| Stable | Unstable |

Assistive devices

| | | |
|---|---|---|
| Crutches | Walker | Prosthesis |
| Cane | Wheelchair | Other |
| Braces | | |

Restrictive devices

| | | |
|---|---|---|
| Cast or splint | Ventilator | IV |
| Traction | Drain | Monitor |
| Braces | Foley | Dialysis |

Range of motion (shoulders, elbows, arms, hips, legs)

| | | |
|---|---|---|
| Full | Limited (specify) | None |

4. Endurance (see *Activity Intolerance* for additional information)
   a. Assess
      Resting pulse, blood pressure, respirations
      BP, respirations, and pulse immediately after activity
      Pulse every 2 minutes until pulse returns to within 10 beats of resting pulse
   b. After activity, assess for the presence of indicators of anoxia (showing intensity, frequency, or duration of activity must be decreased or discontinued) as follows

| | |
|---|---|
| Blood pressure | |
| Failure of systolic rate to increase | Increase in diastolic of 15 mmHg |
| Respirations | |
| Excessive rate increases | Dyspnea |
| Decrease in rate | Irregular rhythm |
| Cerebral and other changes | |
| Confusion | Weakness |
| Incoordination | Pallor |
| Change in equilibrium | Cyanosis |

5. Peripheral circulation
   Capillary refill time (normal less than 3 seconds)
   Skin color, temperature, and turgor
   Peripheral pulses (rate, quality)

| | |
|---|---|
| Brachial | Popliteal |
| Radial | Posterior tibial |
| Femoral | Pedal |

6. Motivation (as perceived by nurse and stated by person)

| | | |
|---|---|---|
| Excellent | Satisfactory | Poor |

## Nursing Goals

Through selected interventions, the nurse will seek to
- Prevent the complications of decreased mobility
- Increase endurance and promote an optimal level of mobility
- Teach methods of adapting to alterations in mobility

## Principles and Rationale for Nursing Care

### Guidelines for range of motion (ROM)

1. There are three ROM categories, passive, active, and functional.

    Passive ROM keeps muscles and joints limber. One person passively moves another person's muscles (*e.g.*, the helper lifts and moves the person's legs).

    Active ROM exercise limbers and strengthens muscles and joints. The person actively uses his muscles, (*e.g.*, while lying down, the person moves his legs).

    Functional ROM strengthens muscles and joints while performing necessary activity (*e.g.*, walking). Performed by individual, himself.

2. Never do range of motion passively if the individual can do it actively.
3. Once the individual can perform active ROM, progress to functional activities.
4. During ROM, the individual's legs and arms should be moved gently to within his pain tolerance; perform ROM slowly to allow the muscles time to relax.
5. Support the extremity above and below the joint.
6. For passive ROM, the supine position is the most effective. The individual who performs ROM himself can use a supine or sitting position.
7. Do range of motion daily with bed bath, 3 to 4 times daily if there are specific problem areas. Try to incorporate into activities of daily living.

### Transfers (Figs. II–2 and II–3)

1. Before transferring anyone, the nurse should assess the number of personnel needed for assistance.
2. The individual should be positioned on the side of the bed. His feet should be touching the floor, and he should be wearing stable shoes or slippers with nonskid soles.
3. For getting in and out of bed, weight-bearing on the uninvolved or stronger side should be encouraged.
4. Wheelchair should be locked before transfer. If using a regular chair, be sure it will not move.
5. The person should be instructed to use the arm of the chair closer to him for support while standing.
6. The nurse should have her arms around the person's rib cage, and her back should be straight, with knees slightly bent.
7. The person should be told to place his arms around the nurse's waist or rib cage, *not her neck.*
8. The nurse should support the person's legs by bracing his with hers. (While facing the person, she should lock his knees with her knees.)
9. Hemiplegic individuals should be instructed to pivot on the uninvolved foot.
10. For individuals with lower limb weakness or paralysis, a sliding board transfer may be used.

    The person should wear pajamas so he will not stick to the board.

    The person needs good upper extremity strength to be able to slide his buttocks from the bed to the chair or wheelchair. (Wheelchairs should have removable arms.)

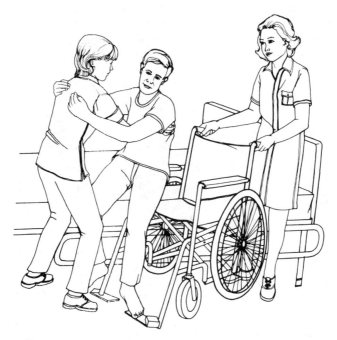

**Figure II–2.** While an assistant brings the wheelchair forward, the nurse swings the patient's legs over the edge of the bed. Next, the nurse helps the patient to lower himself into the wheelchair. Her assistant steadies the chair.

When the person's arms are strong enough, he should progress to a sitting transfer without the board, if he can lift buttocks enough to clear bed and chair seat.

11. If the person's legs give out, the nurse should guide him gently to the floor and *seek additional assistance.*

### Positioning (Fig. II–4)

1. The nurse should assess how frequently position needs to be changed (every 15 minutes to 2 hours, depending on individual's status—*e.g.*, person with spinal cord injury may need his position changed every 15 minutes).
2. People should be positioned with the goal of ambulation in mind (*e.g.*, knees slightly flexed).
3. The nurse should assess problem areas: head, joints, extremities.

If possible, only one pillow should be used under the *head* to prevent flexion contractions of the neck. Shoulder position should be changed throughout the day (adduction, abduction, overhead extension).

*Arms* should be abducted with elbows in slight flexion. The wrist should be neutral position with the fingers slightly flexed and the thumb slightly abducted and flexed. Arms and hands should be elevated to prevent dependent edema.

Prolonged periods of hip flexion (*e.g.*, when head of bed is elevated), should be avoided. The prone position should be encouraged if tolerated by the individual.

External leg rotation should be prevented by placing a small towel lateral to

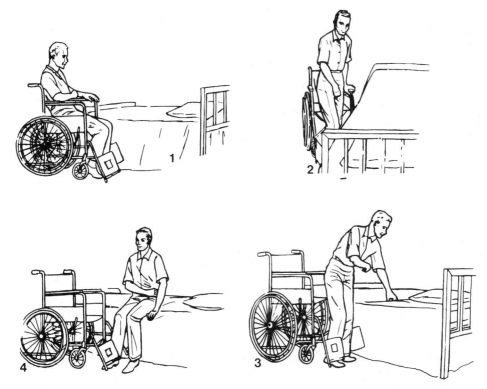

**Figure II-3.** Moving (*clockwise*) from wheelchair to bed. 1. Place wheelchair toward head of bed. Keep front corner of chair (on patient's stronger side) as close to bed as possible (as wheelchair shown in 2). Position the wheelchair so the patient sits near the center of the bed, closer to the foot for a tall person. Lock brakes and lift footrests. 2. Patient assumes standing position from wheelchair. 3. Patient moves stronger hand to edge of bed for support. 4. Patient leans forward, turns on stronger foot, and slowly lowers to sitting position. (From: Up and Around. Reprinted with permission of the American Heart Association)

the leg. Pillows should not be placed under knees. If the lower extremity is to be elevated, pillows should be placed under the calf. (Knee flexion contractures can prevent ambulation.)

*Ankles* should be in the position of 90°. A footboard may be required to prevent prolonged plantar flexion and shortening of the Achilles tendon. Active movement of the ankle during the day is essential.

4. Pillows or soft towel or blanket rolls may be used to protect specific areas from pressure (*e.g.*, bridging by use of rolled blanket under an ankle, preventing weight on heel).

5. Shearing forces should be minimized when changing the person's position. During transfers, the person's buttocks should be lifted, rather than dragged, whenever possible. A turning sheet should be used to assist the individual to change positions.

6. See Principles and Rationale for Nursing Care under *Activity Intolerance* and *Impairment of Skin Integrity* for additional information.

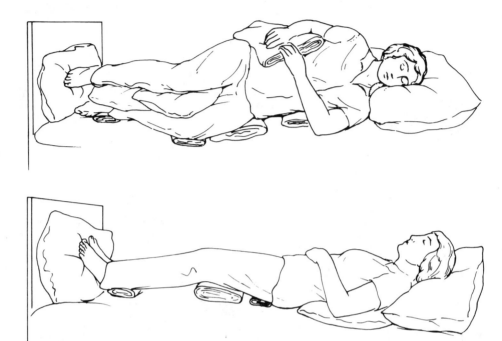

**Figure II–4.**   Positioning. (*Top*) Side-lying position. Pads are used above and below the trochanter and lateral malleolus to relieve pressure. (*Bottom*) Supine position. Pads are used above and below the sacrum and above the heels to relieve pressure. A pad above the knees prevents hyperextension of the knees and relieves pressure on the popliteal space.

# Impaired Physical Mobility
## Related to Alterations in Lower Limbs

### Assessment

Subjective data

| | |
|---|---|
| Pain | Numbness and tingling |
| Fatigue | Weakness |

Objective data

Inability to move or coordinate one or both lower limbs

Limitations in range of motion of lower limbs

Mechanical devices restricting mobility (*e.g.*, cast, traction)

Refusal to acknowledge existence of limbs (*e.g.*, post-CVA)

Impaired ability to transfer with or without adaptive devices (bed–chair, chair–commode)

Impaired ability to perform activities of daily living
Impaired sitting or standing balance
Impaired ability to ambulate with or without assistive devices
Alterations in gait patterns
Partial or total loss of one or both lower limbs
Impaired ability to move within physical environment (*e.g.*, curbs, stairs)

---

**Outcome Criteria**

The person will
  • Demonstrate the use of adaptive devices to increase mobility
  • Utilize safety measures to minimize potential for injury
  • Describe rationale for interventions
  • Demonstrate measures to increase mobility
  • Maintain or increase strength and endurance of upper limbs

---

## Interventions

### A. Assess causative factors

Trauma (*e.g.*, cartilage tears, fractures, amputations)
Surgical procedure (*e.g.*, joint replacement, reduction of fractures, vascular surgery)
Debilitating disease (*e.g.*, diabetes, cancer, rheumatoid arthritis, multiple sclerosis, stroke)

### B. Reduce or eliminate contributing factors

1. Increase limb mobility
   • Perform range-of-motion exercises (frequency to be determined by condition of the individual)
   • Support extremity with pillows to prevent or reduce swelling
   • Medicate for pain as needed, especially before activity* (see *Alterations in Comfort*)
   • Apply heat or cold to reduce pain, inflammation, and hematoma*
   • Apply cold to reduce swelling post-injury (usually first 48 hours)*
   • Encourage the person to perform exercise regimens for specific joints as prescribed by physician or physical therapist
2. Position the person in alignment to prevent complications
   • Avoid pillows under knee; support calf instead
   • Point toes and knees toward ceiling when the client is in a supine position
   • Use footboard to prevent foot drop
   • Avoid prolonged periods of hip flexion (*i.e.*, sitting position)
   • To position hips, place rolled towel lateral to hip to prevent external rotation
   • Change position every 15 minutes to 2 hours depending on individual's skin tolerance to pressure

---

*May require a physician's order.

3. Maintain good body alignment when mechanical devices are used

a. Traction devices
- Assess for correct position of traction and alignment of bones
- Observe for correct amount and position of weights
- Allow weights to hang freely, with no blankets or sheets on ropes
- Assess for changes in circulation; check pulse quality, skin temperature, color of extremities, and capillary refill (should be <2 sec)
- Assess for changes in circulation (numbness, tingling, pain)
- Assess for changes in mobility (ability to flex/extend unaffected joints)
- Assess for signs of skin irritation (redness, ulceration, blanching)
- Assess skeletal traction pin sites for loosening, inflammation, ulceration, and drainage; clean pin insertion sites (procedure may vary with type of pin and physician's order)
- Encourage isometrics* and prescribed exercise program

b. Casts
- Assess for proper fit of casts (they should not be too loose or too tight)
- Assess circulation to the encasted area every 2 hours (color and temperature of skin, pulse quality, capillary refill <2 sec)
- Assess for changes in sensation of extremities every two hours (numbness, tingling, pain)
- Assess motion of uninvolved joints (ability to flex and extend)
- Assess for skin irritation (redness, ulceration, or complaints of pain under the cast)
- Keep cast clean and dry; do not allow sharp objects to be inserted under cast; petal rough edges with adhesive tape; place soft cotton under edges that seem to be causing pressure points
- Allow cast to air dry while resting on pillows to prevent dents
- Observe cast for areas of softening or indentation
- Exercise joints above and below cast if allowed (e.g., wiggle fingers and toes every two hours)
- Assist with prescribed exercise regimens and isometrics of muscles enclosed in casts*
- Keep extremities elevated after cast application to reduce swelling

c. Braces
- Assess for correct positioning of braces
- Observe for signs of skin irritation (redness, ulceration, blanching, itching, pain)
- Assist with exercises as prescribed for specific joints
- Have the person demonstrate correct application of the brace

d. Prosthetic devices
- Observe for signs of skin irritation of the stump before applying prosthetic device (stump should be clean and dry; Ace bandage should be rewrapped and securely in place)
- Have the person demonstrate the correct application of the prosthesis
- Assess the person for gait alterations or improper walking technique
- Proceed with health teaching if indicated

*May require a physician's order.

e. Ace bandages
  - Assess for correct position of Ace bandage
  - Apply Ace bandage with even pressure, wrapping from distal to proximal portions, and making sure that the bandage is not too tight or too loose
  - Observe for "bunching" of the bandage
  - Observe for signs of irritation of skin (redness, ulceration, excessive tightness)
  - Rewrap Ace bandage b.i.d. or as needed, unless contraindicated (*e.g.*, if the bandage is a postoperative compression dressing, it should be left in place)
  - When wrapping lower extremity, leave the heel exposed, using figure 8 technique

**Note**: Some mechanical devices may be removed for exercises, depending on nature of injury or type and purpose of device. Consult with the physician to ascertain when the person may remove the device.

4. Provide progressive mobilization*
  - Assist the person slowly to sitting position
  - Allow the person to dangle his legs over the side of the bed for a few minutes before he stands up
  - Limit time to 15 minutes, three times a day, the first times out of bed
  - Increase the person's time out of bed, as tolerated by 15-minute increments
  - Progress to ambulation with or without assistive devices
  - If unable to walk, assist the person out of bed to a wheelchair or chair
  - Encourage ambulating for short frequent walks (at least 3 times daily), with assistance if unsteady
  - Increase lengths of walks progressively each day

## C. Provide health teaching when indicated

1. Teach the person methods of transfer from bed to chair or commode and to standing position
2. Teach how to ambulate with adaptive equipment (*e.g.*, crutches, walkers, canes)
  a. Instruct the individual in weight-bearing status
  b. Observe and teach the use of
    (1) Crutches
      - No pressure should be exerted on axilla; hand strength should be used
      - Type of gait varies with individual's diagnosis
      - Measure crutches 2 to 3 inches below axilla, and tips 6 inches away from feet
    (2) Walkers
      - Use arm strength to support weakness in lower limbs
      - Gait varies with individual's problems
    (3) Wheelchairs
      - Practice transfers
      - Practice maneuvering around barriers

*May require a physician's order.

       (4) Prostheses (teach about the following)
- Stump wrapping prior to application of the prosthesis
- Application of the prosthesis
- Principles of stump care
- Importance of cleaning the stump, keeping it dry, and applying the prosthesis only when the stump is dry

c. Teach the individual safety precautions
- Protect areas of decreased sensation from extremes of heat and cold
- Practice falling and how to recover from falls while transferring or ambulating
- For decreased perception of lower extremity (post-CVA "neglect"), instruct the individual to check where limb is placed when changing positions or going through doorways; and check to make sure both shoes are tied, that affected leg is dressed with trousers, and that pants are not dragging
- Instruct individuals who are confined to wheelchair to shift position and lift up buttocks every 15 minutes to relieve pressure; maneuver curbs, ramps, inclines, and around obstacles; and lock wheelchairs prior to transferring

d. Practice proper positioning, range of motion (active or passive), and prescribed exercises

e. Practice stair-climbing if individual's condition permits

f. Observe for complications of immobility

    Phlebitis (*i.e.*, redness, tenderness, swelling of calves)

    Decubitus ulcer/pressure sore (*i.e.*, blanching of skin, redness, itching, pain)

    Infection after limb surgery (*i.e.*, pain, swelling, redness)

    Neurovascular compromise (*i.e.*, numbness, tingling, pain, blanching, decreased pulse quality, coolness of skin)

# Impaired Physical Mobility
## Related to Alterations in Upper Limbs

### Assessment

#### Subjective data

The person reports

| | |
|---|---|
| Pain | Fatigue |
| Loss of sensation (numbness, tingling) | Weakness |

#### Objective data

Inability to move one or both upper extremities

Impaired grasp

Limited range of motion of one or more upper limbs

Mechanical devices preventing full range of motion (*e.g.*, traction, cast)

Inability to perform self-care activities
Neglect of one or both upper limbs
Partial or total loss of upper limb(s)
Impaired coordination of upper limb(s)

---

**Outcome Criteria**

The person will
- Demonstrate modes of adaptation to disability, *e.g.*, use of adaptive equipment such as universal cuff
- Relate rationale for interventions
- Maintain or increase strength and endurance of upper limbs

---

## Interventions

### A. Assess causative factors

Trauma (*e.g.*, fractures, crushing injuries, lacerations, amputations)

Surgical procedure (*e.g.*, joint replacement, reduction of fractures, removal of tumors, mastectomy)

Systemic disease (*e.g.*, multiple sclerosis, CVA, Guillain-Barré, rheumatoid arthritis, Parkinson's, lupus)

### B. Reduce or eliminate contributing factors

1. Increase limb mobility if possible
   - Assist with range of motion exercises*
   - Elevate extremity with pillows or sling above level of the heart to prevent or reduce swelling (may be contraindicated in CHF)
   - Medicate for pain as needed, especially before activity* (see *Alterations in Comfort*)
   - Apply cold to reduce swelling post-injury (usually first 48 hours)*
   - Assist with exercise regimens for specific joints as prescribed by physician or physical therapist (*e.g.*, for joint replacements)*
2. Position the person in alignment to prevent complications
   - Arms abducted from the body with pillows
   - Elbows in slight flexion
   - Wrist in a neutral position, with fingers slightly flexed, and thumb abducted and slightly flexed
   - Position of shoulder joints changed during the day (*e.g.*, abduction, adduction, range of circular motion)
3. Prevent injury when mechanical devices are used
   a. Traction devices
      - Assess for correct alignment of bones and position of traction as ordered
      - Observe for correct amount and position of weights
      - Allow weights to hang freely with no blankets or sheets on ropes
      - Assess for changes in circulation; check pulse quality, skin temperature, color of extremities, and capillary refill (should be < 2 sec)
      - Assess for changes in sensation (numbness, tingling, pain)

*May require a physician's order.

- Assess for changes in mobility (ability to flex/extend unaffected joints)
- Assess for signs of skin irritation (redness, ulceration, flaking)
- Assess skeletal traction, pin sites for loosening, inflammation, or skin ulceration; clean pin insertion sites b.i.d. (procedure may vary with type of pin and physician's order)
- Encourage isometrics and prescribed exercise program*

b. Casts
- Assess for tightness of cast
  - Circulation: temperature, color, check pulses, capillary refill should be <2 seconds
  - Sensation: numbness, tingling, increased pain
  - Motion: ability to flex, extend
- Assess for skin irritation: redness, ulceration, complaints of pain under cast
- Keep cast clean and dry; petal edges with adhesive tape if necessary; no sharp objects down into cast
- Allow cast to air dry; observe for areas of softening
- Exercise joints above and below cast; prescribed exercise regimens and isometrics of muscles enclosed in casts
- After application, elevate extremity on pillows to prevent or reduce swelling

c. Slings
- Assess for correct application; sling should be loose around neck and should support elbow and wrist above level of the heart
- Remove slings for range of motion*

d. Ace bandages (care as for lower limbs' bandages)
- Observe for correct position
- Apply with even pressure, wrapping distally to proximally
- Observe for "bunching"
- Observe for signs of skin irritation (redness, ulceration) or tightness (compression)
- Rewrap Ace bandages b.i.d. or as needed, unless contraindicated (*e.g.*, if bandage is postoperative compression dressing, check physician's orders)

4. Encourage use of affected arm when possible (Fig. II–5)
- Encourage the person to use affected arm for self-care activities (*e.g.*, feeding himself, dressing, brushing hair)
- For post-CVA neglect of upper limb
  a. Place objects to affected side to encourage use of "forgotten" limb
  b. Stand to the person's side and encourage him to use all fields of vision
      *Note*: Some mechanical devices may be removed for exercises, depending on nature of injury or type and purpose of device. Physician's orders should be consulted.
- Instruct the person to utilize unaffected arm to exercise the affected arm
- Use appropriate adaptive equipment to enhance the use of arms
  - Universal cuff for feeding in individuals who have poor control in both arms, hands
  - Large-handled or padded silverware to assist individuals with poor fine motor skills

*May require a physician's order.

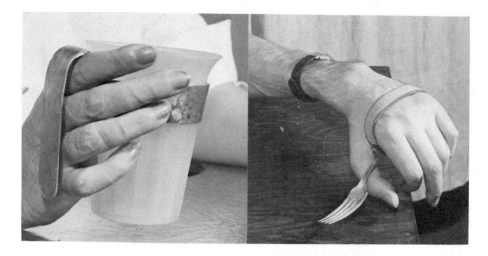

**Figure II–5.**  Adaptive devices.

- Dishware with high edges to prevent food from slipping
- Suction-cup aids to hold dishes in place to prevent sliding of plate
- Use a warm bath to alleviate early morning stiffness and improve mobility
- Encourage the individual to practice handwriting skills, if able
- Allow time for the individual to practice using affected limb

## C. Proceed with health teaching when indicated

- Have the person demonstrate range of motion and prescribed exercises
- Have the person demonstrate the care of adaptive and mechanical devices
- Teach the person safety precautions
- Practice difficult maneuvers (e.g., cooking with one hand)
- For areas of decreased sensation, instruct the person to take precautions with heat, cold, and sharp objects
- For neglect of upper extremity, instruct the person to observe and check for positioning, exposure to irritants, or sharp objects
- Teach person methods of performing self-care activities (see self-care deficits)
- Teach individual when to alternate rest and activity of joints

## Bibliography

Farrell J: Illustrated Guide to Orthopedic Nursing, 2nd ed. Philadelphia, JB Lippincott, 1982

Gartland J: Fundamentals of Orthopedics. Philadelphia, WB Saunders, 1965

Krusen FH, Kottke FJ, Elwood P Jr (eds): Handbook of Physical Medicine and Rehabilitation. Philadelphia, WB Saunders, 1971

Lieberson S, Mendes DG: Walking in bed: Strength and mobility of the lower extremities of bedridden patients. Phys Ther 59:1112–1115, 1979

Meissner JE: Elevate your patient's level of independence. Nursing 10(9):72–73, 1980

Milazzo V: Exercise class for patients in traction. Am J Nurs 81:1843–1844, 1981

Olson EV (ed): The hazards of immobility. Am J Nurs 67:780–797, 1967

Sine R (ed): Basic Rehabilitation Techniques, 2nd ed. Rockville, MD, Aspen Systems Corporation, 1981

# Noncompliance

*Related to* **Anxiety**

*Related to* **Negative Side-Effects of Prescribed Treatment**

*Related to* **Unsatisfactory Relationship with Caregiving Environment or Caregivers**

## Definition

Noncompliance: Personal behavior that deviates from health-related advice given by health care professionals.*

## Etiological and Contributing Factors

Many factors in an individual's life can contribute to noncompliance. Some common ones are listed below.

### Situational

Side-effects of therapy
Impaired ability to perform tasks (poor memory; motor and sensory deficits)
Previous unsuccessful experience with advised regimen
Increasing amount of disease-related symptoms despite adherence to advised regimen
Concurrent illness of family member
Impersonal aspects of the referral process
Nontherapeutic environment
Inclement weather that prevents person from keeping appointment
Complex, prolonged, or unsupervised therapy
Expensive therapy
Nonsupportive family
Nontherapeutic relationship between client and nurse
Knowledge deficit
Lack of autonomy in health-seeking behavior
Health beliefs that run counter to professional advice
Poor self-esteem
Disturbance in body image

## Defining Characteristics

Verbalization of noncompliance or nonparticipation

---

*The use of the nursing diagnosis *Noncompliance* describes the individual who desires to comply, but the presence of certain factors prevents him from doing so. The nurse must attempt to reduce or eliminate these factors for the interventions to be successful. However, the nurse is cautioned against using the diagnosis of noncompliance to describe an individual who has made an informed autonomous decision not to comply.

Associated defining characteristics

Missed appointments

Partially used or unused medications

Persistence of symptoms*

Progression of disease process*

Occurrence of undesired outcomes* (postoperative morbidity, pregnancy, obesity, addiction, regression during rehabilitation)

## Focus Assessment Criteria

### Subjective data

What is the person's general health motivation?

Does client seek help when needed?

Does client accept the diagnosis as valid?

Does client intend to make the advised life-style alterations?

What is the person's perception of his present state of health?

Does client consider himself to be generally well?

Is there fear of a specific illness?

Does client believe his illness is severe?

How does the person view the advised treatment regimen?

Does the person report

Unacceptable side-effects of therapy?

| | |
|---|---|
| Unpleasant taste | Heavy expenses |
| Difficulty swallowing | Time-consuming or inconvenient |
| Pain | |

Inability to repeat or demonstrate the prescribed behavior?

| | |
|---|---|
| Exercise program | Treatment procedure |
| Drug names and schedule | Next appointment date |

Situations that interfere with prescribed behavior?

| | |
|---|---|
| Family demands | Stress |
| Occupation | Lack of transportation |
| Travel (hotels, restaurants) | |

### Objective data

Assess for the presence of

Missed appointments

Obstacles to self-care

| | |
|---|---|
| Inability to read | Musculoskeletal deficits |
| Immaturity | Cognitive deficits |
| Memory lags | Pain |

Evidence of obstacles in caregiving environment

| | |
|---|---|
| Long waiting period | Hurried atmosphere |

Evidence of noncompliance

| | |
|---|---|
| Persistence of symptoms | With medications (pill count, |
| Progression of disease | serum drug levels) |

*When these characteristics are considered to be the result of noncompliance, one is assuming that the therapy prescribed has been proven to be effective and is appropriate.

## Nursing Goals

Through selected interventions, the nurse will seek to
- Determine etiology(ies) of noncompliance
- Identify manifestations of noncompliance that may be detrimental to health
- Promote client understanding of noncompliant behavior
- Determine possible care alternatives that may minimize noncompliant behavior
- Share with client the decision-making process

## Principles and Rationale for Nursing Care

1. Since the diagnosis of noncompliance has a high subjective component, the nurse is cautioned not to utilize the diagnosis as a reflection of the nurse's value judgment but, rather, to seek to identify causative and contributing factors.
2. Both clients and health care professionals share the responsibility for noncompliance and must work together to correct it.
3. There is a gray area between noncompliance and making an informed decision not to adhere to health-related advice. For example, the individual who does not take his medication because he is unable to swallow pills is different from the person who refuses chemotherapy because he is exhausted from previous treatments and is ready to die. In both cases, the nurse intervenes to elicit reasons for this behavior. However, attempts to change the situation may only be directed at the former case.
4. When evaluating noncompliance related to medication, the nurse must consider the following factors that may affect drug absorption, metabolism, effectiveness, side-effects, and excretion: body weight, age, time of administration, route of administration, genetic factors, basal metabolic rate, interactions with other drugs and foods, presence of organ disease (*e.g.*, liver and kidneys), altered body chemistry (*e.g.*, hypokalemia), and infection.
5. When a client reports symptomatic side-effects from a new drug, consider the many manifestations of the human allergic response: hives and the entire spectrum of rashes, respiratory discomfort and distress, pruritus, watery eyes, swelling of mucous membranes, and gastrointestinal discomforts.

# Noncompliance
## Related to Anxiety

### Assessment

#### Subjective data

The person states
    He is anxious or fearful
    He has not followed advice of health care professional

Objective data

The person exhibits nonverbal signs of anxiety

| | |
|---|---|
| Tachycardia | Chest pain |
| Perspiration | Dyspnea |
| Headache | Cold extremities |
| GI discomfort | Tachypnea |
| Insomnia | |

---

**Outcome Criteria**

The person will
- Verbalize fears and anxiety related to health needs
- Identify factors that are contributing to anxiety
- Identify alternatives to present coping patterns

---

## Interventions

### A. Assess causative or contributing factors

Negative experiences with disease or with health care system (either personally or through others)

Stressors

### B. Reduce or eliminate causative or contributing factors if possible

1. Negative experiences with health care system
   - Using open-ended questions, encourage person to talk about previous experiences with health care (*e.g.*, hospitalizations, family deaths, diagnostic tests, blood tests, x-rays)
   - Ask client directly, "What are your concerns about
     . . . taking this drug?"
     . . . following this diet?"
     . . . having a blood test?"
     . . . going through the cystoscopy?"
     . . . having your gallbladder removed?"
     . . . using a diaphragm?"
     . . . paying for the operation?"
   - Encourage client to talk about how the diagnosis and treatment might affect him
   - Acknowledge appropriateness of being fearful
   - Correct any misconceptions
   - Give appropriate instructions
   - Discuss the effects of anxiety on pain, breathing, healing, and general comfort (see also *Anxiety; Fear; Knowledge Deficit*)
2. Stressors
   - Assess person for recent changes in life-style (personal, work, family, health, financial)
   - Facilitate recognition by person of how those factors are affecting his health

- Assist person to manage his stressors; see the appropriate diagnosis that reflects the stressor

| | |
|---|---|
| *Fear* | *Spiritual Distress* |
| *Anxiety* | *Alterations in Thought Processes* |
| *Grieving* | *Ineffective Individual Coping* |
| *Alterations in Nutrition* | *Alterations in Family Processes* |
| *Self-Care Deficit* | *Disturbance in Self-Concept* |

C. Initiate referrals if indicated

Dietician
Nutrition support
Home health
Social service
Other community agencies

---

# Noncompliance
## Related to Negative Side-Effects of Prescribed Treatment

### Assessment

#### Subjective data

The person states that he has altered the prescribed health behavior because of discomforts related to treatment(s)

"Medications make me sick"
"Medications make me tired"

The person describes symptoms such as

| | |
|---|---|
| Dizziness | Indigestion |
| Headache | Drowsiness |
| Dry mouth | Sexual difficulties |
| Pain | Depression |
| Diarrhea | |

The person states that treatments are inconvenient

#### Objective data

Any lab test indicative of treatment effects (*e.g.,* toxic drug levels, hypokalemia due to diuretics)

Physical findings

| | |
|---|---|
| Rashes | Hyperpigmentation |
| Hives | Dehydration |
| Loss or growth of hair | Drowsiness |
| Fat deposits | |

**Outcome Criteria**

The person will

- Describe experiences that cause him to alter prescribed behavior
- Receive appropriate treatment of side-effects, if necessary
- Demonstrate appropriate alternatives to the previous plan

## Interventions

### A. Assess causative or contributing factors of prescribed therapy

Requires prolonged period of time

Is unsupervised

Is complex, with numerous medications, or special equipment is needed

Is very costly

Involves changes in lifelong habits

Is inconvenient in terms of time, place, or side-effects

Is culturally unacceptable

### B. Assess the person's complaints

Onset and duration?

Associated with activity? food? stress?

### C. Review present medication therapy (prescribed and over-the-counter)

- Identify present therapy (names, dosage, time taken)
- Identify possible adverse interactions among drugs (consult pharmacist)
- Establish whether toxicity is present (blood level of drug)*

### D. Assist person to reduce causative factors

- For gastric irritation, suggest that drug be taken with milk or food; may be advisable to eat yogurt (unless contraindicated)
- For drowsiness, take medication at bedtime or late in afternoon; consult physician for dose reduction
- For leg cramps (hypokalemia), increase intake of foods high in potassium (oranges, raisins, tomatoes, bananas)
- For other side-effects, consult pertinent references
- Use long-acting intramuscular preparations whenever possible; this includes some antibiotics and antipsychotic medications
- Suggest that physicians use combination pills if available (*e.g.,* Aldoril [methyldopa and hydrochlorothiazide] and Triavil [perphenazine and amitriptyline])
- When appropriate, be sure client is taking the fewest number of pills possible (check dosages to provide the largest dose available in the fewest number of pills)*
- Instruct client to take pills twice rather than four times per day whenever appropriate*

*May require a physician's order.

- Encourage prescription of generic drugs for persons with financial concerns
- When treatments require more than one set of hands, evaluate home help situation (see *Impaired Home Maintenance Management*)
- When expensive equipment is involved for treatments at home, make appropriate referrals to social workers and local agencies

### E. Initiate health teaching and referrals as indicated

- Teach importance of adhering to prescribed regime
- Teach what to expect (effects of drug or treatment; side-effects)

# Noncompliance
## Related to Unsatisfactory Relationship with Caregiving Environment or Caregivers

### Assessment

### Subjective data
Verbalizes dissatisfaction with setting, caregivers, or treatment regime

### Objective data
Clients seen in waiting areas for long periods of time
Schedules are overbooked
There is a shortage of caregiving personnel
Clients and caregivers are culturally unrelated
Client is seen by a different caregiver at each visit
Physical setting lacks privacy
Setting is located in dangerous or inaccessible area
Prescribed therapies are not provided by caregiving setting
Treatments prescribed are complex or costly

---

**Outcome Criteria**

The person will
- Express anger, frustrations, confusion related to aspects of the clinical setting to nurse
- Identify sources of dissatisfaction
- Offer suggestions of what would be more satisfactory

---

### Interventions

### A. Assess causative or contributing factors
1. Referral process

Prolonged period between referral and scheduled appointment

Referral to a clinic rather than to a specific caregiver

Referral by person other than self

2. Method of scheduling

Block scheduling, or "first come, first serve," rather than individual appointments

Overbooked schedule preventing reasonable amount of time for visit

3. Communication barriers

Presence of language barrier

Teaching center in which a variety of students see clients and disturb continuity

Goals of personnel and clients differ

Personnel lack interest or expertise necessary to develop trust of clients

Personnel make decisions *for* client, rather than *with* him

4. Physical setting

Crowded, impersonal seating in waiting areas

Clients seen in curtained booths rather than individual rooms

Location is not on public transportation lines

Location is in a neighborhood different from client's

## B. Eliminate or reduce contributing factors if possible

1. Referral process

- Whenever possible, allow client to make own appointments
- Shorten referral waiting time
- Personnel handling referral appointments should inquire about transportation and child care, suggesting help available if needed
- Send reminder postcard to client before appointment
- Personnel initiating referral should give client adequate explanations as to why it is indicated and what is expected from the visit

2. Method of scheduling

- If possible, give individual appointments
- Do not schedule unreasonable numbers of clients for a given time period

3. Communication barriers

- Allow person an opportunity to make the decisions about his own health care; assume an advisory approach when counseling, rather than one that is dictatorial
- Consider the use of contracting when behavior modification is indicated; include caregiver in the contract as well as the client
- Schedule interpreters whenever non-English speaking clients are anticipated (consult "language banks" in larger institutions)
- For the caregiver who knows small amounts of a language (Spanish, for example), make note cards inscribed with key words appropriate to the clinical setting
- In teaching centers where clients may see different students at each visit, schedule primary nurses to stop in to see each patient
- Plan patient care conferences, including members of all involved health professions, at regular intervals to promote seeing clients as individuals

4. Physical setting

- Utilize waiting time for teaching (*e.g.*, group classes)

- Use as many resources possible to make waiting and caregiving areas pleasant, welcoming, and nonclinical
- Utilize blank wall space for health education materials, pictorial progress of clients, holiday decorations, original artwork by clients, etc.
- Ensure privacy during interviews, examinations, and procedures
- Causative factors related to the location of the clinical setting, safety, and transportation are difficult problems to correct; nurses may make proposals for
    Special buses
    Enhanced security
    Ramps for wheelchairs
    Improved lighting in parking areas and walkways
    More nearby parking facilities

C. Encourage person to verbalize frustrations with the clinical setting in the context of a therapeutic nursing relationship

## Bibliography

### Books and Articles

Becker H (ed): The Health Belief Model and Personal Health Behavior. Thorofare, NJ, Charles B Slack, 1974

Haynes R, Taylor D, Sackett D: Compliance in Health Care. Baltimore, Johns Hopkins Press, 1979

Komaroff L: The practitioner and the compliant patient. Am J Public Health 66(9):833–835, 1976

Marston MV: Compliance with medical regimes: A review of the literature. Nursing Res 19(4):312–323, 1970

Scherwitz L, Leventhal H: Strategies for increasing patient compliance. Health Values 2(6):301–306, 1978

### Pertinent Literature for the Consumer

Food–drug interactions: Can what you eat affect your medication? Elizabeth, NJ, Wakefern Food Corporation

# Nutrition, Alterations in: Less Than Body Requirements

*Related to* **Chewing or Swallowing Difficulties**

*Related to* **Anorexia**

*Related to* **Difficulty or Inability to Procure Food**

## Definition

Alteration in Nutrition: Less Than Body Requirements: The state in which an individual experiences or is at risk of experiencing reduced weight related to inadequate intake of nutrients.*

## Etiological and Contributing Factors

Pathophysiological

Hyperanabolic/catabolic states
      Burns (post-acute phase)      Cancer
      Infection      Trauma
Chemical dependence
Dysphagia
      Cerebrovascular accident      Muscular dystrophy
      Amyotrophic lateral sclerosis
Absorptive disorders
      Crohn's disease      Intestinal obstruction (ileus)
Stomatitis
    Medications or chemotherapy

Situational

Anorexia
Depression
Stress
Social isolation
Nausea and vomiting
Allergy
Radiation therapy
Parasites
Inability to procure food (physical limitations; financial or transportation problems)
Lack of knowledge of adequate nutrition
Crash or fad diet
Inability to chew (wired jaw, damaged or missing teeth, ill-fitting dentures)

*This diagnostic category should not be used with individuals who are unable to ingest or absorb nutrients.

## Maturational

Infants/children: Congenital anomalies, growth spurts
Adolescent: Anorexia nervosa (post-acute phase)
Elderly: Altered sense of taste

## Defining Characteristics

Weight 10% to 20%+ below ideal for height and frame
Triceps skin fold, mid-arm circumference, and mid-arm muscle circumference less than 60% standard measurement
Reported inadequate food intake less than minimum daily requirement (MDR)
Actual or potential metabolic needs in excess of intake

## Associated defining characteristics (severe deficiencies)

Tachycardia on minimal exercise and bradycardia at rest
Muscle weakness and tenderness
Mental irritability or confusion
Decreased serum albumin
Decreased serum transferrin or iron-binding capacity
Decreased lymphocyte count

## Focus Assessment Criteria

## Subjective data

History of problem (childhood, sociocultural influences)
Diet recall for past 24 hours
    Is that the usual intake pattern?
Diet history
Past diets
Amount weight lost
Weight gained back (how soon? how much?)

## Present dietary patterns

Diet diary (for overweight person)
Instruct person to record for one week
    What, when, where, and why eaten
    Whether doing anything else (e.g., TV, reading)
    Emotions just before eating
    Others present
Food source and preparation
Living arrangements
Financial status

## Activity level

Occupation
Exercise (what? how often?)

## Coping pattern

Response to stress (eat or not eat?)
Perceptions of problem

Perceptions of causation
Desire to change
Support system available (strengths/limitations)

## Knowledge of nutrition

Basic food groups
Foods high in calories
Relationship of activity vs. metabolism

## Physiological alterations

Medication history
Medical/surgical history
Presence of

| | |
|---|---|
| Allergies | Fatigue |
| Nausea | Dsyphagia |
| Vomiting | Pain |
| Anorexia | Stomatitis |

## Objective data

Height and weight
Compare to standardized chart according to sex (see tables under Principles and Rationale for Nursing Care)
Anthropometric measurements (refer to Principles and Rationale for Nursing Care for standard charts)
Triceps skin fold
Mid-arm circumference
Mid-arm muscle circumference
Condition of hair, skin, nails, mouth, and teeth
Ability to chew, swallow, feed self

## Diagnostic studies

Hemoglobin
Serum albumin
Serum transferrin or iron-binding capacity
Lymphocytes
Thyroid function

## Nursing Goals

Through selected interventions, the nurse will seek to assist the person to
- Identify factors that contribute to a decreased nutritional state
- Increase nutritional intake to meet metabolic requirements

## Principles and Rationale for Nursing Care

### General

1. Food habits are influenced by personal preferences, culture and religion, economic factors, family eating patterns, and knowledge of nutrition.
2. The body requires a minimum level of nutrients for health and growth. During the life span, the nutritional needs of individuals vary, as indicated in Table II–5.

Table II-5.   **Age-Related Daily Nutritional Requirements**

| Age | Daily Nutritional Requirements |
| --- | --- |
| **Infants** | |
| Newborn | 12–18 oz milk |
| 2–3 months | 20–30 oz milk |
| 4–5 months | 25–35 oz milk; strained vegetables and fruits; egg yolks |
| 6–7 months | 28–40 oz milk; above solids, plus meat |
| 8–11 months | 24 oz milk; 3 regular meals |
| 1–2 years | 24 oz milk; 1000 calories |
| **Children** | |
| Preschool (3–5 years) | 1500 calories; 40 grams protein |
| | Basic 4 food groups<br>    4–6 servings fruits and vegetables<br>    2 or more servings meat (2 oz portions)<br>    4 servings bread or cereal<br>    4 servings dairy |
| School (6–12 years) | 80 calories/kg; 0.5 gram protein/kg |
| | Basic 4 food groups (as preschool)<br>    1.5–2 grams calcium<br>    400 units vitamin D<br>    1.5–3 liters water |
| Adolescent (13–17 years) | 2200–2400 calories for females<br>3000 calories for males |
| | Basic 4 food groups (as preschool)<br>    50–60 grams protein<br>    3 grams calcium<br>    400 units vitamin D |
| **Adults** | |
| | 1600–3000 calorie range (based on physical activity, emotional state, body size, age, and individual metabolism) |
| | Males need increased protein, ascorbic acid, riboflavin, and vitamins E and $B_6$ |
| | Females need the above and also increased iron and vitamins A and $B_{12}$ |
| Pregnant women<br>  (2nd and 3rd trimesters) | Increase protein 10 grams<br>1.2–3.5 grams calcium<br>Increase vitamins A, B, and C<br>30–60 mg iron |
| Lactating women | 75 grams protein<br>4000 calories<br>Increase vitamin A, niacin, thiamin, and riboflavin |

Table II–5.  **Age-Related Daily Nutritional Requirements** (*continued*)

| Age | Daily Nutritional Requirements |
|---|---|
| **Adults** (*continued*) | |
| Over 65 | Basic 4 food groups |
| | Caloric requirements decrease with age (1600 –1800 for female, 2000–2400 for male) but are dependent on activity, climate, and growth needs |
| | Assure intake of essential amino acids, fatty acids, vitamins, elements, fiber, and water |
| | 60 mg ascorbic acid |
| | 40–60 mg protein |
| | 800 mg calcium |
| | 10 mg iron |

3. Inability to meet metabolic requirements results in loss of weight, poor health, and decreased ability of the body to grow or repair itself.
4. Metabolic needs are increased in the presence of trauma, sepsis, infection, and cancer.
5. To obtain a one-pound weight gain, 3500 calories above metabolic requirements must be acquired.
6. Anorexia is a complex multidimensional problem involving physical, social, and psychological components.
7. Nutritional deficiencies in the elderly can result from chronic disease, anemia, anorexia, dental status, financial problems, loneliness, the inability to procure or prepare foods, and fluid imbalance.
8. The person with cancer experiences nutritional problems that are disease-related and treatment-related, as indicated below.

| *Disease Related* | *Treatment-Related* |
|---|---|
| Malabsorption | Stomatitis |
| Diarrhea | Diarrhea |
| Constipation | Nausea and vomiting |
| Anemia | Anorexia |
| Protein deficits | Fatigue |
| Fatigue | |

9. Tables II–6 and II–7 can be used to compare the individual's weight for height and anthropometric measurements.

Table II-6. **Weight for Height***

**Men**

| Height (cm)† | Weight (kg)† | Height (cm) | Weight (kg) | Height (cm) | Weight (kg) |
|---|---|---|---|---|---|
| 157 | 58.6 | 167 | 64.6 | 177 | 71.6 |
| 158 | 59.3 | 168 | 65.2 | 178 | 72.4 |
| 159 | 59.9 | 169 | 65.9 | 179 | 73.3 |
| 160 | 60.5 | 170 | 66.6 | 180 | 74.2 |
| 161 | 61.1 | 171 | 67.3 | 181 | 75.0 |
| 162 | 61.7 | 172 | 68.0 | 182 | 75.8 |
| 163 | 62.3 | 173 | 68.7 | 183 | 76.5 |
| 164 | 62.9 | 174 | 69.4 | 184 | 77.3 |
| 165 | 63.5 | 175 | 70.1 | 185 | 78.1 |
| 166 | 64.0 | 176 | 70.8 | 186 | 78.9 |

**Women**

| Height (cm) | Weight (kg) | Height (cm) | Weight (kg) | Height (cm) | Weight (kg) |
|---|---|---|---|---|---|
| 140 | 44.9 | 150 | 50.4 | 160 | 56.2 |
| 141 | 45.4 | 151 | 51.0 | 161 | 56.9 |
| 142 | 45.9 | 152 | 51.5 | 162 | 57.6 |
| 143 | 46.4 | 153 | 52.0 | 163 | 58.3 |
| 144 | 47.0 | 154 | 52.5 | 164 | 58.9 |
| 145 | 47.5 | 155 | 53.1 | 165 | 59.5 |
| 146 | 48.0 | 156 | 53.7 | 166 | 60.1 |
| 147 | 48.6 | 157 | 54.3 | 167 | 60.7 |
| 148 | 49.2 | 158 | 54.9 | 168 | 61.4 |
| 149 | 49.8 | 159 | 55.5 | 169 | 62.1 |

* This table corrects the 1959 Metropolitan Standards to nude weight
† 1 centimeter (cm) = 0.39 inch; 1 kilogram (kg) = 2.2 pounds

Table II–7.  **Anthropometric Measurements (adult)***

| Test | Sex | Reference | > 90% Reference | 90%-60% Reference | < 60% Reference |
|------|-----|-----------|-----------------|-------------------|-----------------|
| **Mid-Arm Circumference (MAC) (in cm)** | | | | | |
| | Male | 29.3 | > 26.3 | 26.3-17.6 | < 17.6 |
| | Female | 28.5 | > 25.7 | 25.7-17.1 | < 17.1 |
| **Mid-Arm Muscle Circumference (MAMC) (in cm)** | | | | | |
| | Male | 25.3 | > 22.8 | 22.8-15.2 | < 15.2 |
| | Female | 23.2 | > 20.9 | 20.9-13.9 | < 13.9 |
| **Triceps Skin Fold (TSF) (in mm)** | | | | | |
| | Male | 12.5 | > 11.3 | 11.3-7.5 | < 7.5 |
| | Female | 16.5 | > 14.9 | 14.9-9.9 | < 9.9 |

* If measurements are below 90% reference, nutritional support program may be indicated. (Jelliffe DB: The Assessment of the Nutritional Status of the Community. World Health Organization Monograph No. 53. Geneva, WHO, 1966)

# Alterations in Nutrition: Less Than Body Requirements
## Related to Chewing or Swallowing Difficulties

## Assessment

### Subjective data
The person reports
    Dry mouth
    Sores in mouth
    "Can't chew (swallow)"

### Objective data
    Wired jaw
    Paresis involving muscles required for chewing or swallowing
    Impaired or broken teeth, missing teeth, ill-fitting dentures
    Stomatitis

**Outcome Criteria**
The person will
  · Describe causative factors when known
  · Describe rationale and procedure for treatment
  · Experience adequate nutrition through oral intake

## Interventions

A. Assess causative factors

Mechanical obstruction (wired jaw)
Neurologic condition causing muscle weakness, slowness, uncoordination, paralysis, or a combination of these (CVA, amyotrophic lateral sclerosis, parkinsonian syndrome)
Decreased salivation (radiation therapy)
Dental disorders
Stomatitis (see *Alterations in Oral Mucous Membrane*)

B. Reduce or eliminate causative and contributing factors if possible

1. Mechanical obstruction
   a. Instruct or assist person to
      · Keep a record of intake
      · Perform oral hygiene immediately after eating, *e.g.*
         Water pik-type cleansing (preferred)
         Swishing low-cal carbonated beverage around mouth
         Swishing solution of ½ or ¼ hydrogen peroxide and ½ or ¾ water around mouth (solution can be flavored with mouthwash)
   b. Teach techniques to maintain adequate nutritional intake and stimulate appetite
      · Vary liquids to allow for different textures and tastes (*e.g.*, juices, cream soups)
      · Use commercially prepared or home-made high-protein/calorie supplements (*e.g.*, enrich milk (mix 1 quart fresh milk with 1 cup instant nonfat milk) and blenderize with various flavorings—ripe banana, ice cream, syrups, fresh or frozen fruit)
2. Decreased salivation
   a. Instruct or assist person to
      · Increase liquid intake with meals
      · "Wet" food to make up for lack of saliva
      · Use artificial saliva
      · Suck on lemon immediately before eating to stimulate salivation (overuse can damage tooth enamel)
      · Avoid eating only milk and milk products because they tend to form a tenacious mucus
   b. Check medications person is on for side-effects of dry mouth/decreased salivation
   c. Teach person to rinse mouth whenever needed to remove debris, stimulate gums, or lubricate and refresh mouth

3. Swallowing difficulties
  a. Before beginning feeding, assess that person is adequately alert and responsive, is able to control mouth, has cough/gag reflex, and can swallow own saliva
  b. Have suction equipment available and functioning properly
  c. Position person correctly
     - Have individual sit upright (60°–90°) in chair or dangle feet at side of bed if possible (prop pillows if necessary)
     - Have individual assume position 10 to 15 minutes before and after eating
     - Have individual flex head forward on the midline about 45° to keep esophagus patent
  d. Start with small amounts and progress slowly as person learns to handle each step
     Part of eyedropper filled with water
     Whole eyedropper
     Use juice in place of water
     ¼ teaspoon semi-solid (applesauce)
     ½ teaspoon semi-solid
     1 teaspoon semi-solid
     pureed food
     ½ cracker
     Soft diet
     Regular diet
     - For person who has had a CVA, place food at back of tongue and on side of face he can control
     - Feed slowly, making certain previous bite has been swallowed
  e. Reduce noxious stimuli
     - Minimize distractions by turning off TV or radio and secluding individual for the feeding session
     - Keep patient focused on task by giving directions until he has finished swallowing each mouthful
          "Move food to middle of tongue"
          "Raise tongue to roof of mouth"
          "Think about swallowing"
          "Swallow"
          "Cough to clear airway"
  f. Check that mouth is empty before continuing
     - Make sure food has not collected in the cheek pouches
  g. Instruct or assist person to
     - Administer good oral hygiene before and after feedings
     - Avoid spicy, acid, or salty foods
     - Avoid rough foods (raw vegetables, bran)
     - Soak "dry" foods (toast) to soften
     - If cold foods are soothing to individual, add ice or ice cream to gain extra coldness
     - Avoid smoking and alcohol (they may irritate mouth or throat)

## C. Initiate health teaching and referrals when indicated

 - Consult with speech pathologist for assistance with persons with swallowing difficulties

- Explain to individual and significant others rationale of treatment and how to proceed with it
- See *Alterations in Oral Mucous Membrane Related to Stomatitis* if indicated

# Alterations in Nutrition: Less Than Body Requirements
Related to Anorexia

Anorexia is a lack of appetite for food or fluids.

## Assessment

### Subjective data
The person reports
  He is not hungry
  Nausea
  Cannot concentrate on food

### Objective data
Weight loss
Intake less than Minimum Daily Requirement (MDR)

***

**Outcome Criteria**

The person will
  - Experience an increase in the amount or type of nutrients ingested
  - Describe causative factors when known
  - Describe rationale and procedure for treatments

***

## Interventions

A. Assess causative factors
  Alteration in sense of taste or smell
  Social isolation
  Radiation therapy or chemotherapy
  Alteration in body image or self-concept
  Early satiety
  Noxious stimuli (pain or painful or unpleasant procedures, fatigue, odors, nausea and vomiting)

## B. Reduce or eliminate contributing factors if possible

1. Altered sense of taste or smell
   - Explain to person the importance of consuming adequate amounts of nutrients
   - Teach person to use spices to help improve the taste and aroma of food (lemon juice, mint, cloves, basil, thyme, cinnamon, rosemary, bacon bits)
   - Teach protein sources he may find more acceptable than red meat
        Eggs and dairy products
        Chicken and turkey
        Fish (if not strong-smelling)
        Marinated meat (in wine, vinegar)

2. Social isolation
   - Encourage individual to eat with others (meals served in dining room or group area, at local meeting place such as community center, by church groups)
   - Provide daily contact through phone calls by support system
   - See *Social Isolation* for additional interventions

3. Noxious stimuli (pain, fatigue, odors, nausea, and vomiting)
   a. Pain
      - Plan care so that unpleasant or painful procedures do not take place before meals
      - Medicate individual for pain ½ hour before meals according to physician's orders
      - Provide pleasant, relaxed atmosphere for eating (no bedpans in sight; don't rush); try a "surprise" (*e.g.*, flowers with meal)
      - Arrange plan of care to decrease or eliminate nauseating odors or proceduring near mealtimes
   b. Fatigue
      - Teach or assist individual to rest before meals
      - Teach individual to spend minimal energy in food preparation (cook large quantities and freeze several meals at a time; request assistance from others)
   c. Odor of food
      - Teach him to avoid cooking odors—frying foods, brewing coffee—if possible (take a walk; select foods that can be eaten cold)
      - Suggest using foods that require little cooking during periods of anorexia
   d. Nausea and vomiting
      - Encourage frequent small amounts of ice chips or cool clear liquids (dilute tea, Jell-O water, flat ginger ale or cola) unless vomiting continues (adults 30 to 60 cc q ½–1 hour; children 15 to 30 cc q ½–1 hour)
      - Consider giving medications by suppository rather than by mouth
      - Decrease the stimulation of the vomiting center
        Reduce unpleasant sights and odors
        Provide good mouth care after vomiting
        Teach person to practice deep breathing and voluntary swallowing to suppress the vomiting reflex
        Instruct him to sit down after eating but not to lie down
        Encourage him to eat smaller meals and eat slowly
      - Restrict liquids with meals to avoid overdistending the stomach; also avoid fluids 1 hour before and after meals

- If possible, avoid the smell of food preparation
- Try eating cold foods, which have less odor
- Loosen clothing
- Sit in fresh air
- Avoid lying down flat for at least 2 hours after eating (an individual who must rest should sit or recline so head is at least 4 inches higher than feet)

## C. Promote foods that stimulate eating and increase protein consumption

1. Maintain good oral hygiene (brush teeth, rinse mouth) before and after ingestion of food
2. Offer frequent small feedings (six per day plus snacks) to reduce the feeling of a distended stomach
3. Allow individual to choose food items as close to actual eating time as possible
4. Arrange to have highest protein/calorie nutrients served at the time individual feels most like eating (*i.e.*, if chemotherapy is in early morning, serve in late afternoon)
5. Encourage significant others to bring in favorite home foods
6. Instruct person to
   - Eat dry foods (toast, crackers) upon arising
   - Eat salty foods if permissible
   - Avoid overly sweet, rich, greasy, or fried foods
   - Try clear cool beverages
   - Sip slowly through straw
   - Take whatever he feels he can tolerate
   - Eat small portions low in fat and eat more frequently
7. Try commercial supplements available in many forms (liquid, powder, pudding); keep switching brands until some are found that are acceptable to individual in taste and consistency
8. Teach techniques to individual and family for home food preparation
   - Add powdered milk or egg to milkshakes, gravies, sauces, puddings, cereals, meatballs, or milk to increase protein calorie content
   - Add blenderized or baby foods to meat juices or soups
   - Use fortified milk (*i.e.*, 1 cup instant nonfat milk to fresh 1 quart milk)
   - Use milk or half and half instead of water when making soups and sauces; soy formulas can also be used
   - Add cheese or diced meat whenever able
   - Add cream cheese or peanut butter to toast, crackers, celery sticks
   - Add extra butter or margarine to soups, sauces, vegetables
   - Spread toast while hot
   - Use mayonnaise (100 cal/T) instead of salad dressing
   - Add sour cream or yogurt to vegetables or as dip
   - Use whipped cream (60 cal/T)
   - Add raisins, dates, nuts, and brown sugar to hot or cold cereals
   - Have extra food (snacks) easily available

# Alterations in Nutrition: Less Than Body Requirements
## Related to Difficulty or Inability to Procure Food

Altered ability to procure food is the inability to acquire food because of physical, economic, or sociocultural barriers.

### Assessment

Subjective data

The person reports
"Can't afford to buy food"
"Don't know how to fix foods"
"Too much bother to fix meals for one person"

Objective data

Inability to speak or understand English
Activity restriction

---

**Outcome Criteria**

The person will
• Describe causative factors when known
• Be assisted to acquire food on a regular schedule

---

### Interventions

A. Assess causative factors

Inadequate economic resources to obtain adequate nutrition
Sociocultural barrier
Physical inability to procure food, related to health problem such as COPD, cardiac condition, CVA, or quadriplegia

B. Eliminate or reduce contributing factors if possible

1. Inadequate economic resources
   • Assess eligibility for food stamps, AID, or other government-funded programs for low-income groups; consult with social service
   • Suggest co-ops or local farmers' markets for shopping
   • Buy foods and meats on sale and freeze; utilize cheaper cuts and tenderize
   • Suggest foods that are low in cost and nutritionally high; decrease use of prepackaged or prepared items
      Beans and legumes as protein source
      Powdered milk (alone or mixed half and half with whole milk)
      Seasonal foods when plentiful
   • Encourage growing a small garden or participating in a community plot

- Freeze or can fruits and vegetables in season (refer to county agricultural agent for information on canning and freezing)
2. Sociocultural barrier
   - Introduce individual to locally available foodstuffs and instruct in their preparation
   - Suggest substitutions of locally available foodstuffs for those individual is accustomed to
   - Refer to adult education home economics classes for food preparation
   - Assist individual in recognizing and using additional outlets and sources of food (grocery stores, meat and fruit markets)
   - Encourage peer-group meetings among people of similar backgrounds to allow learning and exchange of ideas
3. Physical deficits
   - Promote alternate methods of food procurement and preparation
     a. Assess support systems for someone willing to purchase or prepare food for individual or take him to store
        Supermarkets that deliver
        Meals on Wheels or similar service
        Homemaker
        Group housing
        Door-to-store bus service
     b. Teach the individual or others to cook enough for six meals at one time and freeze; make own complete "frozen dinners"
   - Aid person in planning daily activities to account for energy need in shopping for food and preparing meals
        Rest periods before and after activity
        Rest periods during activity if needed

## C. Initiate health teaching and referrals when indicated

1. Social worker, occupational therapist, or visiting nurse, as needed
2. Adult education programs
3. Local extension office for information on vegetable gardening, community gardens, and techniques of freezing and canning foods

## Bibliography

### Books and Articles

Buckley JE, Addicks CL, Maniglia J: Feeding patients with dysphagia. Nurs Forum 15(1):69–85, 1976
Cooper KH: The New Aerobics. New York, Bantam Books, 1979
Dansky KM: Assessing children's nutrition. Am J Nurs 77:1610–1611, 1977
Ewald EB: Recipes for a Small Planet. New York, Ballantine Books, 1973
Griffin KM, Stubbert J, Breckenridge K: Teaching the dysphagic patient to swallow. RN 37(9):60–63, 1974
Kaminski MV Jr, Jeejeebhoy KN: Modern clinical nutritional assessment — diagnosis of malnutrition and selection of therapy. American Journal of Intravenous Therapy and Clinical Nutrition 6(3):31–50, 1979
Kornguth ML: Nursing management — when your client has a weight problem. Am J Nurs 81:553–554, 1981
Mitchell HS, Rynbergen HJ, Anderson L et al (eds): Cooper's Nutrition in Health and Disease, 16th ed. Philadelphia, JB Lippincott, 1976
Molleson A: New Dimensions in Nutrition. Columbus, Ohio, Ross Laboratories, 1980

Rang ML: Bibliography for nutrition in pregnancy. Journal of Obstetric and Gynecologic Nursing 9:55–58, 1980

Rouedu JR: Dysphagia: An Assessment and Management Program for the Adult. Minneapolis, Sister Kenny Institute–Abbott-Northwestern Hospital, 1980

Sine R, Liss S, Roush R et al: Basic Rehabilitation Techniques. Germantown, MD, Aspen Systems Corp., 1977

Sussman A, Goode R: Walking for Pleasure, for Health and for Serenity. New York, Famolau, 1977

Worthington B (ed): Symposium on nutrition. Nurs Clin North Am 14(2), 1979

## Pertinent Literature for the Consumer

Chamberlain AS: The Soft Foods Cookbook. Garden City, NY, Doubleday, 19

Chemotherapy and You (N.I.H. Pub. No. 81-1136). These three pamphlets available from U.S. Department of Health, Office of Cancer Communications, National Cancer Institute, Building 31, Room 10A18, Bethesda, Maryland 20205.

Diet and Nutrition (N.I.H. Pub. No. 81-2038). A resource for parents of children with cancer.

Eating Hints (N.I.H. Pub. No. 81-2079). Recipes and tips for better nutrition during cancer treatment.

Goldbeck N: As You Eat So Your Baby Grows: A Guide to Nutrition in Pregnancy. Available from Ceres Press, Box 87, Dept D, Woodstock, NY 12498 ($1.75).

McGill M, Pye, O: The No-Nonsense Guide to Food and Nutrition. Piscataway, NJ, New Century, 1982

List of publications. Society for Nutrition Education, 2140 Shattuck Avenue, Suite 1110, Berkeley, CA 94704.

# Nutrition, Alterations in: More Than Body Requirements

*Related to* **Imbalance of Intake vs. Activity Expenditures**

## Definition
Alterations in Nutrition: More Than Body Requirements: The state in which the individual experiences or is at risk of experiencing weight gain related to an intake in excess of metabolic requirements.*

## Etiological and Contributing Factors

### Pathophysiological
Altered satiety patterns
Decreased sense of taste and smell

### Situational
Anxiety, depression, stress, loneliness, boredom, guilt
Sedentary life-style
Pregnancy (at risk to gain more than 25–30 pounds)
Lack of basic nutritional knowledge
Ethnic or cultural values and expectations that emphasize hearty eating and a hefty body weight

### Maturational
Adult/elderly: Decreased activity patterns; decreased metabolic needs

## Defining Characteristics
Overweight (weight 10% over ideal for height and frame)
Obese (weight 20% or more over ideal for height and frame)
Triceps skin fold greater than 15 mm in men and 25 mm in women
Reported undesirable eating patterns
Intake in excess of metabolic requirements
Sedentary activity patterns

## Focus Assessment Criteria
See *Alterations in Nutrition: Less Than Body Requirements*

## Nursing Goals
Through selected interventions, the nurse will seek to assist the individual to
- Identify factors that contribute to intake in excess of metabolic needs
- Identify alternative behaviors to replace excess intake
- Lose weight

*The individual *at risk* for weight gain can be described by the label Alteration in Nutrition: Potential for More Than Body Requirements.

## Principles and Rationale for Nursing Care

### Obesity

1. Intake must be reduced to 500 calories per day less than requirement to obtain a one-pound-per-week weight loss.
2. The desirable weight loss rate is 1 to 2 pounds per week.
3. Overeating is complex multidimensional problem with physical, social, and psychological components.
4. Overweight persons are usually nutritionally deprived.
5. Exercise produces weight loss by increasing the caloric requirements of the body. Exercise does not have to occur in one time period to lose weight but may be spread out over a period of days and still be successful.
6. Internal motivation is essential for a successful weight-loss program.
7. An individual's body image and coping patterns influence the weight-loss program's success or failure.
8. Childhood obesity is influenced by genetic factors; cellular structure; general body build; metabolic and endocrine factors (pancreatic insufficiency, hypothyroidism, hypersecretion of adrenal cortex); activity level; infantile obesity; and the psychological, social, or cultural use of food for comfort, reward, or solace or as a symbol of affluence.
9. See *Alterations in Nutrition: Less Than Body Requirements* for additional principles.

# Alterations in Nutrition: More Than Body Requirements
## Related to Imbalance of Intake vs. Activity Expenditures*

## Assessment

### Subjective data

> Client states, "I like to eat"
> "Eating calms my nerves"
> "I don't have time for exercise"
> "I don't like sports or exercise"

### Objective data

> Weight > 10% over ideal for height and frame
> Triceps skin fold greater than 15 mm in men and 25 mm in women

*This specific diagnosis describes the individual who ingests calories in excess of metabolic need.

**Outcome Criteria**

The person will
- Experience increased activity expenditure with weight loss
- Describe relationship between activity level and weight
- Identify eating patterns that contribute to weight gain
- Lose weight

## Interventions

A. Assess causative factors

Stress response (increased oral intake)

Lack of basic nutritional knowledge

Low body image or self-concept (see *Ineffective Individual Coping Related to Depression*)

Ethnic or cultural values

Boredom

Sedentary life-style or work

B. Increase individual's awareness of those actions that contribute to excessive oral intake
- Request him to write down all the food he has eaten for the past 24 hours
- Instruct him to keep a diet diary for one week

    What, when, where, and why eaten?

    Whether doing anything else (*e.g.*, watching TV, preparing dinner)

    Emotions just before eating

    Others present (snacking with spouse, children)
- Review diet diary with individual to point out patterns (*i.e.*, time, place, persons, emotions, foods) that affect intake

C. Assist person to set realistic goals (i.e., decreasing oral intake by 500 calories will result in a 1-to-2-lb loss each week)
- Calculate requirements for actual weight minus 15 pounds and recalculate every two months or as necessary (actual weight in pounds $-15 \times 10 =$ maximum daily calories allowed if there is to be a weight loss)
- Plan balanced acceptable diet (remember cultural and personal preferences and use exchange lists; diet should provide choices)
- Plan for extra calories on weekends or as a special treat
- Select non-food rewards such as new clothes or a night out

D. Alter identified patterns of eating (i.e., if Friday night is the time when excess eating occurs, plan to be out on Friday night; if the person eats while watching TV, keep hands occupied in another manner such as knitting or crocheting, limit TV watching, or eat low-calorie snacks such as unbuttered popcorn, raw celery, and carrots)

E. Teach behavior modification techniques
- Eat only at a specific spot at home (*i.e.*, kitchen table)

- Do not eat while doing other activities such as reading or watching TV; eat only when sitting
- Drink 8-oz glass of water immediately before eating
- Decrease second helpings, fat and fatty foods, sweets and sugar and alcohol
- Use small plates (portions look bigger)
- Prepare small portions, just enough for meal, and throw away leftovers
- Never eat from another person's plate
- Eat slowly and chew thoroughly
- Put down utensils and wait 15 seconds between bites
- Eat low-calorie snacks that need to be chewed to satisfy oral need (carrots, celery, apples)
- Decrease liquid calories; drink diet sodas or water
- Plan eating splurges (save a number of calories a day and have a treat once a week) but eat only a small amount of splurge foods

## F. Increase activity level*

- Use stairs instead of elevator
- Park at outer edge of parking lot
- Plan a daily walking program and gradually increase rate and length of walk
  1. Start out at 5 to 10 blocks for 0.5 to 1.0 mile/day; increase 1 block or 0.1 mile/week
  2. Remember, progress slowly
  3. Avoid straining or pushing too hard and becoming overly fatigued
  4. Stop immediately if any of the following signs occur:

  | | |
  |---|---|
  | Lightness or pain in chest | Dizziness |
  | Severe breathlessness | Loss of muscle control |
  | Lightheadedness | Nausea |

  5. If pulse is 120 beats per minute (BPM) 5 minutes after stopping exercise, or if pulse is 100 BPM 10 minutes after stopping exercise, or if short of breath 10 minutes after exercise, slow down either the rate of walking or the distance
  6. If unable to walk 5 blocks or 0.5 mile without signs of overexertion appearing, decrease length of walking for one week to before signs appear and then start to add 1 block/0.1 mile each week
  7. Walk at same rate; time self with stopwatch or second hand on watch; after reaching 10 blocks (1 mile) try to increase speed
  8. Remember, increase only the rate *or* the length of walk at one time
  9. Establish a regular time of day to exercise, with the goal of 3 to 5 times per week for a duration of 15 to 45 minutes and with a heart rate of 80% of stress test or gross calculation (170 BPM for 20–29 age group; decrease 10 BPM for each additional decade of life—*e.g.*, 160 BPM for ages 30–39, 150 BPM for ages 40–49, etc.)
- Encourage significant others to engage in walking program also

## G. Add additional exercise as tolerated

| | |
|---|---|
| TV or tape cassette exercise program | Dancing |
| | Swimming |
| Exercycle | Bicycling |
| Spa/gym/YMCA | |

*Caution: If health problem exists, consult physician before increasing activity.

## H. Initiate health teaching and referrals as indicated
- Explain basic nutritional knowledge
- Explain health hazards of overweight
- Explain the benefits of exercise, *e.g.*, consumes calories, reduces stress
- Refer to support groups, *e.g.*, Weight Watchers, Overeaters Anonymous, TOPS, trim clubs, The Diet Workshop, Inc.

## Bibliography

See *Alterations in Nutrition: Less Than Body Requirements* for additional sources of information.

Hoepfel HJ: Improving compliance with an exercise program. Am J Nurs 80:449–450, 1980

Jacobson P: Help for fat teenagers. Pediatric Nursing 5(2):49–50, 1979

Kaufmann NA: Eating habits and opinions of teenagers on nutrition and obesity. J Am Diet Assoc 66:264–268, 1975

Overeaters anonymous: A self-help group. Am J Nurs 81:560–563, 1981

# Oral Mucous Membrane, Alterations in

*Related to* **Inadequate Oral Hygiene**

*Related to* **Stomatitis**

## Definition

Alterations in oral mucous membrane: The state in which an individual experiences or is at risk of experiencing disruptions in the oral cavity.

## Etiological and Contributing Factors

### Pathophysiological

Diabetes mellitus
Oral cancer
Periodontal disease
Infection
Herpes simplex                    Gingivitis

### Situational

Chemical trauma
Acidic foods              Alcohol
Drugs                     Tobacco
Noxious agents

Mechanical trauma
Broken or jagged teeth    Endotrachial tube
Ill-fitting dentures      Nasogastric tube
Braces

Radiation to head or neck
Malnutrition
Dehydration
Mouth breathing
NPO > 24 hours
Inadequate oral hygiene
Lack of knowledge
Fractured mandible
Prolonged use of steroids or other immunosuppressives
Antineoplastic drugs

## Defining Characteristics

Coated tongue             Leukoplakia
Xerostomia (dry mouth)    Edema

Stomatitis                          Hemorrhagic gingivitis
Oral tumors                         Purulent drainage
Oral lesions

## Focus Assessment Criteria

### Subjective data

1. The person complains of
   Mouth pain, irritation, or burning
   Xerostomia (dry mouth)
   Bad taste or odor in mouth
   Chewing difficulties
   Change in tolerance to temperatures of food (cold, hot)
   Change in tolerance to acidic or highly seasoned food
   Change in taste
   Poorly fitting dentures
2. History
   Medical/surgical
   Medication use (prescribed, over the counter)
   Use of tobacco
       Type (cigarettes, pipe, cigars, snuff)
       Frequency (packs per day, how many years)
   Use of alcohol
       Type
       Amount (daily, weekly)
3. Oral hygiene
   Frequency of dental checkups
   Personal hygiene
       "Describe your oral care procedure"
       Type of equipment (brush, floss)
       Frequency
   Possible barriers to performing oral care
       Unable to hold standard brush
       Unable to close hand
       Limited arm movement
       Semicomatose
       Lack of knowledge
4. Nutritional status (refer to *Alterations in Nutrition* for specific assessment criteria)
   Daily intake of basic four food groups
   Daily fluid intake
   Difficulty in chewing or swallowing
   Are certain foods avoided? Why?

### Objective data

1. Lips
   Color
   Presence of
           Cracks                          Blisters
           Fissures                        Ulcers/lesions

  2. Tongue
       Color
       Presence of
          Masses                         Cracks, dryness
          Lesions                         Exudates
          Hairy extensions
  3. Oral mucosa (gums, floor of mouth, inner cheeks, palate)
       Color
       Presence of
          Bleeding                     Plaques
          Swelling                     Lesions
  4. Teeth
       Presence of
          Sharp edges              Looseness
          Chips                       Missing teeth
          Cracks
  5. Dentures/prosthetics
       Condition
       Fit
       Presence of
          Sharp edges              Cracks
          Loose parts               Chips

## Nursing Goals

Through selected interventions, the nurse will
  • Assess for and prevent potential mouth problems
  • Teach the person self-care when appropriate
  • Give effective mouth care or supervise the performance of other personnel

## Principles and Rationale for Nursing Care

  1. Oral health directly influences many activities of daily living (eating, fluid intake, breathing) and interpersonal relations (appearance, self-concept, communication).
  2. The frequency of oral health maintenance will vary according to an individual's health status and self-care ability. All persons should have their teeth and mouths cleaned at least once after meals and at bedtime. High-risk persons (*e.g.*, persons with cancer and poorly nourished persons) should have oral assessments daily. Persons in chronic care settings should have oral assessments *at least* once a month.
  3. Factors that contribute to oral disease are alcohol and tobacco (excessive use), microorganisms, inadequate nutrition (quantity, quality), inadequate hygiene, and trauma (ill-fitting dentures, sharp-edged teeth, sharp-edged prostheses, improper use of cleaning devices).
  4. Many oral diseases begin quietly and are painless until significant involvement has taken place.
  5. Plaque is microbial flora found in the mouth and is the primary factor contributing to dental cavities and periodontal disease. Daily removal of plaque through brushing and flossing can help prevent dental decay and disease.
  6. Decreased salivary flow and increased viscosity of saliva reduce the removal of debris (food, bacteria) from the mouth.

7. Common causes of decreased salivation are dehydration, anemia, radiation treatment to head and neck, vitamin deficiencies, removal of salivary glands, allergies, and side-effects of drugs (*e.g.*, antihistamines, anticholinergics, phenothiazines, narcotics, chemotherapy).

8. Excessive use of hydrogen peroxide for mouth care may predispose to an oral yeast infection. Rinse afterward with normal saline.

9. Lemon and glycerine swabs should be used only on clean, healthy mouths as a source of refreshment for an NPO client.

10. Alcohol and tobacco are chronic irritants to oral mucosa and may lead to oral carcinoma.

# Alterations in Oral Mucous Membrane
Related to Inadequate Oral Hygiene

## Assessment

### Subjective data
The person reports
   Does not practice oral hygiene
   Cannot perform oral hygiene

### Objective data
   Pain
   Burning
   Coated tongue

---

**Outcome Criteria**

The person will
   • Maintain or be assisted to maintain the integrity of the oral cavity
   • Débride or be débrided of harmful plaque to prevent secondary infection
   • Be free of oral discomfort during food and fluid intake

---

## Interventions

A. Assess for the presence of causative or contributing factors
   Lack of knowledge
   Lack of motivation
   Impairment of use of hands
   Fatigue
   Altered consciousness

B. Discuss the importance of daily oral hygiene and periodic dental exams
  - Explain the relationship of plaque to dental and gum disease
  - Evaluate the person's ability to perform oral hygiene
  - Allow person to perform as much of his oral care as possible

C. Teach correct oral care
  1. Have person sit or stand upright over sink (if unable to get to sink, place an emesis pan under the chin)
  2. Remove and clean dentures and bridges daily
     - Fill wash bowl half full of water (place washcloth on bottom to keep denture from breaking if dropped)
     - Brush dentures with a denture brush or stiff hard toothbrush inside and outside; rinse in cool water before replacing
     - Stains and odors can be removed from dentures by soaking them overnight in 8 oz of water and 1 teaspoon of laundry bleach (avoid bleach on any appliance with metal)
     - Hard deposits can be removed by soaking dentures in white (not brown) vinegar overnight
     - If commercial liquid denture cleaners are used, brushing is still required
  3. Floss teeth (q 24 hr)
     - With a piece of dental floss approximately 25 inches long, floss each tooth by wrapping the floss around the second and third fingers of each hand
     - Beginning with the back teeth, insert the floss between each tooth gently to prevent injuring the gum
     - Wrap floss around tooth, making a C, and gently pull floss up and down over the back of each tooth
     - Repeat this in reverse to floss the front of the tooth
     - Remove the floss by either pulling straight up or by releasing one end and pulling the floss through (minor bleeding may occur)
     - Allow the person to rinse
     - Floss holders can be used by the person or the nurse to make flossing easier (back teeth cannot be reached with a floss holder)
  4. Brush teeth (after meals and before sleep)
     - Use a soft toothbrush (avoid hard brushes) with a nonabrasive toothpaste or sodium bicarbonate (1 teaspoon in 8 oz of water; may be contraindicated in persons with sodium restrictions)
     - Brush back and forth or in a small circle, starting at the back of the mouth and brushing one or two teeth at a time
     - Gently brush tongue and inner sides of cheeks
     - Rinse with water
  5. Inspect mouth for lesions, sores, or excessive bleeding

D. Perform oral hygiene on person who is unconscious or at risk for aspiration as often as needed
  1. Preparation
     - Tell person what you are going to do
     - Turn person on his side, supporting back with pillow (protect bed with an absorbent pad)
     - Place a tongue blade or bite block to keep mouth open
     - Wear gloves to protect hands

2. Brushing procedure
  - For persons with their own teeth, brush following the procedure outlined in Nos. 3 and 4 above
  - Use a solution instead of toothpaste: hydrogen peroxide and water (1 to 4), sodium bicarbonate (1 tsp to 8 oz water), or normal saline (may be contraindicated in persons with sodium restrictions)
  - For persons with dentures, remove dentures and clean according to procedure in No. 2
  - Leave dentures out for persons who are semicomatose and store in water (in denture cup)
  - If gums are inflamed, use moist cotton tipped applicators or soft foam Toothettes
  - Use a bulb syringe to rinse mouth; aspirate rinse with suction or use an aspirating toothbrush
  - Move tongue blade or bite block for access to other areas; do not put fingers on tops or edges of teeth
  - Brush tongue and inner cheek tissue gently
  - Pat mouth dry and apply lip lubricant
  - Gums and teeth should be lightly wiped four to six times a day to prevent drying (*e.g.*, swab with mineral oil or saline but use sparingly to prevent aspiration)

E. Initiate health teaching and referrals as indicated
  1. Identify individuals who need toothbrush adaptations to perform own mouth care (Fig. II–6)
     a. Difficulty closing hand tightly
        - Tape a wide elastic band to toothbrush tight enough to hold brush snugly in hand
     b. Limited hand mobility
        - Enlarge toothbrush handle with a sponge hair roller, wrinkled aluminum foil, or a bicycle handbar grip attached with a small amount of plaster of paris
     c. Limited arm movement
        - Extend handle of standard toothbrush by attaching handle of an old toothbrush (after cutting off bristle end) to a new toothbrush with strong cord or plastic cement, or by attaching toothbrush to a plastic rod (the toothbrush can be curved by gently heating and then bending it)
  2. Refer individuals with tooth and gum disorders to a dentist
  3. Teach parents to
     - Provide their child with fluoride supplements if not present in concentrations over 0.7 parts per million (ppm) in drinking water
     - Avoid taking tetracycline drugs during pregnancy or giving to child during infancy
     - Refrain from putting an infant to bed with a bottle of juice or milk
     - Provide child with safe objects for chewing during teething
     - Replace toothbrushes frequently (q 3 months)
     - Schedule dental checkups every 6 months after the age of 2 years
  4. Teach child to
     - Avoid highly sugared liquids and foods
     - Drink water as an extra fluid
     - Brush teeth using fluoride toothpaste

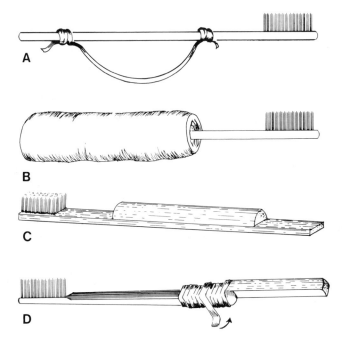

**Figure II–6.** Toothbrush adaptations. (*A*) Toothbrush handle with elastic band. (*B*) A sponge hair roller enlarging the toothbrush handle. (*C*) A short piece of plastic tubing glued to the toothbrush handle. (*D*) The handle of an old toothbrush attached to the present toothbrush to provide a longer handle.

# Alterations in Oral Mucous Membrane
## Related to Stomatitis

Stomatitis is inflammation of the mucous membrane of the mouth, ranging from redness to ulcerations to hemorrhage.

### Assessment

#### Subjective data
The person reports
    Oral burning or pain
    Change in tolerance to food temperatures (cold, hot)
    Change in tolerance to acidic or highly seasoned food

#### Objective data
    Erythema of oral mucosa (mild)
    Small areas of ulcerations or white patches (moderate)

White patches over 25% of oral mucosa (moderate to severe)
Hemorrhagic ulcerations (severe)

---

**Outcome Criteria**

The person will
  • Be free of oral mucosa irritation or exhibit signs of healing with decreased inflammation
  • Demonstrate knowledge of optional oral hygiene
  • Maintain adequate hydration and nutrition

---

## Interventions

### A. Assess for the presence of causative or contributing factors

Lack of oral hygiene
Malnourishment
History of high alcohol intake and tobacco use
Chemotherapeutic drugs with mucous membrane toxicity
Radiation to head or neck
Immunosuppression
Dehydration
Steroid therapy

### B. Teach individuals at risk to develop stomatitis preventive oral hygiene

1. Refer to *Alterations in Oral Mucous Membrane Related to Inadequate Oral Hygiene* for specific instructions on brushing and flossing
2. Instruct person to
    • Perform the regimen after meals and before sleep (if there is excessive exudate, perform regimen before breakfast also)
    • Avoid mouthwashes with high alcohol content, lemon/glycerine swabs, or prolonged use of hydrogen peroxide
    • Use an oxidizing agent to loosen thick, tenacious mucus (gargle and expectorate), *e.g.*, hydrogen peroxide and water ¼ strength (avoid prolonged use) or sodium bicarbonate 1 tsp in 8 oz warm water (can flavor these with mouthwash or one drop of oil of wintergreen)
    • Rinse mouth with saline after gargling
    • Apply lubricant to lips q 2 hours and PRN (*e.g.*, lanolin, A&D ointment, petroleum jelly)
    • Inspect mouth daily for lesions and inflammation and report alterations
3. For person who is unable to tolerate brushing or swabbing, teach to irrigate mouth (q 2 hours and PRN)
    • With baking soda solution (4 teaspoons in 1 liter warm water) using an enema bag (labeled for oral use only) with a soft irrigation catheter tip
    • By placing catheter tip in mouth and slowly increasing flow while standing over a basin or having a basin held under chin
    • Remove dentures prior to irrigation and do not replace in person with severe stomatitis
4. Consult with physician for possible need of prophylactic antifungal or antibacterial agent

## C. Promote healing and progression of stomatitis

1. Inspect oral cavity three times daily with tongue blade and light; if stomatitis is severe, inspect mouth q 4 hours
2. Ensure that oral hygiene regimen is done q 2 hours while awake and q 6 hours (q 4 if severe) during the night
3. Use normal saline as a mouthwash unless crusts and debris are present; then use
   - Hydrogen peroxide and water ¼ strength; then rinse with saline
   - Sodium bicarbonate solute, 1 tsp in 8 oz water; then rinse with water
   - Alternate one of the above q 2 hours with saline rinses
4. Floss teeth only once in 24 hours
5. Omit flossing if excessive bleeding occurs and use extreme caution with persons with platelet counts of less than 50,000

## D. Reduce oral pain and maintain adequate food and fluid intake

1. Assess person's ability to chew and swallow
2. Administer mild analgesic q 3–4 hours as ordered by physician
3. Instruct individual to
   - Avoid commercial mouthwashes, citrus fruit juices, spicy foods, extremes in food temperature (hot, cold), crusty or rough foods
   - Eat bland, cool foods (sherbets)
   - Drink cool liquids q 2 hours and PRN
4. Consult with dietitian for specific interventions
5. Refer to *Alterations in Nutrition: Less Than Body Requirements Related to Anorexia* for additional interventions
6. Consult with physician for an oral pain relief solution
   - Xylocaine Viscous 2% oral swish and expectorant q 2 hours and before meals (if throat is sore, the solution can be swallowed; if swallowed, Xylocaine produces local anesthesia and may affect the gag reflex)
   - Mix equal parts of Xylocaine Viscous, 0.5 aqueous Benadryl solution, and Maalox; swish and swallow 1 oz of mixture q 2–4 hours PRN
   - Mix equal parts of 0.5 aqueous Benadryl solution and Kaopectate; swish and swallow q 2–4 hours PRN

## E. Initiate health teaching and referrals as indicated

1. Teach person and family the factors that contribute to the development of stomatitis and its progression
2. Teach diet modifications to reduce oral pain and to maintain optimal nutrition

**Bibliography**

Ariaudo A: How frequently must patients carry out effective oral hygiene procedures in order to maintain gingival health? J Periodontol 42:309–313, 1971
Beck S: Impact of a systematic oral care protocol on stomatitis after chemotherapy. Cancer Nursing 2:185–199, 1979
Bennett J: Oral health maintenance. In Carnevale D, Patrick M: Nursing Management for the Elderly, pp 111–135. Philadelphia, JB Lippincott, 1981
Bruya M, Maderia N: Stomatitis After Chemotherapy. Am J Nurs 75:1349–1352, 1975
Daeffler R: Oral hygiene measures for patients with cancer. Cancer Nursing 3:347–355, 1980; 3:427–432, 1980; 4:29–36, 1981
DeWalt E: Effect of timed hygienic measures on oral mucosa in a group of elderly subjects. Nurs Res 24:104–108, 1975

DeWalt E, Haines S: Effects of specified stressors on healthy oral mucosa. Nurs Res 18:22–27, 1969

Kloch J, Seidduth A: Oral hygiene instruction and plaque formation during hospitalization. Nurs Res 18:124–130, 1969

Lovelock DJ: Oral hygiene for patients in hospitals. Nursing Mirror 61(6):39–42, 1973

O'Leary TJ: Oral hygiene agents and procedures. J Periodontol 41:625–629, 1970

Passos J, Brand L: Effects of agents for oral hygiene. Nurs Res 15:196–202, 1966

Reitz M, Pope W: Mouth care. Am J Nurs 73:1728–1730, 1973

Schweiger J, Lang JW, Schweiger JW et al: Oral assessment: How to do it. Am J Nurs 80:654–657, 1980

Wiley S: Why lemon and glycerol? Am J Nurs 69:342–348, 1969

# Parenting, Alterations in

*Related to* **Impaired Parental–Infant Attachment (Bonding)**

*Related to* **Child Abuse/Neglect**

*Related to* **Breast-Feeding Difficulties**

## Definition

Alterations in parenting: The state in which one or more individuals experiences a real or potential inability to provide a constructive environment which nurtures the growth and development of his/her/their child (children).*

## Etiological and Contributing Factors

Individuals or families who may be at high risk for developing or experiencing parenting difficulties:

Parent(s)

| | |
|---|---|
| Single | Addicted to drugs |
| Adolescent | Terminally ill |
| Abusive | Acutely disabled |
| Emotionally disturbed | Accident victim |
| Alcoholic | |

Child

| | |
|---|---|
| Of unwanted pregnancy | Mentally handicapped |
| Of undesired sex | Hyperactive |
| With undesired characteristics | Terminally ill |
| Physically handicapped | Rebellious |

### Situational

Separation from nuclear family

Lack of extended family

Lack of knowledge

Economic problems

| | |
|---|---|
| Inflation | Unemployment |

Relationship problems

| | |
|---|---|
| Marital discord | Step-parents |
| Divorce | Live-in boy/girl friend |
| Separation | Relocation |

Change in family unit

| | |
|---|---|
| New child | Relative moves in |

### Other

History of ineffective relationships with own parents

Parental history of abusive relationship with parents

Unrealistic expectations of child by parent

*A family's ability to function is at a high risk to develop problems when the child or parent has a condition that increases the stress of the family unit.

Unrealistic expectations of self by parent
Unrealistic expectations of parent by child
Unmet psychosocial needs of child by parent
Unmet psychosocial needs of parent by child

## Defining Characteristics

Lack of parental attachment behavior
Diminished or inappropriate visual, tactile, or auditory stimulation of infant
Frequent verbalization of dissatisfaction or disappointment with infant/child
Verbalization of frustration of role
Verbalization of perceived or actual inadequacy
Evidence of abuse or neglect of child
Growth and development lag in infant/child
Inappropriate parenting behaviors

## Focus Assessment Criteria

Applies to each individual (mother and father) and to family unit
1. Attachment Behavior
   Pregnancy
   Planned?                          Was an abortion considered?
   Desired?                          If yes, why was decision
                                        changed?

   Prenatal
   Verbalizes anticipation           Seeks prenatal care
   Selects name                      Follows the regimen
   Plans layette                     Decides about infant feeding
                                        (breast or bottle)

   Intrapartum
   Participates in the decision and the birthing process
   Verbalizes positive feelings
   Attempts to see infant as soon as delivered
   Responds positively (happy) or negatively (sad, apathetic, disappointed, angry, ambivalent)
   Holds and talks to infant
   Uses baby's name
   Talks to baby's father

   Postpartum
   Verbalizes positive feelings
   Seeks proximity by holding infant closely; touches and hugs
   Smiles and gazes at infant; seeks eye-to-eye contact
   Seeks family resemblance (*i.e.*, "has my eyes," "sleeps like his father")
   Refers to infant by name and sex
   Expresses interest in learning infant care
   Performs nurturing behavior (*i.e.*, feeding, changing)
2. Support system
   Location of most relatives
   Frequency of visits with relatives
   Length of time lived at present residence
   Patterns of parental socialization with friends and relatives
   Interrelationship between parents

3. Parenting knowledge/experience

Parents' recall of their relationship with their parents or caretakers and types of discipline and punishment used

Experiences with previous pregnancies

Knowledge of developmental needs

Parental expectations of child

4. Parent/child relationship

Subjective

Parental level of satisfaction with child

Amount of play activities between mother and child

Amount of play activities between father and child

Amount of caretaking activities between mother and child

Amount of caretaking activities between father and child

Provisions for child development (toys, verbal stimulation)

Reasons for disciplining

Methods of discipline or punishment

Objective

Child's affect (animated, warm, apathetic, cold, withdrawn)

Presence of touching/holding behavior

Presence of injuries

Explanation by child and parent

Correlation of explanation to injury

History of injuries (type, causes)

5. High-risk individuals (parent, child)

Assess for presence of at-risk factors in parent and child (see Etiological and Contributing Factors)

## Nursing Goals

Through selected interventions, the nurse will seek to

- Promote parent/child attachment
- Identify families at risk for potential parenting difficulties
- Provide support to families in crisis
- Protect the child from further abuse, when abuse or neglect has been determined or suspected

## Principles and Rationale for Nursing Care

In the past, because of living in extended families, young children observed and frequently assisted in the birth and care of infants. Today in the United States, due to our mobile society and the more isolated nuclear family living style, young men and women often approach parenthood with only a vague recollection of their own childhood, no knowledge of the birthing process, and limited, if any, experience in infant and child care.

### General

1. Parenting is a learned behavior, and in general people parent as they were parented.
2. Support groups partially replacing the extended family have become very popular and useful in providing knowledge regarding the birth process and in developing parenting skills.
3. Parents need confidence, as well as skill, in order to be comfortable in their new

role. The nurse is in the enviable position of being able to assist families by providing them with information on parenting.

4. Situations that contribute to potential or actual alteration in parenting are often related to ineffective individual or family coping

5. See Appendix VIII for age-related developmental tasks with related interventions

## Bonding/attachment

1. Research indicates that there is a "sensitive period" during the newborn's first minutes and hours of life during which the child is beautifully equipped to meet and interact with the parents. Close contact at this time and in the days to follow is most beneficial to the bonding process.

2. The process of bonding begins before conception by planning the pregnancy and its conception as described by the following steps (Josten): planning the pregnancy, confirming the pregnancy, accepting the pregnancy, feeling fetal movement, accepting the fetus as an individual, giving birth, hearing and seeing the baby, touching and holding the baby, and caring for the baby.

3. The period from birth to three days is an important period for father-child bonding.

4. Bonding is promoted by seeing, touching, and caring for the infant.

5. Participation of the father in caregiving activities in American society has increased. Fathers who choose the traditional role (allowing the mother to be totally responsible for caretaking activities) must be assessed in their socio-cultural context.

6. Attachment during the postpartum period is influenced by three factors: the characteristics of the baby—its appearance (attractive) and behavior (alert); the characteristics of each parent (satisfaction with baby, beliefs about ability to care for baby, ability to console and comfort baby, frequency of interactions with baby); and support—the availability of a positive resource person (relative, neighbor) and the availability of follow-up for high-risk families.

7. The bonding process is impeded when the parent(s) and child are separated because of the condition of the infant or a parent.

8. Parents are reluctant to form attachments to a sick infant because of their fear of loss. This reluctance creates tremendous guilt.

9. Parents must be given the opportunity for grief work in the case of an ill or defective infant before attachment can begin.

10. No single behavior during pregnancy or in the postpartem period can be a conclusive sign of attachment difficulty. The presence of several characteristic signs should direct the nurse to gather more data.

11. The use of birthing rooms enhances the bonding process because of the decrease in interruptions.

## Child abuse and neglect

1. Approximately half a million cases of suspected abuse and neglect were reported in 1975, and the estimated number of cases of actual abuse and neglect was 2 to 4 million.

2. The discrepancy between the reported cases of child abuse and the estimated number is related to the failure of professionals to report suspected cases, the misdiagnosis of inflicted injuries as accidental, and the lack of listing of child abuse in the International Classification of Disease.

3. The nurse should consult the legislation mandating the reporting of child abuse for the specifics of legal definition, penalties for failure to report, reporting procedure, and legal immunity for reporting.

4. The nurse may come in contact with an abused child in an emergency room, school, or physician's office or in her personal life.

5. The identification of child abuse is dependent on the nurse's recognizing the physical signs, specific parent behavior, specific child behavior, inconsistencies in the history of the injury, and contributing factors (familial, environmental).

6. The first priority of care for the abused child is preventing further injury.

7. Reporting child abuse is a means of getting help to the child and the family. The purpose of protective services is to preserve the family. Only after all other possibilities have failed is the child removed from the home. All states have laws regarding child abuse; everyone who comes in contact with children in their normal working day has a legal responsibility to report suspected child abuse.

8. Child abuse is a symptom of a family in crisis or a family dysfunction. The crisis can be illness, financial difficulties, or any recent change in the family unit (new members, loss of a member, relocation).

9. Separation of the infant from its parents, as in the case of prematurity, can reduce the attachment and nurturing behaviors of the mother toward her child. A disproportionate number of abused children were premature or ill at birth.

10. Children are usually abused by someone they know: a parent, a babysitter, a relative, or a friend of the family. It must be remembered that the majority of people who abuse a child are well-intentioned adults who know the child and care about its welfare. Their intent was to punish or teach the child a lesson. The abusing parent usually feels extremely guilty and is often relieved when help is offered. The child also may feel guilt, sensing that he is "bad" and therefore required the discipline.

11. Factors that contribute to child abuse are:
    - Lack of or unavailability of the extended family
    - Economic conditions (inflation, unemployment)
    - Lack of role model as a child
    - High-risk children (unwanted, of undesired sex or appearance, physically or mentally handicapped, hyperactive, or terminally ill)
    - High-risk parents (single, adolescent, emotionally disturbed, alcoholic, drug addicted, or physically ill)

12. Characteristic personal patterns of abusers are:
    - No dominant ethic or socioeconomic characteristics
    - History of abuse by their parents and lack of warmth and affection from them
    - Social isolation (few friends or outlets for tensions)
    - Marked lack of self-esteem, with low tolerance for criticism
    - Emotional immaturity and dependency
    - Distrust of others
    - Inability to admit the need for help
    - High expectations for/of child (perceiving child as a source of emotional gratification)
    - Desire for the child to give them pleasure

13. The nonabusing parent, who is usually passive and compliant in the abuse, must be included in the treatment plan.

# Alterations in Parenting
Related to Impaired Parental—Infant Attachment (Bonding)

Bonding is the strong attachment formed between parent and child.

## Assessment

### Subjective data
The parent verbalizes
  Feelings of inadequacy
  Disgust at infant's bodily functions
  Resentment toward infant
  Disappointment in sex or physical characteristics of infant

### Objective data
  Does not hold infant close
  Does not seek eye-to-eye contact
  Does not talk to infant or call infant by name
  Inattentive to infant's needs
  Asks no questions about care
  Cries, appears sad
  Is hostile to father

---

**Outcome Criteria**

The parent will
  • Demonstrate increased attachment behaviors, such as holding infant close, smiling and talking to infant, and seeking eye contact with infant
  • Initiate an active role in the infant's care
  • Begin to verbalize positive feelings regarding the infant

---

## Interventions

A. Assess causative or contributing factors
  1. Maternal
      Unwanted pregnancy
      Prolonged or difficult labor and delivery
      Postpartum pain or fatigue
      Lack of positive support system (mother, spouse, friends)
      Lack of positive role model (mother, relative, neighbor)
  2. Parental inadequate coping patterns (one or both parents)
      Alcoholic
      Drug addict
      Marital difficulties (separation, divorce, violence)
      Change in life-style related to new role

Adolescent parent
Career change (*e.g.*, working woman to mother)
Illness in family
3. Infant
Premature, defective, ill
Multiple birth

## B. Eliminate or reduce contributing factors if possible

1. Illness, pain, fatigue
   - Establish with mother what infant-care activities are feasible
   - Provide mother with uninterrupted sleep periods of at least 2 hours during the day and 4 hours during the night
   - Provide relief for discomforts
   a. Episotomy
      - Evaluate degree of pain
      - Assess for hematomas and abscesses
      - Provide with comfort measures (ice, warm compresses, analgesics*)
   b. Hemorrhoids
      - Prevent and treat constipation
      - Provide comfort measures (compresses with witch hazel, suppositories,* analgesics*)
   c. Breast engorgement of nursing mother
      - Nurse as frequently as possible
      - Apply warm compresses (shower) before nursing
      - Apply cold compresses following nursing
      - Try hand massage, hand expressing, or breast pump between nursing
      - Offer mild analgesics
      - See *Alterations in Parenting Related to Breast-Feeding Difficulties*
   d. Breast engorgement of non-nursing mother
      - Offer analgesics as ordered
      - Apply ice packs
      - Encourage use of a good supporting brassiere that covers the entire breast
2. Lack of experience or lack of positive mothering role model
   - Explore with mother her feelings and attitudes concerning her own mother
   - Assist her to identify someone who is a positive mother and encourage her to seek that person's aid
   - Outline the teaching program available to her during hospitalization
   - Determine who will assist her at home initially
   - Identify community programs and reference material that can increase her learning about child care after discharge (see Bibliography)
3. Lack of positive support system
   a. Identify mother's support system and assess its strengths and weaknesses
   b. Assess the need for counseling
      - Encourage the parent(s) to express feelings about the experience and about the future
      - Be an active listener to the parent(s)
      - Observe the parent(s) interacting with the infant

*May require a physician's order.

- Assess for resources (financial, emotional) already available to the family
- Be aware of resources available both within the hospital and in the community
- Counsel the parent(s) on assessed needs
- Refer to hospital or community services

## C. Provide opportunities for the bonding process

1. Promote bonding in the immediate postdelivery phase
   - Encourage mother to hold infant following birth (may need a short recovery period)
   - Provide skin-to-skin contact if desired; keep room warm (72° to 76°) or use a heat panel over the infant
   - Provide mother with an opportunity to breast-feed if desired
   - Delay the administration of silver nitrate to allow for eye contact
   - Give family as much time as they need together with minimum interruption from the staff (the "sensitive period" lasts from 30 to 90 minutes)
   - Encourage father to hold infant
2. Facilitate the bonding process during the postpartum phase
   - Check mother regularly for signs of fatigue, especially if she had anesthesia
   - Offer flexible rooming-in to the mother; establish with her the amount of care she will assume initially and support her requests for assistance
   - Discuss the future involvement of the father in the infant's care (if desired, plan opportunities for father to participate in his child's care during visits)
3. Provide support to the parent(s)
   - Listen to the mother's replay of her labor and delivery experience
   - Allow for verbalization of feelings
   - Indicate acceptance of feelings
   - Point out the infant's strengths and individual characteristics to the parent(s)
   - Demonstrate the infant's responses to the parents
   - Have a system of follow-up following discharge, especially for families considered at risk, *e.g.,* a phone call or a home visit by the community health nurse
   - Be aware of resources and support groups available within the hospital and the community and refer the family as needed
4. Assess the need for teaching
   - Observe the parent(s) interacting with the infant
   - Support each parent's strengths
   - Assist each parent in those areas where they are uncomfortable (role modeling)
   - Offer classes in infant care
   - Have handouts and audiovisual aids available for parent(s) to view at odd hours
   - Assess for level of knowledge in the area of growth and development and provide information as needed
   - See Bibliography for recommended printed material on parenting and child care

## D. Initiate referrals as needed

- Consult with community agencies for follow-up visits if indicated
- Refer parents to pertinent organizations (see Bibliography)

# Alterations in Parenting
Related to Child Abuse/Neglect

Child abuse is an action or inaction that brings injury to a child, including physical and psychological injury, neglect, and sexual abuse.

## Assessment

### Subjective data (Kempe, Heifer)
The parent or caretaker
  Cannot explain the source of injury
  Gives an explanation that is in conflict with the developmental ability of the child (*e.g.*, six-month-old spilled pot on stove)
  Gives an explanation that is inconsistent with injury (*e.g.*, concussion and broken leg from falling out of bed)
  Has delayed seeking medical attention
  Describes frequent injuries and accidents
  Blames someone else for causing the injury
  Verbalizes family discord, feelings of inadequacy; says that the child is different in some way or that his anger cannot be controlled
The child
  Reports an incident of abuse
  Tells a story that conflicts with the caretaker's story

### Objective data
The parent or caretaker
  Does not comfort the child
  Is detached
  Is out of control or highly controlled
The child
  Has a developmental lag
  Appears poorly cared for
  Is fearful of adults
  Seeks to comfort the parent
  Remains stoic during painful procedures
  Has a lack of social initiative

### Findings and reports
Of abuse
  Multiple injuries in various stages of healing
  Injury to genital area
  Gonorrhea
  Marks on skin from straps, buckles, rope, cigarette burns
  Subdural hematoma
  Bruising around the eye
  Contusions
  Ruptured abdominal organs
  Early pregnancy ( < 12–14)

Of neglect
> Malnourished
> Unbathed
> Inadequately dressed for weather
> Frequently left unsupervised

---

**Outcome Criteria**

The child will
- Be protected from injury or neglect by caretaker
- Establish a trusting relationship with a caretaker
- Be free from injury or neglect

The parent will
- Seek assistance for his abusive behavior
- Demonstrate nurturing behavior toward the child

---

## Interventions

### A. Identify families at risk for child abuse
- Refer to Principles and Rationale for Nursing Care

### B. Intervene prior to abuse with families at risk
- Establish a relationship with parents that encourages them to share difficulties ("Being a parent is sure hard [frustrating] work, isn't it?")
- Provide parents with access to information about parenting and child development (see Appendix VII)
- Provide anticipatory guidance relative to growth and development (*e.g.*, the need to cry in early months; toilet training)
- Stress the importance of support systems (*e.g.*, encourage parents to exchange experiences with other parents)
- Encourage parents to allow time for their own needs (*e.g.*, attend an exercise class 3 times a week)
- Discuss with parents how they respond to parental frustrations (share feelings with other parents?) and instruct them not to discipline children when very angry
- Explore other methods of discipline aside from physical punishment
- Refer parents to expert help
  - Inform parents of community services (telephone hotlines, clergy)
- See Appendix VII for age-related needs

### C. Identify suspected cases of child abuse
1. Assess for and evaluate
   a. Evidence of maltreatment (refer to Assessment data)
   b. History of incident or injury
   > Conflicting stories
   > Story improbable for age of child
   > Story not consistent with injury

    c. Parental behaviors

        Care sought for a minor complaint (*e.g.*, cold) when other injuries are seen

        Exaggerated or absent emotional response to the injury

        Unavailable for questioning

        Fails to show empathy for child

        Angry or critical of child for being injured

        Demands to take child home if pressured for answers

    d. Child behaviors

        Does not expect to be comforted

        Adjusts inappropriately to hospitalization

        Defends parents

        Blames self for inciting parents to rage

## D. Report suspected cases of child abuse

1. Know your state's child abuse laws and procedures for reporting child abuse (*e.g.*, Bureau of Child Welfare, Department of Social Services, Child Protective Services)
2. Maintain an objective record

    Description of injuries

    Conversations with parents and child in quotes

    Description of behaviors, not interpretation (*e.g.*, avoid "angry father"; instead, "father screamed at child, 'If you weren't so bad this wouldn't have happened' ")

    Description of parent–child interactions (*e.g.*, shies away from mother's touch)

    Nutritional status

    Growth and development compared to age-related norms

## E. Promote a therapeutic environment during hospitalization for child and parent

1. Provide the child with acceptance and affection
   - Show child attention without reinforcing inappropriate behavior
   - Use play therapy to allow child self-expression
   - Provide child with consistent caregivers and reasonable limits on behavior; avoid pity
   - Avoid asking too many questions and criticizing parent's actions
   - Ensure that play and educational needs are met
   - Explain in detail all routines and procedures
2. Assist child with grieving if foster home placement is necessary
   - Acknowledge that child will not want to leave parents despite how severe the abuse was
   - Allow opportunities for child to ventilate feelings
   - Explain the reasons for not allowing child to return home; dispel belief that this is a punishment
   - Encourage foster parents to visit child in hospital
3. Provide interventions that promote parents' self-esteem and sense of trust
   - Tell them it was good that they brought the child to the hospital
   - Welcome parents to the unit and orient them to activities
   - Promote their confidence by presenting a warm, helpful attitude and acknowledging any competent parenting activities
   - Provide opportunities for parents to participate in their child's care (*e.g.*, feeding, bathing)

F.  Initiate health teaching and referrals as indicated

1. Provide anticipatory guidance for families at risk
   - Assist individuals to recognize stress and to practice techniques to manage stress (see Appendix IV) (*e.g.*, planning for time alone away from child)
   - Discuss the need for realistic expectations of the child's capabilities (see Appendix VII)
   - Teach child development and constructive methods for handling developmental problems (enuresis, toilet training, temper tantrums); refer to literature in Bibliography
   - Discuss methods of discipline other than physical (*e.g.*, deprive the child of his favorite pastime: "May not ride your bike for a whole day"; "May not play your stereo")
   - Emphasize rewarding positive behavior
2. Refer abusive parents to community agencies and professionals for counseling
3. Disseminate information to the community about the problem of child abuse (*e.g.*, parent-school organizations, media: (radio, TV, newspaper)
   - Discuss with parents and parents-to-be the problems of parenting
   - Teach those who are at risk of being future abusers
   - Discuss constructive stress management
   - Teach the signs and symptoms of abuse and the method for reporting
   - Focus on abuse as a problem that results from child-rearing difficulties, not parental deficiencies
   - Relay your understanding of stresses but do not condone abuse
   - Focus on the parents' needs; avoid an authoritative approach
   - Take opportunities to demonstrate constructive methods for working with children (give the child choices; listen carefully to the child)

# Alterations in Parenting
## Related to Breast-Feeding Difficulties

Breast-feeding difficulties include lack of knowledge, feeding problems, breast discomfort, and maternal/infant separation.*

## Assessment

### Subjective data

The mother verbalizes

Feelings of inadequacy (*e.g.*, "I suppose my breasts [nipples] are too small"; "I guess I don't have enough milk")

Lack of knowledge—or belief in myths (*e.g.*, "I would like to nurse my baby, but I would not be able to lose any weight")

Fear of the unknown (*e.g.*, "I would like to nurse my baby, but I don't know anybody who does")

Negative social pressure (*e.g.*, "My husband is against it")

*Minor breast-feeding difficulties can also be stated as *Alterations in Comfort Related to Breast Discomfort.*

Concerns about the intimacy of contact with the child
Discomfort

## Objective data
First baby or first time breast-feeding
The mother is uncomfortable holding or putting baby to her breast
The mother is obviously in pain during nursing
The baby is not contented following feedings

---

**Outcome Criteria**

The mother will
- Make an informed decision related to the method of feeding child (breast or bottle)
- Identify activities that deter and promote successful breast-feeding

---

## Interventions

### A. Assess causative or contributing factors
Lack of knowledge
Lack of role model
Lack of support from significant other(s)
Separation of mother and child
Sore or engorged breasts
Presence of stress
Fatigue
Lack of conviction regarding the decision to breast-feed
Sleepy, unresponsive infant

### B. Promote open dialogue
- Assess knowledge base and reasons for choice to breast-feed
- Explore myths and clarify misconceptions regarding breast-feeding
- Build on the mother's knowledge and provide written and visual material to support your statements
- Support the mother in her decision to breast- or bottle-feed

### C. Assist the mother during the first feeding
- Help the mother to be comfortable and relaxed, use relaxation techniques, warm bath, deep breathing exercises, or glass of wine
- Explain different positions to nurse the infant (sitting, lying, football hold)
- Use pillows for support of baby and mother (one under the arm that is supporting baby)
- Demonstrate and explain the rooting reflex
- Demonstrate the scissor hold to assist infant in grasping the breast
- Make sure the baby's gums are well back on the areola
- Stay with the mother until the baby has successfully started to nurse
- Demonstrate how to use a finger on the breast during nursing to keep breast tissue from obstructing baby's airway (nose)
- Advise the mother to limit each nursing time to 5 to 7 minutes per side the first day, and gradually increase time daily

- Both breasts should be offered each feeding, alternating the beginning side each time; infant should be burped between breasts
- Demonstrate methods to awaken the baby (usually necessary before offering the second breast)

### D. Support the mother throughout hospitalization
- Allow for flexibility in scheduling of feedings
- Provide for privacy during the feedings
- Be positive even if a feeding experience is unsuccessful

### E. Assist mother with specific nursing problems
1. Sore nipples
   - Decrease time baby breast-feeds at each breast to 5 minutes at each feeding
   - Increase the number of feedings
   - Allow breasts to air dry after nursing
   - Use cream only after breasts are dry
   - Change nursing pads at each feeding
   - Use breast shields as a last measure (remove following milk let-down)
2. Engorgement
   - Wear a well-fitting support bra day and night
   - Apply warm compresses 15 to 20 minutes before nursing
3. Difficulty with baby grasping nipple
   - Use the scissor hold
   - Apply ice to nipple to cause it to become erect
   - Hand-express some milk onto the baby's mouth
   - Use breast shields as a last measure (remove following milk let-down)
4. Separation
   - Make the mother aware of the availability of a breast pump (helps to establish a milk supply and to relieve engorgement)
   - Provide a comfortable, private location for nursing during mother's visits

### F. Initiate referrals if indicated
- Advise of the use of organizations for assistance and support following discharge
  La Leche League
  The Nursing Mothers of the Childbirth Education Association

## Bibliography

### General

Admire G, Byer L: Counseling the pregnant teenager. Nursing 11(4):62–63, 1981

Bishop B: A guide to assessing parenting capabilities. Am J Nurs 75:1784–1787, 1975

Brink R: How serious is the child's behavioral problem? Matern Child Nurs J 7(1):33–36, 1982

Cameron J: Year-long classes for couples becoming parents. Matern Child Nurs J 4(5):358–362, 1979

Dressen S: The young adult: Adjusting to single parenting. Am J Nurs 76:1286–1289, 1976

Hawkins-Walsh E: Diminishing anxiety in parents of sick newborns. Matern Child Nurs J 5(1):30–34, 1980

Johnson SH: High-Risk Parenting. Philadelphia, JB Lippincott, 1979

Johnston M: Cultural variations in professional and parenting patterns. Journal of Obstetric and Gynecologic Nursing 8(4):9–15, 1980

Malinowski JS: Answering a child's questions about sex and a new baby. Am J Nurs 79:1956–1968, 1979

McKeever P: Fathering the chronically ill child. Matern Child Nurs J 6(2):124–128, 1981

Melichar M: Using crisis theory to help parents cope with a child's temper tantrums. Matern Child Nurs J 5(3):181–185, 1980

Mercer RT: Teenage motherhood: The first year. Journal of Obstetric and Gynecologic Nursing 9(1):16–29, 1980

Moore ML: Newborn, Family, and Nurse. Philadelphia, WB Saunders, 1981

Nelms B: What is a normal adolescent? Matern Child Nurs J 6(6):402–406, 1981

Petrillo M, Sangay S: Emotional Care of the Hospitalized Child. Philadelphia, JB Lippincott, 1980

Stranik MK, Hogberg, BL: Transition into parenthood. Am J Nurs 79:90–93, 1979

Waley L, Wong D: Nursing Care of Infants and Children. St. Louis, CV Mosby, 1979

Woolery L, Barkley N: Enhancing couple relationship during prenatal and postnatal classes. Matern Child Nurs J 6(3):184–188, 1981

## Abuse

Helfer RE, Kempe CH: Helping the Battered Child and His Family. Philadelphia, JB Lippincott, 1972

Olson RJ: Index of suspicion: Screening for child abusers. Am J Nurs 76:108–110, 1976

Symposium on child abuse and neglect. Nurs Clin North Am 16(2), 1981

Tagg PI: Nursing interventions for the abused child and his family. Pediatric Nursing 2(5):36–39, 1976

Wegmann M, Lancaster J: Child neglect and abuse. Family and Community Health 11(2):11–17, 1981

## Bonding

Dean P, Morgan P, Towle JM et al: Making baby's acquaintance a unique attachment. Strategy 7(1):37–41, 1982

Jenkins R, Westhus NK: The nurse role in parent-infant bonding: Overview, assessment, intervention. Journal of Obstetric and Gynecologic Nursing 10(2):114–118, 1981

Josten L: Prenatal assessment guide for illuminating possible problems with parenting. Matern Child Nurs J 6(2):113–117, 1981

Klaus MH, Kennell JH: Maternal/Infant Bonding. St. Louis, CV Mosby, 1976

Mercer R: Nursing Care for Parents at Risk. Thorofare, NJ, Charles B Slack, 1977

# Pertinent Literature and Organizations for Parents

## Books

Child Care Manual.
ROCOM Press, P.O. Box 1577, Newark, New Jersey 07101

Christophersen ER: Little people: Guidelines for common sense childrearing. Lawrence, KS: H & H Enterprises, 1977

Mash EJ: Behavior Modification Approaches to Parenting. New York, Brunner/Mazel Publishers, 1976

Salk L, Kramer R: How to Raise a Human Being. New York, Warner Books, 1973

Your Child From 1 to 6, U.S. Department of Health, Education, and Welfare, Children's Bureau, Publication No. 30, Washington, D.C. 20014

## Organizations

Parents Without Partners, 7910 Woodmount Avenue, #1000 Washington, D.C. 20014; also local chapters

LaLeche League International, 9616 Minneapolis Avenue, Franklin Park, Illinois 60131; also local chapters

Parent Effectiveness Training, 531 Stevens Avenue, Solana Beach, California 92075

## Local Counseling Services

Catholic Charities, Jewish Family Services, Christian Family Services, community agencies, and mental health centers

# Powerlessness

*Related to* **Hospitalization**

## Definition

Powerlessness: The state in which an individual perceives a lack of personal control over certain events or situations.*

## Etiological and Contributing Factors

### Pathophysiological

Any disease process, acute or chronic, can cause or contribute to powerlessness. Some common sources are

Inability to communicate (CVA, Guillain-Barré, intubation)

Inability to perform activities of daily living (CVA, cervical trauma, myocardial infarction, pain)

Inability to perform role responsibilities (surgery, trauma, arthritis)

Progressive debilitating disease (multiple sclerosis, terminal cancer)

### Situational

Lack of knowledge

Personal characteristics that highly value control (*e.g.*, internal locus of control)

Hospital or institutional limitations

| | |
|---|---|
| Some control relinquished to others | Not consulted regarding decisions |
| No privacy | Social displacement |
| Altered personal territory | Relocation |
| Social isolation | Insufficient finances |
| Lack of explanations from caregivers | Sexual harassment |

### Maturational

Adolescent: Dependence on peer group, independence from family

Young adult: Marriage, pregnancy, parenthood

Adult: Adolescent children, physical signs of aging, career pressures

Elderly: Sensory deficits, motor deficits, losses (money, significant others)

## Defining Characteristics

Expresses dissatisfaction over inability to control situation (*e.g.*, illness, prognosis, care, recovery rate)

Refuses or is reluctant to participate in decision-making

---

*Most individuals are subject to feelings of powerlessness in varying degrees in various situations. This diagnostic category can be used to describe individuals who respond to loss of control with apathy, anger, or depression.

## Associated defining characteristics

| | |
|---|---|
| Apathy | Uneasiness |
| Aggressive behavior | Resignation |
| Violent behavior | Acting-out behavior |
| Anxiety | Depression |

## Focus Assessment Criteria

Since powerlessness is a subjective state, all inferences made regarding a person's feelings of powerlessness must be validated. The nurse will assess each individual to determine his usual level of control and decision-making and the effects that losing elements of control has had on him.

### Subjective data

1. Decision-making patterns
   "How would you describe your usual method of making decisions (career, financial, health care)?"
   Make them alone
   Consult with others for advice (who?)
   Allow others to make them for me (spouse? children? others?)
2. Individual and role responsibilities
   "What responsibilities did you have
   . . . as a school child and adolescent?"
   . . . at home?"
   . . . at work?"
   . . . in community and religious organizations?"
3. Perception of control
   a. "How would you describe your ability—high, moderate, fair, or poor—to control or cure your present health problem?" (*e.g.*, diabetes mellitus, aphasia, activity intolerance, obesity)
   b. "To what do you attribute your (high, moderate, fair, poor) ability to control?"

      Preventive measures
      | | |
      |---|---|
      | Good nutrition | Stress management |
      | Weight control | Exercise program |

      Others
      | | |
      |---|---|
      | Physician | Significant others |
      | Nurses | |

      No control
      | | |
      |---|---|
      | Fate | Luck |

### Objective data

1. Participation in grooming and hygiene care (when indicated)

   | | |
   |---|---|
   | Actively seeks involvement | Reluctant to participate |
   | Requires encouragement | Refuses to participate |

2. Information-seeking behaviors

   | | |
   |---|---|
   | Actively seeks information and literature from others concerning condition | Requires encouragement to ask questions |
   | | Expresses lack of interest |

3. Response to limits placed on decision-making and self-control behaviors

   | | |
   |---|---|
   | Acceptance | Depression |
   | Apathy | Anger |

## Nursing Goals
Through selected interventions, the nurse will seek to
- Identify factors that contribute to a sense of powerlessness
- Provide opportunities for the individual to make decisions

## Principles and Rationale for Nursing Care
1. One manifestation of alienation is powerlessness. Powerlessness is a subjective feeling.
2. An individual's response to loss of control depends on the meaning of the loss, individual patterns of coping, personal characteristics (psychological, sociological, cultural, spiritual), and the response of others.
3. Each individual, whether well or ill, has a desire for control.
4. Feelings of powerlessness are sometimes appropriate.
5. Powerlessness can have a negative effect on learning.
6. Powerlessness exists with a constant feeling of anxiety.
7. Children can gain control (mastery) over threatening situations by participating in play therapy (see Appendix III).
8. Attempting to meet the developmental needs of the child can reduce the anxiety of powerlessness (see Appendix VII for specific interventions)
9. Health care providers may frequently deny economically, socially, or educationally deprived individuals opportunities for decision-making.
10. Powerlessness is very closely related to but not synonymous with the concept of external vs. internal locus of control.
11. A person with internal locus of control believes he can affect his outcome by actively manipulating himself or the environment. Examples of internal behavior are participating in a regular exercise program, acquiring printed literature about a new diagnosis, or learning assertive skills.
12. A person with external locus of control believes that affecting his outcome is outside his control and attributes what happens to him to others or to fate. Examples of external behavior are losing weight because of fear of physician's response and blaming others for his present position (*e.g.*, depression, anger).
13. Internally controlled persons motivate themselves, while externally controlled persons usually need others to motivate them. Young children are usually externally controlled but can be taught to be internally controlled. For example, a child can be taught to keep a daily chart record of the nutrients needed daily and his intake of them to assist him to understand the concept of good nutrition and to encourage him to take responsibility for his eating patterns.
14. Individuals possessing internal locus of control may experience the loss of decision-making ability more profoundly than individuals possessing external locus of control.

# Powerlessness
## Related to Hospitalization*

### Assessment

Subjective data

The person reports
Feelings of lack of control

Objective data

| | |
|---|---|
| Anger | Hostility |
| Sadness | Lack of participation in regimen |
| Apathy | |

---

**Outcome Criteria**

The person will
- Identify factors that can be controlled by him
- Make decisions regarding his care, treatment, and future when possible

---

### Interventions

A. Assess for causative and contributing factors

Lack of knowledge

Previous inadequate coping patterns (*e.g.*, depression; for discussion, see *Ineffective Individual Coping Related to Depression*)

Unsatisfactory health care provider's routines

Locus of control (internal or external)

B. Eliminate or reduce contributing factors if possible

1. Lack of knowledge
   - Increase effective communication between person and health care provider
   - Explain all procedures, rules, and options to person
   - Allow time to answer questions; ask him to write questions down so as not to forget them
   - Provide children with
     a. Opportunities to make decisions (*e.g.*, setting time for bath, holding still for injection)
     b. Specific play therapy (see Appendix III) before and after a traumatic situation (refer to Appendix VII for specific interventions for age-related developmental needs)
   - Provide a specific time (10–15 minutes) each shift that person knows can be used to ask questions or discuss subjects as desired
   - Keep person informed about condition, treatments, and results

*This specific diagnosis should be restricted to use for individuals exhibiting objective data, not all hospitalized persons.

- While being realistic, point out positive changes in person's condition, such as serum enzymes decreasing after myocardial infarction or surgical incision healing well
- Be an active listener by allowing person to verbalize concerns and feelings; assess for areas of concern
- Provide consistent staffing
- Single out one nurse to be responsible for 24-hour plan of care, and provide opportunities for person and family to identify with this nurse

2. Unsatisfactory health care provider's routines
   a. Provide opportunities for individual to control decisions
      - Allow person to manipulate surroundings, such as deciding what is to be kept where (shoes under bed, picture on window)
      - Keep needed items within reach (call bell, urinal, tissues)
      - Do not offer options if none exist (*e.g.*, a deep IM Z-tract injection must be rotated)
      - Discuss daily plan of activities and allow person to make as many decisions as possible about it
      - Increase decision-making opportunities as person progresses
      - Respect and follow individual's decision if you have given him options
      - Record person's specific choices on care plan to ensure that others on staff acknowledge preferences ("Dislikes orange juice," "Takes showers," "Plan dressing change at 7:30 prior to shower")
      - Keep promises
      - Provide opportunity for person and family to express feelings
      - Provide opportunities for person and family to participate in care
      - Be alert for signs of paternalism/maternalism in health care providers (*e.g.*, making decisions for patients)
      - Plan a care conference to allow staff to discuss methods of individualizing care; encourage each nurse to share at least one action that she discovered a particular individual liked

3. Locus of control
   a. Assess the person's usual response to problems (see Focus Assessment Criteria)
      Internal control (seeks to change own behaviors or environment to control problems)
      External control (expects others or other factors—fate, luck—to control problems)
   b. Provide person with internal locus of control the needed information to alter behavior or environment
      - Explain the problem as explicitly as the individual requests
      - Explain the relationship of prescribed behavior and outcome (*e.g.*, need for salt restriction, the physiological effects of exercise, the effects of bedrest on impaired cardiac function)
   c. Monitor a person with external locus of control to encourage participation
      - Have him keep a record for you (*e.g.*, his food intake for 1 week; weight loss chart; exercise program—type and frequency; medications taken)
      - Use telephone contact to monitor if feasible
      - Provide explicit written directions to follow (*e.g.*, meal plans; exercise regimen—type, frequency, duration; speech practice lessons—for aphasia)

C. Initiate health teaching and referrals as indicated (social worker, psychiatric nurse/physician, visiting nurse)

## Bibliography

Carlson C, Blackwell B: Behavioral Concepts and Nursing Interventions, 2nd ed. Philadelphia, JB Lippincott, 1978

Current Practice in Critical Care, vol 1. St. Louis, CV Mosby, 1979

Feather NT: Attribution of responsibility and valence of success and failure in relation to initial confidence and task performance. J Pers Soc Psychol 13:129–144, 1969

Hickey T: Powerlessness. In Carnevali DL, Patrick M (eds): Nursing Management for the Elderly. Philadelphia, JB Lippincott, 1979

Johnson DE: Powerlessness: A significant determinant in patient behavior. Journal of Nursing Education 6(2):39–44, 1967

Kritek PB: Patient power and powerlessness. Supervisor Nurse 12(6):26–34, 1981

Lowerly B, DuCutte J: Disease-related learning and disease control in diabetes as a function of locus of control. Nurs Res 25(5):358–362, 1976

Roberto SL: Behavioral Concepts and Nursing Throughout the Life Span. Englewood Cliffs, NJ, Prentice-Hall, 1978

Rotter JB: Generalized expectancy for internal vs. external control of reinforcement. Psychology Monograph 80(609):1–28, 1966

Seeman M: On the meaning of alienation. Am Sociol Rev 24(6):783–791, 1959

Stephenson CA: Powerlessness and chronic illness: Implications for nursing. Baylor Nursing Educator 1(1):17–23, 1979

Wilkinson MB: Power and the identified patient. Perspect Psychiatr Care 17(6):248–253, 1979

# Rape Trauma Syndrome

## Definition

Rape trauma syndrome: A state in which the individual experiences a forced, violent sexual assault (vaginal or anal penetration) against his or her will and without his or her consent. The trauma syndrome that develops from this attack or attempted attack includes an acute phase of disorganization of the victim and family's life-style and a long-term process of reorganization of life-style.*

## Defining Characteristics

If the victim is a child, parent(s) may experience similar responses

### Acute phase

Somatic responses
    Gastrointestinal irritability (nausea, vomiting, anorexia)
    Genitourinary discomfort (pain, pruritus)
    Skeletal muscle tension (spasms, pain)
Psychological responses
    Denial
    Emotional shock
    Anger
    Fear—of being alone or that the rapist will return (a child victim will fear: punishment, repercussions, abandonment, rejection)
    Guilt
    Panic on seeing assailant or scene of the attack
Sexual responses
    Mistrust of men (if victim is a woman)
    Change in sexual behavior

### Long-term phase

Any response of the acute phase may continue if resolution does not occur.
Psychological responses
    Phobias
    Nightmares or sleep disturbances
    Anxiety
    Depression

## Focus Assessment Criteria

### Subjective data (must be recorded)

1. History of the assault
    Time and place of rape
    Identity or description of assailant
    Sexual contact (type, amount, coercion, weapon)

*Holmstrom L, Burgess AW: Development of diagnostic categories: Sexual traumas. Am J Nurs 75:1288–1291, 1975.

Witnesses, if any

Activities that may alter evidence (changing clothes, bathing, urinating, douching)

2. Sexual history

| | |
|---|---|
| Date of last menses | Contraceptive use |
| Menstrual history | Date of last sexual contact |
| History of venereal disease | |

3. Response to the assault during acute phase

Assess person and family for

Somatic symptoms

Psychological symptoms

Sexual reactions

Assess child for

Understanding of the event

Knowledge of the identity of the molester

Possibility of previous assaults

Assess parent(s), spouse, others for

Understanding of the event

Ability to help the victim cope

Ability to cope

4. Response to the assault during long-term phase

Assess person and family for psychological symptoms and sexual reactions

### Objective data

1. Observe for injury (ecchymoses, lacerations, abrasions)

| | |
|---|---|
| Gastrointestinal system | Genitourinary system |
| (mouth, anus, abdomen) | Skeletal muscle system |

2. Assess the emotional responses

| | |
|---|---|
| Crying | Detachment |
| Hysterical | Composure |
| Withdrawal | |

## Principles and Rationale for Nursing Care

### General

1. Rape is an act of physical violence rather than sexual passion.
2. Rape is a crime that must be reported by health care providers.
3. The medicolegal examination serves to assess the condition of the victim and to gather documentary evidence. It consists of a thorough general physical exam; a pelvic exam, with smears for semen and cultures for venereal disease; a urine sample for pregnancy test; scrapings from fingernails; and combing and samples of victim's pubic hair.
4. Rape Crisis Centers provide rape victims and significant others with information regarding the medical examination, police interrogation, and court procedures; with escort service to hospital, police department, and courts; and with counseling.
5. Rape Crisis Centers work in the community to educate the public on rape and rape prevention, improve the response of hospitals and the police to rape victims, and improve rape-related legislation.
6. Nurses need to explore their own feelings about rape before attempting to intervene effectively with rape trauma victims.
7. The nurse may not see every symptom of rape trauma syndrome with each rape victim.

8. Short-term rape crisis intervention should begin during the acute phase.
9. During the acute phase, hospital emergency rooms and crisis intervention centers are two places where the nurse may encounter the rape victim.
10. Nurses should consider pre-existing conditions of the rape trauma victim (*i.e.*, physical or psychiatric illnesses; substance abuse) that may lead to compound reactions.
11. Acute symptoms overlap with long-term symptoms of rape trauma syndrome
12. Follow-up intervention is usually counselor-initiated.
13. Nurses in community settings can teach primary prevention concepts by reviewing with clients measures to take to reduce the possibility of rape.
14. The rape victim will resolve the rape trauma event at her/his own readiness.

## Children

1. When working with young rape trauma victims, nurses should be cognizant of individual developmental levels, since the impact of the event will vary according to the child's developmental stage.
2. The child's reaction is dependent on age, degree of physical trauma, relationship to assailant, and parental (caretaker) reaction.
3. The assailant of a child is most likely someone the child knows, and the assaults have occurred for a period of time within the child's own home or neighborhood.
4. The pelvic exam can be more traumatic than the assault. Explaining the procedure and allowing the child to handle the equipment (speculum) may reduce the fear.
5. Play therapy should be an integral part of the treatment regime. Guidelines for play therapy are presented in Appendix III. Use dolls that have genitalia for play therapy for rape victims; rag dolls can have genitalia attached. The child will then act out the assault with dolls of appropriate sex (a boy victim can use two male dolls). Puppets are also beneficial for play therapy.

---

**Outcome Criteria**

### Short-term goals

The person will
- Experience decreased symptoms
- Describe rationale and treatment procedures
- Identify members of support system and utilize them appropriately

### Long-term goals

The person will
- Experience optimal psychosocial adjustment to the rape trauma event
- Return to pre-crisis level of functioning

The child will
- Discuss the assault
- Express feelings concerning the assault and the treatment

The parent(s), spouse, or significant other will
- Discuss their response to the assault
- Experience optimal psychosocial adjustment to the event
- Return to pre-crisis level of functioning

---

## Interventions

The interventions for rape trauma syndrome are listed for usefulness under the three types of responses: psychological, sexual, and somatic. The nurse must assess and intervene with each response for each victim.

### Psychological responses

A. Assess for psychological responses

1. General
   Phobias, nightmares
   Denial, emotional shock
   Anger, fear, anxiety
   Depression, guilt
2. Subjective
   Expressions of numbness, shame, self-blame
3. Objective
   Crying
   Silence
   Trembling hands
   Excessive bathing (seen particularly with child or adolescent)
   Avoiding interaction with others (staff, family)

B. Eliminate or reduce psychological responses where possible

1. Promote trusting relationship
   - Stay with person during acute stage or arrange for other support
   - Brief person on police and hospital procedures during acute stage
   - Assist person during medical examination and explain all procedures in advance
   - Help person to meet personal needs (bathing *after* examination and evidence has been acquired)
   - Listen attentively to person's requests
   - Maintain unhurried attitude toward person and family
   - Avoid rescue feelings toward person
   - Maintain nonjudgmental attitude
   - Support person's beliefs and value system and avoid labeling
   - Initiate play therapy with a child to explain treatments and allow child to express feelings
2. Whenever possible, provide crisis counseling within one hour of rape trauma event
   - Ask permission to contact the rape crisis counselor
   - Be flexible and individualize approach according to person's needs
   - Observe person's behavior carefully and record objective data
   - Encourage victim to verbalize thoughts/feelings/perceptions of the event
   - Discuss her/his treatment as victim; express empathy
   - Assess person's verbal style (expressive, controlled)
   - Discuss with person previous coping mechanism
   - Explore available support system; involve significant others if appropriate
   - Assess stress tolerance
   - Reassure person about manner in which she/he reacted
   - Explore with person her/his strengths and resources

- Convey to person confidence in her/his ability to return to prior level of functioning
- Assist person in decision-making and problem-solving; involve patient in own treatment plan
- Help restore person's dignity by calmly exploring basis for feelings together
- Reassure person that these feelings/symptoms—fear of rapist, fear of death, guilt, loss of control, shame, short attention span, anger, anxiety, phobias, depression, flashbacks, embarrassment, and eating/sleeping pattern disturbances—are often experienced by rape trauma victims
- Respect victim's rights; honor wishes to restrict unwanted visitors and offer privacy when appropriate
- Explain to person that this experience will disrupt his/her life and feelings that occurred during acute phase may reoccur; encourage person to proceed at his/her own pace
- Offer explanation of any papers that need to be signed
- Briefly counsel family and friends at their level
    a. Share with them the immediate needs of the victim for love and support
    b. Encourage them to express their feelings and ask questions

3. Support person's efforts to overcome feelings
   - Change residence and/or telephone number
   - Use objects that symbolize safety (nightlight)
   - Take a trip
   - Turn to support system
   - Plan one day at a time
   - Avoid highly stressful situations
   - Engage in diversional activities
   - Use previous coping mechanisms that proved effective

## C. Proceed with follow-up until victim is in control of reactions and feelings

1. Before person leaves hospital, provide card with information about follow-up appointments and names and telephone numbers of local crisis and counseling centers
2. Plan home visit or telephone call
3. Arrange for legal or pastoral counseling if appropriate
4. Recommend and make referrals to psychotherapist, mental health clinic, citizen action and community group, advocacy related services
5. Fulfill legal responsibilities
    a. Document physical and psychological signs and symptoms
    b. Record all objective data, omitting any subjective impressions and opinions (may be subpoena)
    c. Complete required forms

## Sexual responses

## A. Assess for sexual responses

1. General
     Fear of intercourse
     Parents' fear that assault will affect child's future sexual health
2. Subjective
     Mistrust of men

3. Objective

  Change in sexual behavior

  Lack of sexual desire (especially if victim never had intercourse before)

## B. Promote helping relationship

- Encourage person to express feelings openly
- Provide accepting atmosphere
- Reassure person that her/his symptoms are frequently experienced by rape trauma victims
- Offer feedback to person on feelings verbalized
- Encourage person to recognize positive responses or support from sexual partner or members of opposite sex
- Discuss with person possible fear of rejection by significant others
- Discuss potential anxiety about resuming sexual relations with partner
- Explore sexual concerns with patient

## C. Proceed with referrals

- Recommend couple therapy
- Recommend sexual counseling

## Somatic responses

## A. Assess for somatic responses

  Gastrointestinal irritability

  Genitourinary discomfort

  Rectal discomfort

  Skeletal muscle tension

  Vaginal discharge

  Bruising and edema

  Reports of

|  |  |
|---|---|
| Headaches | Nausea |
| Fatigue | Pain |
| Itching | Burning on urination |
| Anorexia | |

## B. Eliminate or reduce somatic symptomatology

1. Gastrointestinal irritability
   a. Anorexia
      - Offer small, frequent feedings
      - Provide appealing foods
      - Record intake
      - Refer to *Alterations in Nutrition* if anorexia is prolonged
   b. Nausea
      - Avoid gas-forming foods
      - Restrict carbonated beverages
      - Observe for abdominal distention
      - Offer antiemetic as per physician's order
2. Genitourinary discomfort
   a. Pain
      - Assess pain for quality and duration
      - Monitor intake and output

- Inspect urine and external genitalia for bleeding
- Listen attentively to person's description of pain
- Give pain medication as per physician's order (see *Alterations in Comfort: Pain*)

b. Discharge
- Assess amount, color, and odor of discharge
- Allow person time to wash and change garments after initial examination has been completed

c. Itching
- Encourage bathing in cool water
- Avoid use of detergent soaps
- Avoid touching area causing discomfort

3. Skeletal muscle tension

a. Headaches
- Avoid any sudden change of person's position
- Approach person in calm manner
- Slightly elevate bed (unless contraindicated)
- Discuss with person pain-reducing measures that have been effective in the past

b. Fatigue
- Assess present sleeping patterns if altered (see *Sleep Pattern Disturbance*)
- Discuss with person precipitating factors for sleep disturbance and try to eliminate these factors if possible
- Provide frequent rest periods throughout the day
- Avoid interruptions during sleep
- Avoid stress-producing situations

c. Labile emotional responses
- Provide person with emotionally secure environment
- Discuss person's daily routines and adhere to them as much as possible
- Avoid any sudden movements and approach in calm manner
- Provide frequent quiet periods throughout the day

4. Generalized bruising and edema
- Avoid constrictive garments
- Handle affected body parts gently
- Elevate affected body part if edema is present
- Apply cool, moist compress to edematous area the first 24 hours, then warm compress after 24 hours
- Encourage person to verbalize discomfort
- Record presence and location of bruises, lacerations, edema, or abrasions

## C. Proceed with health teaching with person and family

A. Gastrointestinal irritability
- Explain to person side-effects of DES (diethylstilbestrol) (nausea and vomiting; vaginal spotting when discontinued)

B. Genitourinary discomfort
- Advise person against scratching area causing discomfort

C. Skeletal muscle tension
- Explain to person potential causes of discomfort
- Explain to person measures that may help release tension
- Teach person relaxation methods (see Appendix IV)
- Explain to person that these symptoms are often experienced by rape trauma victims

# Bibliography

## General

Burgess AW: Applying flight education principles to rape prevention. Family and Community Health 4(2):45–51, 1981

Burgess AW, Holmstrom L: Crisis and counseling requests of rape victims. Nurs Res 23(3):196, 1974

Burgess AW, Holmstrom L: Rape Trauma Syndrome. Am J Psychiatry 131:981–986, 1974

Holmstrom L, Burgess AW: Development of diagnostic categories: Sexual traumas. Am J Nurs 75:1288–1291, 1975

Holmstrom L, Burgess A: Rape—Victims of Crisis. Bowie, MD, Robert J Brady, 1974

Notman MT, Nadelson CC: The rape victim: Psychodynamic considerations. Am J Psychiatry 133:408, 1976

Stuart, Sundeen SJ: Counseling the victims of rape. In Principles and Practice of Psychiatric Nursing. St. Louis, CV Mosby, 1979

## Children

Brant R, Tisza V: The sexually misused child. Am J Orthopsychiatry 47(1):80–90, 1977

Burgess AW, Holmstrom L: Sexual trauma of children and adolescents. Nurs Clin North Am 10(3):551–563, 1975

Goldstein F: Practical care for the victim of rape. Patient Care 12:20–45, 1978

Gorline L, Ray M: Examining and caring for the child who has been sexually assaulted. Med Clin North Am 4(2):110–114, 1979

Leaman K: The sexually abused child. Nursing 7(5):68–72, 1977

Medenwald N: Children's liberation—in a hospital! Matern Child Nurs J 5(4):231–234, 1980

Petrillo M, Sanger S: Emotional care of hospitalized children. Philadelphia, JB Lippincott, 1972

Vipperman J, Rager P: Childhood coping: How nurses can help. Pediatric Nursing 6(2):11–18, 1980

Whaley L, Wong D: Nursing care of infants and children. St. Louis, CV Mosby, 1979

# Respiratory Function, Alterations in

Related to **Smoking**

Related to **Immobility**

Related to **Chronic Allergy**

## Ineffective Airway Clearance

Related to **(Specify)**

## Ineffective Breathing Patterns

Related to **Hyperpnea or Hyperventilation**

## Impaired Gas Exchange

Related to **Chronic Tissue Hypoxia**

### Definitions

Alterations in respiratory function (AIRF):* The state in which the individual experiences a real or potential threat to the passage of air through the respiratory tract, and to the exchange of gases ($O_2$–$CO_2$) between the lungs and the vascular system.

Ineffective airway clearance (IAC): The state in which the individual experiences an actual or potential threat to the passage of air through the respiratory tract related to partial or complete airway obstruction.

Ineffective breathing patterns (IBP): The state in which the individual experiences an actual or potential loss of adequate ventilation resulting from an altered breathing pattern.

Impaired gas exchange (IGE): The state in which the individual experiences an actual or potential decreased passage of gases ($O_2$–$CO_2$) between the alveoli of the lungs and the vascular system.

### Etiological and Contributing Factors

The codes IGE (Impaired Gas Exchange), IAC (Ineffective Airway Clearance), and IBP (Ineffective Breathing Patterns) are used to indicate factors specific to that diagnosis. Factors without a code relate to all four diagnostic categories.

---

*This diagnostic category has been added by the author to describe a state in which the entire respiratory system is affected, not just isolated areas such as airway clearance or gas exchange. Smoking, allergy, and immobility are examples of factors that affect the entire system and thus make it incorrect to say Impaired Gas Exchange Related to Immobility, since immobility also affects airway clearance and breathing patterns. The three diagnoses *Ineffective Airway Clearance, Ineffective Breathing Patterns,* and *Impaired Gas Exchange* can be used when the contributing factor affects a specific respiratory function. The nurse is cautioned not to use this diagnostic category to describe acute respiratory disorders, which are the primary responsibility of medicine and nursing.

## Pathophysiological

Excessive or thick secretions (IAC, IGE)
Infection (IAC, IGE)
Neuromuscular impairment

| | |
|---|---|
| Diseases of the nervous system | CNS depression |
| (*e.g.*, Guillain-Barré syndrome, | CVA (stroke) |
| MS, myasthenia gravis) | |

Loss of lung elasticity

| | |
|---|---|
| COPD (chronic bronchitis, | Aging process |
| asthma) | |

Decreased lung compliance
Loss of functioning lung tissue (IGE)

| | |
|---|---|
| Emphysema | Tumor |
| Atelectasis | Surgery |

Allergic response
Hypertrophy or edema of upper airway structures—tonsils, adenoids, sinuses
    (IAC)


## Situational

Surgery or trauma
Pain, fear, anxiety
Fatigue
Mechanical obstruction (IAC, IGE)
Improper positioning (IAC)
Altered anatomic structure (IAC, IGE)

| | |
|---|---|
| Tracheostomy | Congenital deformity |

Medications (narcotics, sedatives, analgesics)
Anesthesia, general or spinal (IAC, IBP)
Aspiration
Extreme high or low humidity (IAC, IGE)
Smoking
Suppressed cough reflex (IAC)
Bedrest or immobility
Severe nonrelieved cough (IAC, IBP)
Exercise intolerance
Decreased oxygen in the inspired air (IGE)
Mouth breathing (IAC, IBP)
Perception/cognitive impairment (IAC)


## Maturational

Neonate: Complicated delivery, prematurity, cesarian birth, low birth weight
Infant/child: Asthma or allergies, increased emesis (aspiration), croup, cystic
    fibrosis, small airway
Elderly: Decreased surfactant in the lungs, decreased elasticity of the lungs,
    immobility, slowing of reflexes

# Alterations in Respiratory Function (AIRF)

## Defining Characteristics

Asymmetrical expansion of chest
Changes in rate of respiration (from baseline).
Changes in depth of respiration (from baseline).
Changes in pattern of respiration (from baseline).
Cyanosis
Rales, rhonchi, fremitus, heaves, wheezes
Alterations in blood gases
Cough
Report of dyspnea
Report of orthopnea
Nasal flaring
Anxiety or restlessness
Also see *Ineffective Breathing Patterns, Impaired Gas Exchange, Ineffective Airway Clearance*

## Focus Assessment Criteria

### Subjective data

1. History of symptoms (*eg.*, pain, dyspnea, cough)
    Onset? Precipitated by what?
    Description? Relieved by what?
    Effects on other body functions
        Gastrointestinal (nausea, vomiting, anorexia, constipation)?
        Genitourinary (impotence, kidney function)?
        Circulatory (angina, tachycardia/bradycardia, fluid retention)?
        Neurosensory (thought processes, headache)?
        Musculoskeletal (muscle fatigue, atrophy)?
    Effects on life-style
        Occupation                      Social/sexual functions
        Role functions                  Financial status
2. Presence of contributing or causative factors
    Smoking ("pack years": number of packs per day times number of smoking years)
    Allergy (medication, food, environmental factors—dust, pollen, other)
    Trauma, blunt or overt (chest, abdomen, upper airway, head)
    Surgery/pain
        Healing incision of chest/neck/head/abdomen
        Recent intubation
    Environmental factors
        Toxic fumes (cleaning agents, smoke)

Extreme heat or cold
Daily inspired air, work and home (humid, dry, level of pollution, level of pollens)
Infection
3. Current drug therapy
What? How often? When was last dose taken?
Effect on symptoms?
4. Medical/surgical history
Cardiac disease
Pulmonary disease
5. For infants only, History of:
Immaturity? Low birth weight?
Cesarean birth? Complicated delivery?
Family history of Sudden Infant Death Syndrome (SIDS)?

## Objective data

### Respiratory
1. Description
Rate (per minute)
Slowed                                   Increased
Rhythm
Regular                              Smooth
Irregular                            Uneven
Depth
Decreased                            Symmetrical
Increased                            Variable
Asymmetrical                         Even
Type (see Table II–8)
Regular                              Hyperpnea
Tachypnea                            Splinted/guarded
Bradypnea                            Kussmaul
Apnea                                Cheyne-Stokes
2. Cough
Raspy                                Productive
Barking                              Dry
Painful
3. Sputum

| Color | Character | Amount | Odor |
|---|---|---|---|
| Clear | Frothy | Small | None |
| Yellow | Watery | Moderate | Foul |
| White | Tenacious | Copious | Yeastlike |
| Greenish | Hemoptysic (bloody) | | |
| Reddish (bloody) | | | |
| Brown specks | | | |

4. Breath sounds (detected by auscultation: compare right upper and lower lobes to left upper and lower lobes; list to all four quadrants of the chest)
Diminished                           Rales (crackles)
Absent                               Rhonchi (wheezes)
Abnormal                             Rubs (squeaks)

Table II–8.   **Types of Respirations**

| Respiration | Rate | Rhythm | Depth |
|---|---|---|---|
| Normal | Adult, 15 to 25 | Even | Variable |
| | Child, 15 to 25 | Variable | Variable |
| | Infant, 25 to 40 | Variable | Variable |
| | Newborn, 30 to 80 | Variable | Variable |
| Tachypnea | Rapid | Variable | Decreased |
| Bradypnea | Slowed | Variable | Normal to increased |
| Apnea | Variable or absent | Irregular | Variable |
| Hyperpnea | Increased | Regular | Increased |
| Splinted/guarded | Increased | Variable | Decreased |
| Kussmaul | Usually variable | Variable | Increased |
| Cheyne-Stokes* | Variable | Variable | Cyclic periods of apnea alterating with hyperpnea |

*Normal in children and the elderly at rest.

5. Vital capacity
   a. Test ability to blow out lit match 2 to 3 inches in front of mouth without pursing lips (failure to do this indicates significant obstructive problem)
   b. Measure timed vital capacity (maximum forced expiration following maximum forced inspiration); values over 5 seconds indicate significant obstructive problem
      Inspiratory phase (normal/diminished/prolonged)
      Expiratory phase (normal/diminished/prolonged)
      Inspiratory/expiratory ratio should be 1:2
6. Associated signs
      Use of accessory muscles of respiration (neck, chest, abdomen)
      Clubbing of fingers
      Crepitus (subcutaneous air; note location)
      Nasal flaring
      Retractions with respiratory effort
         Suprasternal (indentation of space above sternum)
         Sternal (indentation of sternum—in infants only)
         Intercostal (indentation of space between ribs)

Circulatory
   Pulse

| | Rate | Rhythm | Quality | Baseline |
|---|---|---|---|---|

   Blood pressure

| | Usual | Present | Pulse pressure | Baseline |
|---|---|---|---|---|

   Skin color
         Within normal limits                Ruddy
         Pale                                Cyanotic (central/peripheral)
         Ashen

## Diagnostic studies

Pulmonary functions
> Tidal volume                  Vital capacity
> Minute volume

Arterial blood gases
Complete blood count/electrolytes
Pulmonary function studies
Chest x-ray
CT scan
Exercise tolerance (treadmill)
Protein ion phoresis (sweat test for cystic fibrosis)
Bronchoscopy

## Nursing Goals

Through selected nursing interventions, the nurse will seek to
- Promote optimal movement of air in and out of the lungs
- Prevent atelectasis, infection, and stasis of air and secretions in the lungs
- Establish a good pulmonary toilet regime, in order to remove pulmonary secretions
- Assist the individual to accomplish effective coughing practices with minimal discomfort

## Principles and Rationale for Nursing Care

### General

1. Ventilation requires synchronous movement of the walls of the chest and abdomen. (Coordination and conscious control of breathing are key elements in teaching a person to breathe efficiently.) With *inspiration* the diaphragm moves downward, the intercostal muscles contract, the chest wall lifts up and out, the pressure inside the thorax lowers, and air is drawn in. *Expiration* occurs as air is forced out of the lungs by the elastic recoil of the lungs and the relaxation of the chest and diaphragm. Expiration is diminished in the elderly and with chronic pulmonary disease.
2. There are two phases of respiration. *External respiration* occurs in the lungs at the alveolar level (outside air to bloodstream). *Internal respiration* occurs between the systemic capillaries and the interstitial fluid (bloodstream to tissues; optimum perfusion needed).
3. A cough ("the guardian of the lungs") is accomplished by closure of the glottis and the explosive expulsion of air from the lungs by the work of the abdominal and chest muscles.
4. Lying flat causes the abdominal organs to shift toward the chest, thus crowding the lungs and making it more difficult to breathe.
5. Breath-holding can result in a "Valsalva" maneuver: a marked increase in intrathoracic and intra-abdominal pressure, with profound circulatory changes (decreased heart rate, cardiac output, and blood pressure).
6. Hyperventilation (blowing off of $CO_2$) causes an acid–base imbalance and may result in temporary loss of consciousness (fainting).
7. The terms tachypnea, hyperpnea, hyperventilation, bradypnea, and hypoventilation are frequently confused. For our purposes, these terms will be defined as follows:
   > *Tachypnea*: rapid, shallow respiratory rate

*Hyperpnea*: rapid respiratory rate with increased depth

*Hyperventilation*: increased rate or depth of respirations causing an alveolar ventilation that is above the body's normal metabolic requirements

*Bradypnea*: Slow respiratory rate

*Hypoventilation*: decreased rate or depth of respiration, causing a minute alveolar ventilation that is less than the body's requirements

## Smoking

1. Smoking has immediate and long-term effects upon the respiratory system.
2. Immediate effects are paralysis of the ciliary cleansing mechanism of the lungs (which should keep breathing passages free of inhaled irritants and bacteria); irritation of the lining of the lungs, causing an inflammatory response; increased production of mucus; and decreased oxygenation.
3. Long-term effects are *permanent* disabling of the ciliary cleansing mechanism; reduction of the number of macrophages in the airways; a *permanent* decrease in the lung's ability to fight infection; increased production of mucus cells; a significant increase in the risk of developing pulmonary disease (a history of 15 to 20 "pack years" indicates a high risk); possible enlargement of the distal air passages; and chronic $CO_2$ retention, which results in hypoxia's becoming the drive to breathe, rather than hypercarbia (increased $CO_2$).
4. Smoking has immediate and long-term effects upon the cardiovascular system.
5. Immediate effects are vasoconstriction and decreased oxygenation of the blood; elevated blood pressure; increased heart rate and possible arrhythmias; and an increase in the work of the heart.
6. Long-term effects include an increased risk for coronary artery disease and myocardial infarction. Smoking also contributes to hypertension, to peripheral vascular disease (*e.g.*, leg ulcers), and to chronically abnormal arterial blood gases (low oxygen, or $pO_2$, and high carbon dioxide, or $pCO_2$).

## Oxygen needs

1. An insufficient supply of oxygen reaching the tissues is called *hypoxia*. The effects of hypoxia upon vital signs are:

| *Vital Sign* | *Early Hypoxia* | *Late Hypoxia* |
|---|---|---|
| Blood pressure | Rising systolic/falling diastolic | Falling |
| Pulse | Rising, bounding, arrhythmic | Falling, shallow, arrhythmic |
| Pulse pressure | Widening | Widened/narrowed |
| Respirations | Rapid | Slowed/Rapid |

2. The clinical manifestations of hypoxia are:

| *Early Hypoxia* | *Late Hypoxia* |
|---|---|
| Irritability | Seizures |
| Headache | Coma or brain tissue swelling |
| Confusion | Decreased cardiac output |
| Agitation | Oliguria or anuria |
| Pain | |
| Oliguria | |

3. Infants consume three times more $O_2$ per Kg of body weight than adults.
4. Hypoxia contributes to coma and shock. Oxygen demand is greater during febrile illness, exercise, pain, and physical and emotional stress.
5. Oxygen should be administered carefully (less than 3 liters per minute) to people with a history of chronic $CO_2$ retention, for their drive to breath is hypoxia.

6. Oxygenation is dependent upon the ability of the lungs to deliver oxygen to the blood and upon the ability of the heart to pump enough blood to deliver the oxygen to the microcirculation of the cells.

## Chronic diseases of the lung (asthma, bronchitis, emphysema, COPD)

1. The normal range of arterial blood gases for a person with chronic lung disease may be much different from the range of the normal individual because of body adaptation to chronically high $CO_2$ levels. (*Baseline* normals are of utmost importance.)
2. Sustained moderate breathlessness from supervised exercise improves accessory muscle strength and respiratory function.
3. In normal individuals, the work of breathing is very limited. In people with obstructive lung disease, however, the work of breathing may be increased 5 to 10 times above normal. Under such conditions, the amount of oxygen consumed *just for breathing activities* may be a large fraction of total oxygen consumption.
4. Consciously controlled breathing techniques can improve alveolar gas exchange and prevent air entrapment in the lungs, thus causing each breath to be more efficient.

   *Pursed-lip breathing* causes expiratory resistance, which helps air passages to stay open longer, allows for more movement of air, and prevents air entrapment within the lungs.

   *Diaphragmatic breathing* is accomplished by lifting the walls of the abdomen up and out, which causes decreased pressure within the abdomen and easier downward movement of the diaphragm.
5. People who suffer from chronic lung disease experience permanent effects on every body system, due to chronic hypoxemia (Table II–9).

Table II–9.   **Effects of Chronic Hypoxia**

| | |
|---|---|
| **Thought Processes** | Confusion and lethargy |
| | Mood swings, anxiety, depression |
| | Sleep disturbances |
| | Headache |
| **Respiratory System** | Tachypnea, bradypnea, arrythmic breathing |
| | Abnormal flow rates (increased inspiratory/expiratory [I/E] ratio) |
| | Pursed-lip breathing |
| | Use of accessory muscles (neck, shoulders, abdomen) |
| | Gasping before speech effort |
| | Inability to speak or cry |
| | Orthopnea (assumption of 3-point position) |
| | Cough, shortness of breath, exercise intolerance |
| | Increased sputum production |
| | Inability to move secretions |
| | Mouth breathing |
| | Abnormal breath sounds (rales, rhonchi) |
| | Decreased breath sounds |
| | Fremitus |

*(continued)*

Table 11–9.  **Effects of Chronic Hypoxia** *(continued)*

| | |
|---|---|
| **Circulatory System** | Neck vein distention<br>Edema, decreased cardiac output, enlarged heart<br>Cyanosis<br>Chest pain |
| **Gastrointestinal System** | Decreased bowel sounds<br>Constipation<br>Anorexia, nausea, vomiting |
| **Genitourinary System** | Decreased kidney function<br>Decreased urinary output<br>Decreased libido |
| **Skeletal System** | Hypertrophy of accessory breathing muscles (neck and shoulders)<br>Atrophy or weakness of extremity muscles<br>Barrel chest, horizontal sloping of ribs<br>Cachexia (malnutrition)<br>Skeletal muscle pain or weakness |

# Alterations in Respiratory Function
## Related to Smoking

### Assessment

Subjective data

History of smoking (pack years: number of packs per day times number of years person has smoked)

Objective data

Overt smoking
Odor of smoke on breath
Staining of teeth, fingernails, and fingertips
Cough
Increased sputum production

**Outcome Criteria**

The person will
- Relate the immediate effect that inhaling smoke has upon the body (*e.g.,* increasing blood pressure, vasoconstriction, and inflammatory response of the lining of the lung)
- Relate the long-term effects of chronic smoking upon the respiratory system
- Stop smoking during periods of increased physical stress (*e.g.,* before and after strenuous exercise, during a respiratory illness, during pregnancy)
- Stop smoking altogether and find alternative adaptive coping mechanisms

## Interventions

A. Assess for the following
  1. Type of smoking
     Cigarettes (filter or nonfilter; packs per day)
     Cigar
     Pipe
     Number of years of chronic smoking
     Whether or not smoke is inhaled
  2. Knowledge of effects of smoking on the respiratory and cardiovascular system (proceed with health teaching as indicated)
  3. Situations when the person feels a desire to smoke
  4. Whether the person has a desire to change his smoking habits
  5. Whether the person has tried to stop smoking in the past, what method was used, and at what time

B. Initiate health teaching as indicated
  - Teach to avoid factors that aggravate symptoms and advance disease (excessive allergens, pollution, smoking)
  - If the person does not want to stop smoking, instruct
    1. Not to smoke immediately before or after meals or activity
    2. Try to reduce the number of cigarettes smoked daily
    3. Where to go for assistance if he ever decides to stop smoking
  - If the person wants to stop smoking, instruct to
    1. Contact a community agency for a stop smoking program, *e.g.*
       American Cancer Society
       American Heart Association
       American Lung Association
    2. Make a list of all the reasons he wants to stop smoking
    3. Begin an exercise program slowly (see *Alterations in Health Maintenance* for an exercise program)

# Alterations in Respiratory Function
## Related to Immobility

### Assessment

Subjective data
Fatigue, weakness, or pain

Objective data
Inability to turn self
Inability to ambulate
Presence of respiratory rales and diminished respiratory depth

---

**Outcome Criteria**

The person will
- Perform hourly deep breathing exercises (sigh) and cough sessions as needed
- Achieve maximum pulmonary function
- Relate importance of daily pulmonary exercises

---

### Interventions

A. Assess causative factors

Pain, lethargy
Medical order of bedrest
Neuromuscular impairment
Lack of motivation (to ambulate; to cough and deep-breathe)
Decreased level of consciousness
Lack of knowledge

B. Eliminate or reduce causative factors if possible

1. Assess for optimal pain relief with minimal period of fatigue or respiratory depression
2. Encourage ambulation as soon as consistent with medical plan of care
   - If unable to walk, establish a regime for being out of bed in a chair several times a day (*i.e.*, one hour after meals and one hour before bedtime)
   - Increase activity gradually, explaining that respiratory function will improve and dyspnea will decrease with practice
3. For neuromuscular impairment
   - Vary the position of the bed, thus gradually changing the horizontal and vertical position of the thorax, unless contraindicated
   - Assist to reposition, turning frequently from side to side (hourly if possible)
   - Encourage deep breathing and controlled coughing exercises five times every hour
   - Teach individual to use blow bottle or incentive spirometer every hour while awake (with severe neuromuscular impairment, the person may have to be awakened during the night as well)

- For child, use colored water in blow bottle; have him blow up balloons
- Auscultate lung fields every 8 hours; increase frequency if altered breath sounds are present
4. For the person with a decreased level of consciousness
   - Position from *side to side* with set schedule (*e.g.,* left side even hours, right side odd hours); do not leave person lying flat on back
   - Position on right side after feedings (nasogastric tube feeding, gastrostomy) to prevent regurgitation and aspiration
   - Keep head of bed elevated 30° unless contraindicated

## C. Prevent the complications of immobility

See specific diagnoses for interventions to prevent or treat the complications of immobility:

> *Impairment of Skin Integrity*
> *Alterations in Bowel Elimination: Constipation*
> *Sensory-Perceptual Alterations*
> *Activity Intolerance*
> *Diversional Activity Deficit*

# Alterations in Respiratory Function
## Related to Chronic Allergy

## Assessment

### Subjective data

The person states
> "I'm allergic to ———"
> "——— gives me a rash"
> "I have trouble breathing"
> "I feel short of breath"
> "I feel itchy"
> "Something bit (stung) me"
> "I have asthma"

History of ingestion of new food or drugs
> Frequent ear infections

### Objective data

> Hoarseness, wheezing/dyspnea
> Coughing and sneezing, watery eyes and nose
> Hives/rashes
> Presence of stinger (bee)
> Erythema
> Edema

**Outcome Criteria**

The person will
- State causative allergens, if known
- State methods of avoiding allergens
- Relate the emotional aspects of the allergic response
- State the need to seek immediate medical attention for severe allergic response and demonstrate the use of hypodermic injection (for administration of epinephrine) if applicable

## Interventions

### A. Assess causative factors

Chronic allergy (known allergens such as molds, dust, pollen, food, others)
Stinging insect
Nonspecific (unknown) allergen

### B. Provide the following health teaching

1. For chronic allergy to molds
   a. Avoid barns, cut grass, leaves, weeds, decaying or rotting vegetation, firewood, house plants, damp basements, attics, and crawl spaces
   b. Avoid eating marinated or aged foods (bread, flour, cheese, fruits, vegetables)
   c. Maintain household walls clean and dry
      - Be sure that there is adequate house drainage to keep walls dry
      - Check walls for black or grayish-blue mold spots
      - Wash walls with chlorine bleach solution to remove mold
   d. Maintain a dust-free environment, especially in the bedroom*
      - Empty room to the bare walls, including closets (store contents elsewhere if possible)
      - Scrub woodwork and floors
      - Thereafter, dust and vacuum well daily and clean thoroughly once a week
      - Keep bedroom furniture to a minimum (preferably wood, rather than stuffed furniture)
      - Choose waxed, hardwood floors (no carpets)
      - Use pull shades rather than venetian blinds at windows; do not use curtains or draperies
      - Use closet to a minimum; keep it as dust free as the bedroom, and keep the door closed
      - Use bedroom for sleeping only; if it is a child's bedroom, encourage play elsewhere
      - Do not use stuffed toys
      - Keep animals of fur or feathers out of the area
      - Do not use fuzzy blankets or feather comforters; cotton bedspreads are preferred
      - Launder bed linens frequently

*It is difficult to keep one's home and work environment dust free, but special efforts can readily be made to keep the area where one sleeps free of dust.

   e. Keep dust down throughout the entire house
- Use steam or hot-water heat if available
- Maintain a clean filter in furnace; use air conditioning if possible
- Cover hot-air furnace outlets with cheesecloth or have a filter installed; change filter frequently
- Avoid any room while it is being cleaned and do not handle any objects that may be dust collectors (such as books)
- Wear a mask while cleaning

2. For chronic allergy to pollen
- Reduce exposure as much as possible to trees (April–May), grass (May–July), weeds (mid-May to first frost)
- Use air conditioning with electrostatic filters
- Stay inside on windy days, avoiding drafts and cross-ventilation
- Use air conditioning in cars, and avoid extended rides
- Wear a dampened mask while cutting lawn
- Avoid strong odors (scents and perfumes)
- Do not drink ice-cold beverages or food (can cause spasms)
- Avoid granaries, barns, decaying materials, cut grass, weeds, dry leaves, firewood
- Try to arrange vacations during high pollen season in a low-pollen area such as the eastern seashore
- Be sure over-the-counter drugs such as antihistamines are approved by physician, for some may give the opposite intended effect

3. To avoid stinging insects (bees, wasps, yellow jackets, hornets)
- Do not wear brightly colored clothing (choose lighter colors such as white, light green, khaki)
- Keep hair short or tied back; avoid hair sprays, perfumes, and flappy clothing
- Wear shoes and socks
- Avoid riding horses or bicycles in areas where bees or wasps are plentiful (*e.g.,* fields of clover, flowers)
- Avoid mowing lawns, trimming hedges, or pruning trees during the insect season
- Carry an insect spray in the glove compartment of the car and keep one handy at home (attempts to swat or kill bees must be well planned, for a missing blow may infuriate the insect and make it more dangerous)
- If approached by a bee or wasp in the open, stay still or move back very slowly
- Each spring, have home and garden searched for new hornet or bees' nests and obtain professional assistance from an exterminator or fire department in eliminating them

4. For a severe allergic reaction where hives or any respiratory symptoms appear, or *if one has had a previous severe reaction to any kind of sting,* carry out the following procedure
- Remove stinger if possible
- Keep as quiet as possible (avoid panic)
- Apply ice immediately
- Use emergency beesting kit injection if available
- Be driven to the nearest emergency room for *immediate* medical treatment and further observation (the person who merely suspects that a severe reaction may occur need not actually register, but should stay close by in case of an anaphylactic reaction)

5. General instructions for unknown or nonspecific allergies
- Assess for introduction of new food or medication
- Eliminate

    Fish and fish oils (cod-liver oil products)

    All kinds of nuts

    All fresh fruits and fresh vegetables (this elimination does not apply to cooked fruits and vegetables)

    Chocolate

    Eggs and foods containing eggs

    Milk and foods containing milk

    Wheat and foods containing wheat
- If you have an asthmatic response, practice conscious control of breathing (see *Ineffective Breathing Patterns* for technique)

# Ineffective Airway Clearance

## Definition
Ineffective airway clearance: The state in which the individual experiences a real or potential threat to the passage of air through the respiratory tract related to partial or complete airway obstruction.

## Defining Characteristics
Abnormal respiratory rate, rhythm, or depth
Nasal flaring
Ineffective cough
Dyspnea, shortness of breath
Cyanosis, pallor, diaphoresis
Asymmetrical expansion of the chest
Inability to remove secretions
Absence of or abnormal breath sounds

## Associated characteristics
Fremitus (palpable vibrations felt on chest wall when person speaks)
Rising temperature
Change in pulse rate, rhythm, quality
Changes in blood pressure
Irritability/agitation
Abnormal arterial blood gases
Decreased tidal volume/vital capacity
Restlessness or anxiety

## Nursing Goals
Through selected nursing interventions, the nurse will seek to
- Promote optimal movement of air in and out of the lungs
- Prevent aspiration
- Prevent atelectasis, infection, and stasis of air and secretions in the lungs
- Establish a good pulmonary toilet regime, thus removing pulmonary secretions
- Assist the individual to accomplish effective coughing practices with minimal discomfort

## Principles and Rationale For Nursing Care
See *Alterations in Respiratory Function*

# Ineffective Airway Clearance
Related to (*specify*)

---

**Outcome Criteria**

The person will
- Have a decreased risk of aspiration
- Demonstrate effective coughing and increased air exchange in his lungs

---

## Interventions

The nursing interventions for the diagnosis *Ineffective Airway Clearance* represent interventions for any individual with this nursing diagnosis, regardless of the etiological and contributing factors.

### A. Assess for causative or contributing factors

Inability to maintain proper position
Ineffective cough
Pain or fear of pain
Viscous secretions (dehydration)
Fatigue, weakness, drowsiness
Lack of knowledge (of how to cough, and why it is important)
Chronic, nonrelieved cough

### B. Reduce or eliminate factors if possible

1. Inability to maintain proper position
   - Maintain a side-lying position if not contraindicated by injury
   - If the person cannot be positioned on his side, open oropharyngeal airway by lifting the mandible up and forward, with the head tilted backward (for a small infant, hyperextension of the neck may not be effective)
   - Assess for position of the tongue, assuring that it has not dropped backward, occluding the airway
   - Keep the head of the bed elevated, if not contraindicated by hypotension or injury
   - Maintain good oral hygiene: Clean teeth and use mouthwash on cotton swab; apply petroleum jelly to lips, removing encrustations gently
   - Prevent aspiration
     a. Clear secretions from mouth and throat with a tissue or gentle suction
     b. Reassess frequently for presence of obstructive material in mouth and throat
     c. Re-evaluate frequently for good anatomic positioning
     d. Maintain side-lying position after feedings
2. Ineffective cough
   - Instruct person on the proper method of controlled coughing
     a. Breathe deeply and slowly while sitting up as high as possible
     b. Use diaphragmatic breathing

  c. Hold the breath for 3 to 5 seconds and then slowly exhale as much of this breath as possible through the mouth (lower rib cage and abdomen should sink down)

  d. Take a second breath, hold, and cough forcefully from the chest (not from the back of the mouth or throat), using two short forceful coughs

3. Pain or fear of pain

 a. Assess present analgesic regime

  &bull; Administer pain medication as needed

  &bull; Assess its effectiveness: Is the individual too lethargic? Is the individual still in pain?

  &bull; Note time when person appears to have best pain relief with optimal level of alertness and physical performance: *This is the time for active breathing and coughing exercises*

 b. Provide emotional support

  &bull; Stay with person for the entire coughing session

  &bull; Explain the importance of coughing after pain relief

  &bull; Reassure person that suture lines are secure and that splinting by hand or pillow will minimize pain of movement

 c. Use appropriate comfort measures for site of pain

  &bull; Splint abdominal or chest incisions with hand, pillow, or both

 d. For sore throat

  &bull; Assess for adequate humidity in the inspired air

  &bull; Consider warm saline gargle every 2 to 4 hours

  &bull; Consider use of anesthetic lozenge or gargle, especially before coughing sessions*

  &bull; Examine throat for exudate, redness, and swelling and note if it is associated with fever

  &bull; Explain that a sore throat is common after anesthesia and should be a short-term problem

 e. Maintain good body alignment to prevent muscular pain and strain

  &bull; Acquire and use extra pillows on both sides of person, especially the affected side, for support

  &bull; Position person to prevent slouching and cramping positions of the thorax and abdomen; reassess positioning frequently

 f. Assess person's understanding of the use of analgesia to enhance breathing and coughing effort

  &bull; Teach person during periods of optimal level of consciousness

  &bull; Continually reinforce rationale for plan of nursing care ("I will be back to help you cough when the pain medicine is working and you can be most effective")

4. Viscous (thick) secretions

  &bull; Maintain adequate hydration (increase fluid intake to 2–3 quarts a day if not contraindicated by decreased cardiac output or renal disease)

  &bull; Maintain adequate humidity of inspired air

5. Fatigue, weakness, drowsiness

  &bull; Plan and bargain for rest periods ("Work to cough well now; then I can let you rest")

*May require a physician's order.

- Vigorously coach and encourage coughing, using positive reinforcement ("You worked hard; I know it's not easy, but it is important")
- Be sure coughing session occurs at peak comfort period after analgesics, but not peak level of sleepiness
- Allow for rest after coughing and before meals
- For lethargy or decreased level of consciousness, stimulate person to breathe ("Take a deep breath")

6. Lack of understanding or motivation (of how and why to cough)
    - Assess knowledge of reasons and method for coughing
    - Proceed with health teaching with constant reinforcement in principles of care
    - Acknowledge and encourage good individual effort and progress

7. For chronic, nonrelieved coughing
    - Minimize irritants in the inspired air (*e.g.,* dust, allergens)
    - Provide periods of uninterrupted rest
    - Administer Rx—cough suppressant, expectorant—as ordered by physician (hold food and drink immediately after administration of meds for best results)
    - Relieve mucous membrane irritation through humidity (inhaling steam from shower, or sitting over pot of steaming water with a towel over the head, will loosen thick secretions and soothe the membranes)

## C. Initiate health teaching and referrals as indicated

- Instruct parents on the need for child to cough, even if painful
- Allow adult and older child to listen to lungs; describe if clear or if rales are present
- Consult with respiratory therapist for assistance if needed

# Ineffective Breathing Patterns

### Definition
Ineffective breathing patterns: The state in which the individual experiences an actual or potential loss of adequate ventilation related to an altered breathing pattern.

### Etiological and Contributing Factors
See *Alterations in Respiratory Function*

### Defining Characteristics (See also *Alterations in Respiratory Function*)
Orthopnea
Bradypnea
Tachypnea, hyperpnea, hyperventilation
Arrhythmic respirations
Splinted/guarded respirations
Periodic apnea (Cheyne-Stokes respirations)

### Nursing Goals (See also *Alterations in Respiratory Function*)
Through selected nursing interventions, the nurse will seek to
- Identify contributing factors
- Decrease the work of breathing by teaching appropriate breathing exercises
- Maintain optimal air exchange by teaching the proper use of accessory muscles and body posture

### Principles and Rationale for Nursing Care
See *Alterations in Respiratory Function*

# Ineffective Breathing Patterns
## Related to Hyperpnea or Hyperventilation

Hyperpnea or hyperventilation is rapid, unsatisfactory breathing.

### Assessment

Subjective data

The person states
"I can't catch my breath"
"My fingers tingle and my heart beats fast"
"I feel dizzy (faint)"
History of existing emotional or physical stress
Fear or anxiety

Objective data
Tachypnea (forceful)
Tachycardia
Bounding pulse
Rising blood pressure
Anxious facial expression

---

**Outcome Criteria**

The person will
- Demonstrate an effective respiratory rate and experience improved gas exchange in the lungs
- Relate the causative factors, if known, and relate adaptive ways of coping with them

---

## Interventions

A. Assess causative factors
Fear
Pain
Exercise/activity

B. Remove or reduce causative factors
1. Fear
   - Remove cause of fear, if possible
   - Reassure person that measures are being taken to ensure his safety
   - Distract person from thinking about his anxious state by having him maintain eye contact with you (or perhaps with someone else he trusts); say, "Now, look at me and breathe slowly with me like this"
   - Consider use of paper bag as means of rebreathing expired air (expired $CO_2$ will be reinspired, thereby slowing respiratory rate)
   - See *Fear.*
2. Pain
   - Determine location of discomfort
   - Use appropriate comfort measures (see *Alterations in Comfort*)
   - Encourage displacement of pain perception through concentration on more efficient breathing (*e.g.,* concentrating completely on air going in and out of lungs, giving plentiful oxygen to the body)
   - Stay with person and coach in taking slower, more effective breaths
3. Exercise/activity
   - Encourage slow deep breaths, pausing when ambulating for the first time after immobility or surgery
   - Encourage conscious control of breathing during exercise (slower, deeper, abdominal breathing)
   - See *Activity Intolerance* for additional interventions

C. Proceed with health teaching
- Explain that one can learn to overcome hyperventilation through conscious control of breathing even when the cause is unknown
- Discuss possible causes, physical and emotional, and methods of coping effectively (see *Anxiety*)

# Impaired Gas Exchange

### Definition
Impaired gas exchange: The state in which the individual experiences an actual or potential decreased passage of gases (oxygen and carbon dioxide) between the alveoli of the lungs and the vascular system.

### Etiological and Contributing Factors
See *Alterations in Respiratory Function*

### Defining Characteristics (See also *Alterations in Respiratory Function*)
Tendency to assume three-point position (sitting, one hand on each knee, bending forward)

Pursed-lip breathing with prolonged expiratory phase

Increased anteroposterior chest diameter, if chronic

Lethargy and fatigue

Increased pulmonary vascular resistance (increased pulmonary artery/right ventricular pressure)

Decreased gastric motility, prolonged gastric emptying

Decreased oxygen content, decreased oxygen saturation, increased $pCO_2$, as measured by blood gases

Cyanosis

### Nursing Goals (See also *Alterations in Respiratory Function*)
Through selected nursing interventions, the nurse will seek to
- Teach the person to conserve energy and control his symptoms
- Prevent infection and preserve pulmonary function
- Prevent "pulmonary crippling" by maintaining the person's optimal level of daily activity
- Decrease the work of breathing by helping the person to master conscious, controlled breathing techniques (*e.g.*, pursed-lip breathing) and maintaining strength of accessory muscles and optimal body posture

### Principles and Rationale of Nursing Care
See *Alterations in Respiratory Function*

# Impaired Gas Exchange
## Related to Chronic Tissue Hypoxia

Chronic hypoxia—insufficient oxygen in the tissues—with hypercarbia ($CO_2$ retention) results in permanent tissue damage.

## Assessment

### Subjective data

Because chronic tissue hypoxia affects all body systems, data are presented by systems.

Respiratory history
      Lung disease (chronic)
      Shortness of breath or dyspnea on exertion

Chronic cough
Orthopnea (sleeping with extra pillows)

Circulatory history
      Chest pain aggravated by activity

Enlarged heart

Gastrointestinal history
      Anorexia
      Nausea and vomiting

Constipation

Mental history
      Confusion or lethargy
      Mood swings, anxiety, depression

Sleep disturbances
Headache

Skeletal history
      Skeletal muscle pain aggravated by activity

Muscle weakness
Chronic fatigue

Genitourinary history
      Decreased kidney function

Decreased libido or impotence

### Objective data

Respiratory
    Tachypnea, bradypnea, arrhythmic breathing
    Abnormal chest film
    Abnormal flow rates; increased inspiratory/expiratory (I/E) ratio
    Pursed-lip breathing
    Abnormal blood gases ($\downarrow PO_2 \uparrow CO_2$)
    Use of accessory muscles (neck, shoulders, abdomen)
    Gasping before speech effort/inability to speak or cry
    Orthopnea/assumption of 3-point position (sitting, leaning forward with one hand on each knee)
    Cough
    Increased sputum production and inability to remove secretions
    Mouth breathing
    Abnormal breath sounds (rales and rhonchi)
    Decreased breath sounds
    Fremitus
Circulatory
    Neck vein distention
    Edema
    Cyanosis
Gastrointestinal
    Decreased bowel sounds
Genitourinary
    Decreased kidney function ($\uparrow$ Creatinine, $\uparrow$ BUN)
    Decreased urinary output

Skeletal system
   Hypertrophy of accessory breathing muscles (neck and shoulder)
   Atrophy or weakness of extremity muscles
   Barrel chest/horizontal sloping ribs
   Cachexia (malnutrition)

---

**Outcome Criteria**

The person will
- Preserve pulmonary function by maintaining optimal activity level and preventing infection
- Demonstrate methods of effective coughing, breathing, and conserving energy
- Relate relief of symptoms of pain, weakness, and dyspnea
- Relate the rationale of working to prevent further pulmonary problems
- Demonstrate improved vital signs and diagnostic studies

---

## Interventions

### A. Assess causative or contributing factors

Inadequate pulmonary hygiene regimen
Maladaptive breathing techniques
Inadequate nutritional intake
Insufficient level of activity
Lack of knowledge
Smoking or inhaling other irritants or allergens

### B. Eliminate or reduce causative factors

1. Inadequate pulmonary hygiene routine
   - Instruct person to practice controlled coughing four times a day, ½ hour before meals and at bedtime (allow 15–30 minutes' rest after coughing session and before meals)
   - Consider use of inhaled humidity and postural drainage, chest clapping before coughing session (assess for use of prescribed aerosol bronchodilators to dilate airways and thin secretions)
   - Explain the importance of adhering to daily coughing schedule for clearing the lungs (this is a lifetime commitment)
   - Teach the proper method of coughing
     a. Breathe deeply and slowly while sitting up as upright as possible
     b. Use diaphragmatic breathing
     c. Hold the breath for 3 to 5 seconds and then slowly exhale as much of this breath as possible through your mouth (lower rib cage and abdomen should sink down as you inhale)
     d. Take a second deep breath, hold, and cough forcefully from deep in the chest (not from the back of the mouth or throat); use two short forceful coughs
     e. Rest after session

2. Maladaptive breathing techniques
   - Encourage conscious controlled breathing techniques during increased activity and times of emotional and physical stress (techniques include pursed-lip and diaphragmatic breathing)
   - For pursed-lip breathing, the person should breathe in through his nose; then he should breathe out slowly through partially closed lips while counting to seven and making a "pu" sound (often this is learned naturally by person with progressive lung disease)
   - For diaphragmatic breathing
     a. The nurse should place her hands on the person's abdomen below the base of the ribs and keep them there while he inhales
     b. To inhale, the person should relax his shoulders, breathe in through his nose, and push his stomach outward against the nurse's hands, holding his breath for 1 to 2 seconds to keep the alveoli open
     c. To exhale, the person should breathe out slowly through his mouth while the nurse applies slight pressure at the base of the ribs
     d. This breathing technique should be practiced several times with the nurse; then the person should place his own hands at the base of the ribs and practice on his own
     e. Once the person has learned, he should practice this exercise a few times each hour
3. Inadequate nutritional intake
   - Suggest that person brush teeth and use mouthwash before meals (and especially after coughing session, because there is frequently an associated bad taste in the mouth, causing a decreased appetite and a decrease in tasting ability)
   - Encourage smaller, more frequent meals (large portions require more oxygen/energy to digest and also limit the downward movements of the diaphragm during inspiration)
   - Choose foods that are easy to chew and swallow (food that must be chewed extensively will require more work, causing fatigue); assist in food preparation (*e.g.*, cutting meat) if person is extremely fatigued
   - Avoid gas-producing foods or liquids
   - Discourage talking while eating; encourage thorough chewing and slow eating
   - Encourage drinking 2 to 3 quarts of liquid a day (minimum) if sodium and fluids are unrestricted (consult with physician for desired daily fluid intake)
   - Assure satisfactory bowel elimination (See *Alterations in Nutrition* for additional interventions)
4. Insufficient level of activity
   - Encourage gradual increase in daily activity to prevent "pulmonary crippling"
   - Encourage person to use adaptive breathing techniques to decrease the work of breathing
   - Discuss physical barriers at home and at work (*e.g.*, number of stairs) and ways of alternating expenditure of energy with rest pauses (place a chair in bathroom near sink to rest during daily hygiene)
   - Encourage verbalization of feelings about disease and limitations and discuss methods of coping with daily stressors (see *Ineffective Individual Coping*)
   - Encourage socialization with others and methods of reducing depression (taking a walk, visiting with a friend)

- Give calm, consistent emotional support in time of increased respiratory distress, in hopes of reducing oxygen demands
- Support person by suggesting that he follow your breathing pattern and by demonstrating pursed-lip and diaphragmatic breathing

5. Lack of knowledge
- Assess person's understanding of the prescribed therapeutic regimen; proceed with health teaching, using simple clear instructions and including family members*
- Explain that the person with chronic pulmonary disease is susceptible to infection and must detect symptoms early and consult with physician for treatment (frequently, early antibiotic therapy is necessary)
- Discuss the need for annual immunizations (against flu, bacteria)
- Instruct person to wear warm dry clothing; avoid crowds, heavy smoke, fumes, and irritants; avoid exertion in cold, hot, or humid weather; and balance work, rest, and recreation to conserve energy
- Teach person to observe his sputum, note changes in color, amount, and odor, and seek professional advice if sputum changes
- Emphasize importance of maintaining a good wholesome diet (high calorie, high vitamin C, high protein, and 2 to 3 quarts of liquid a day, unless on fluid restriction)
- Specifically assess
  a. Knowledge and skill of adaptive breathing techniques
  b. Knowledge of medicines (when taken, why, how much, how often, and food and drug interactions)
  c. Knowledge of the care, cleansing, and use of inhalatory equipment
  d. Awareness of fire hazards (if on oxygen therapy, especially at home); explain need for home extinguisher

6. Smoking
- Teach person to avoid factors that aggravate symptoms and advance disease (excessive allergens, pollution)
- Discourage smoking
- If person insists on smoking, discourage smoking immediately before meals or activity
- See further interventions under *Alterations in Respiratory Function Related to Smoking* if person wishes to reduce or stop smoking

## C. Initiate health teaching and referrals as indicated

- Give clear, written and verbal instructions; be specific
- Reassess knowledge of skills and rationale frequently; keep clear progress notes on strengths and weaknesses of person's knowledge
- Encourage person to keep a daily written log of his activities and symptoms and of measures that relieve symptoms
- Refer to community nurse for follow-up if needed
- Refer to organizations and pertinent literature for the person with lung disorders

---

*A person who is chronically hypoxic should always be taught in simple terms and assured of support by family and caretakers, because thought processes frequently become confused during periods of hypoxia.

# Bibliography

## Books and Articles

Aashika T: Evaluation of a community-based educational program for individuals with C.O.P.D. J Rehabil 46(2):23–27, 1980

Bates B: A Guide to Physical Examination. Philadelphia, JB Lippincott, 1979

Ellmyer P: A guide to your patient's safe home use of oxygen. Nursing 12(1):54–57, 1982

Harimon A: Anaphylaxis can mean sudden death. Nursing 10(10):40–43, 1980

Harper RW: A Guide to Respiratory Care. Philadelphia, JB Lippincott, 1981

Hungel D, Madsen L: Acute and chronic asthma: A guide to intervention. Am J Nurs 80:1791–1795; 1980

Jacobs M: Protocol for C.O.P.D. Nurse Pract 4(6):11–28, 1979

Jecklin J: Positioning, percussion, and vibrating patients for effective bronchial drainage. Nursing 9(3):64–70, 1979

Kaufman J, Woody J: C.O.P.D.—better living through teaching. Nursing 10(3):57–61, 1981

Largerson J: The cough: Its effectiveness depends on you. Respiratory Care 27(4):418–434, 1982

Larter N: Cystic fibrosis. Am J Nurs 81:527–532, 1981

McCaully E: Breathing exercises as play for asthmatic children. Matern Child Nurs J 5(5):340–345, 1979

McCreary C, Watson J: Pickwickian syndrome. Am J Nurs 81:555, 1981

Mechanical ventilation: Patient assessment and nursing care—a programmed unit. Am J Nurs 80:2191–2217, 1980

Pinney M: Foreign body aspiration. Am J Nurs 81:521–522, 1981

Pinney M: Pneumonia. Am J Nurs 81:517–518, 1981

Richard E, Shephard A: Giving up smoking: A lesson in loss theory. Am J Nurs 79:755–757, 1979

Rice V: Clinical hypoxia. Critical Care Nurse. 1(6):21–29, 1980

Rifas E: How you and your patient can manage dyspnea. Nursing 10(6):34–41, 1980

Simkins R: Asthma: Reactive airway disease. Am J Nurs 81:523–526, 1981

Simkins R: The crisis of bronchiolitis. Am J Nurs 81:515–516, 1981

Simkins R: Croup and epiglottitis. Am J Nurs 81:519–520, 1981

Stroud S: Ammonia inhalation, a case report. Critical Care Nurse 1(1):23–26, 1981

Webber J: OTC (Over the Counter) Bronchodilators: What are the risks of relief in seconds? Nursing 10(1):34–39, 1980

Woolf CR: The Clinical Core of Respiratory Medicine. Philadelphia JB Lippincott, 1981

## Pertinent Organizations and Literature for the Consumer

American Cancer Society, 777 3rd Avenue, New York, NY 10017

American Heart Association, 7320 Greenville Avenue, Dallas, TX 75231

American Lung Association, 1740 Broadway, New York, NY 10019

Cystic Fibrosis Foundation, 3091 Mayfield Road, Cleveland, OH 44118

SIDS Clearing House, Suite 600, 1555 Wilson Boulevard, Rosslyn, VA 22209

Tuhy J, Bither S: Breathing easy: Living with emphysema and chronic bronchitis. A manual for patients with chronic obstructive disease. Portland, Oregon Lung Association, 1977. Write for a copy: 830 Medical Arts Building, 1020 Southwest Taylor Street, Portland, Oregon 97205.

## Sources of Information on Allergy Control

Dickey Enterprises (environmentalists), 635 Gregory Road, Fort Collins, CO 80524; (303) 482-6001

Meridian, Bio-Medical (for pollen guide), 3278 Wadsworth Boulevard South, Denver, CO 80227; (303) 986-5555

Hollister-Stier Laboratories, Division of Cutter Laboratories, Inc., Box 3145, Terminal Annex, Spokane, WA 99220

# Self-Care Deficit

*Related to* **Inability to Feed Self**

*Related to* **Inability to Bathe Self**

*Related to* **Inability to Dress Self**

*Related to* **Inability to Toilet Self**

## Definition

Self-care deficit: The state in which the individual experiences an impaired motor function or cognitive function, causing a decreased ability to feed, bathe, dress, or toilet oneself.

## Etiological and Contributing Factors

Pathophysiological

Neuromuscular impairment
    Autoimmune alterations (arthritis, multiple sclerosis)
    Metabolic and endocrine alterations (diabetes mellitus, hypothyroidism)
    Nervous system disorders (Parkinsonism, myasthenia gravis, muscular dystrophy)
    Lack of coordination
    Spasticity or flaccidity
    Muscular weakness
    Partial or total paralysis (spinal cord injury, stroke)
    CNS tumors
    Increased intracranial pressure
Musculoskeletal disorders
    Atrophy
    Muscle contractures
    Connective tissue diseases (systemic lupus erythematosus)
    Edema (increased synovial fluid)
Visual disorders
    Glaucoma
    Cataracts
    Diabetic/hypertensive retinopathy
    Ocular histoplasmosis
    Cranial nerve neuropathy
    Visual field cuts

Situational

Immobility
Trauma or surgical procedures
            Fractures                          Jejunostomy
            Tracheotomy                        Ileostomy
            Gastrostomy                        Colostomy

Nonfunctioning or missing limbs
External devices (casts or splints, braces, IV equipment)

## Maturational

Elderly: Decreased visual and motor ability, muscle weakness

## Defining Characteristics

1. Self-feeding deficits
   Is unable to cut food
   Is unable to bring food to mouth
2. Self-bathing deficit (includes washing entire body, combing hair, brushing teeth, attending to skin and nail care, and applying makeup)
   Is unwilling or unable to

|  |  |
|---|---|
| Wash body or body parts | Regulate temperature or water |
| Obtain a water source | flow |

3. Self-dressing deficit (including donning regular or special clothing, not nightclothes)
   Has impaired ability to

|  |  |
|---|---|
| Groom self satisfactorily | Fasten clothing |
| Put on or take off clothing | Obtain or replace articles of clothing |

4. Self-toileting deficit
   Is unable or unwilling to

|  |  |
|---|---|
| Get to the toilet or commode | Handle clothing |
| Transfer to and from toilet or commode | Carry out proper hygiene |
|  | Flush toilet or empty commode |

## Focus Assessment Criteria

Self-feeding abilities

|  |  |
|---|---|
| Swallowing | Selecting foods |
| Chewing | Seeing |
| Using utensils and cutting food |  |

Self-bathing abilities

|  |  |
|---|---|
| Undressing to bathe | Obtaining equipment (water, |
| Reaching water source | soap, towels) |
| Differentiating water temperatures | Washing body parts |

Self-dressing abilities

|  |  |
|---|---|
| Putting on or taking off necessary clothing | Retrieving appropriate clothing |
| Selecting appropriate clothing | Fastening clothing |

Self-toileting ability

|  |  |
|---|---|
| Getting to toilet and undressing | Cleaning self/flushing toilet |
| Sitting on toilet | Redressing |
| Rising from toilet | Performing proper hygiene (wash hands) |

## Nursing Goals

Through selected interventions, the nurse will seek to
- Help the individual to cope with deficits by accepting realistic long-term goals
- Teach the individual how to use adaptive devices to facilitate all areas of self-care
- Minimize the potential for injury through the use of safety measures
- Preserve or promote optimal function of all body systems
- Help the individual to maintain a positive self-esteem

## Principles and Rationale for Nursing Care

### General

1. The concept of self-care emphasizes each person's right to maintain individual domain over his own pattern of living. (This applies to both the ill individual and the well individual.)
2. Regardless of handicap, people should be given privacy and treated with dignity while performing self-care activities.
3. Self-care does not imply allowing the person to do things for himself as planned by the nurse but, rather, encouraging and teaching the person to make his own plans for optimal daily living.
4. Mobility is necessary to meet one's self-care needs and to maintain good health and self-esteem. (Fig. II–7)
5. Cleanliness is important for comfort, for positive self-esteem, and for social interactions with others.
6. Inability to care for oneself produces feelings of dependency and poor self-concept. With increased ability for self-care, self-esteem increases.
7. Disability often causes denial, anger, and frustration. These are valid emotions that must be recognized and addressed.
8. It is acceptable for a limited period of time to be dependent on others to provide basic physiological and psychological needs.
9. Regression in ability to perform self-care activities may be a defense mechanism to threatening situations.
10. Neglect of an extremity refers to the memory loss of the presence of an extremity (*e.g.*, a person who has had a stroke or head trauma resulting in partial paralysis may ignore the arm or leg on the affected side of the body).

### Endurance

1. The endurance or ability of the individual to maintain a given level of performance is influenced by the ability to use oxygen to produce energy (related to the optimal functioning of the heart, respiratory, and circulatory systems) and the functioning of the neurological and musculoskeletal systems. Thus, individuals with alterations in these systems have increased energy demands or a decreased ability to produce energy.
2. Stress is energy consuming; the more stressors an individual has, the more fatigue he will experience. Stressors can be personal, environmental, disease-related, and treatment-related. Examples of possible stressors follow.

| *Personal* | *Environmental* | *Disease-Related* | *Treatment-Related* |
|---|---|---|---|
| Age | Isolation | Pain | Walker |
| Support system | Noise | Anemia | Medications |
| Life-style | Unfamiliar setting | | Diagnostic studies |

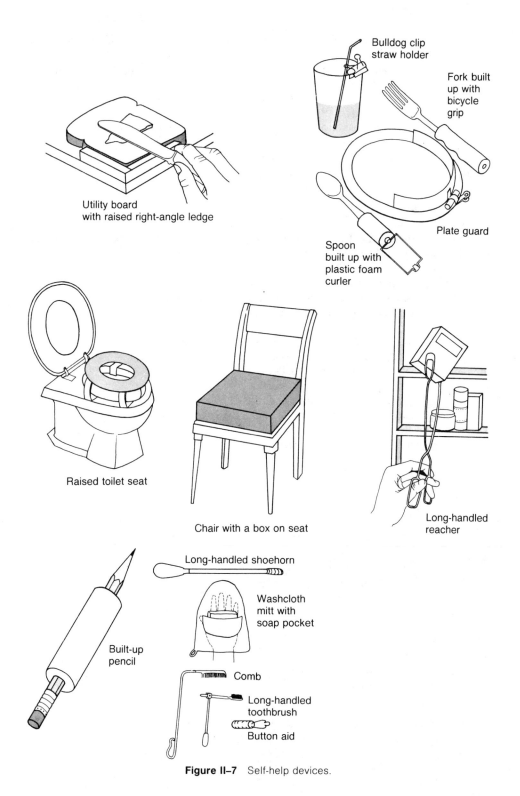

**Bulldog clip straw holder**

**Fork built up with bicycle grip**

**Utility board with raised right-angle ledge**

**Plate guard**

**Spoon built up with plastic foam curler**

**Raised toilet seat**

**Chair with a box on seat**

**Long-handled reacher**

**Long-handled shoehorn**

**Washcloth mitt with soap pocket**

**Built-up pencil**

**Comb**

**Long-handled toothbrush**

**Button aid**

**Figure II–7** Self-help devices.

3. The signs and symptoms of decreased oxygen in response to an activity—*e.g.*, self-care, mobility—are:
    Sustained increased heart rate 3 to 5 minutes after ceasing the activity or a change in the pulse rhythm
    Failure of systolic blood pressure reading to increase with activity, or a decrease in value
    Decrease or excessive increase in respiratory rate and dyspnea
    Weakness, pallor, cerebral anoxia (confusion, incoordination)
4. Refer to Principles of Nursing Care under *Activity Intolerance* for additional information.

## Teaching/relearning

1. Optimal patient education promotes self-care. To teach effectively the nurse must determine what the learner perceives as his own needs and goals, determine what the nurse feels are his needs and goals, and then work to establish mutually acceptable goals.
2. Offering the individual choices and including him in planning his own care reduces feelings of powerlessness; promotes feelings of freedom, control, and self-worth; and increases the person's willingness to comply with therapeutic regimens.
3. The following key elements promote relearning of self-care tasks:
    Providing a structured, consistent environment and routine
    Repeating instructions and tasks
    Teaching and practicing tasks during periods of least fatigue
    Maintaining a familiar environment and teacher
    Using patience, determination, and a positive attitude (by both person and teacher)
    Practicing, practicing, practicing

# Self-Care Deficit
## Related to Inability to Feed Self

### Assessment

### Subjective data
The person reports
    Problems with eating ("I can't feed myself"; "I'm too tired to eat"; "Could you help me with my food?")
    Pain

### Objective data
    Impaired visual acuity
    Mental lethargy

Poor oral hygiene (lack of teeth or poorly fitting dentures; oral injury, ulcer, deformity)
Drooling or facial paralysis
Uncoordination
Inability to use hands to move food to mouth
Absence of gag reflex

---

**Outcome Criteria**

The person will
- Demonstrate increased ability to feed self *or*
- Demonstrate that he is coping with inability to feed self
- Demonstrate ability to make use of adaptive devices, if indicated
- Demonstrate increased interest and desire to eat
- Describe rationale and procedure for treatment
- Describe causative factors for feeding deficit

---

## Interventions

### A. Assess causative factors

Visual deficits (blindness, field cuts, poor depth perception)
Affected or missing limbs (casts, amputations, paresis, paralysis)
Cognitive deficits (aging, trauma, CVA)

### B. Provide opportunities to relearn or adapt to activity

1. Common nursing interventions for feeding
   - Ascertain from person or family members what foods the person likes or dislikes
   - Have meals taken in the same setting: pleasant surroundings that are not too distracting
   - Maintain correct food temperatures (hot foods hot, cold foods cold)
   - Provide pain relief, since pain can affect appetite and ability to feed self
   - Provide good oral hygiene before and after meals
   - Encourage person to wear dentures and eyeglasses
   - Place person in the most normal eating position suited to his physical disability (best is sitting in chair at a table)
   - Provide social contact during eating
   - See *Alterations in Nutrition: Less Than Body Requirements*
2. Specific interventions for people with sensory/perceptual deficits
   - Encourage the person to wear prescribed corrective lenses
   - Describe location of utensils and food on tray or table
   - Describe food items to stimulate appetite
   - For perceptual deficits, choose different-colored dishes to help distinguish items (*e.g.,* red tray, white plates)
   - Ascertain person's usual eating patterns and provide food items according to preference (or arrange food items in clocklike pattern); record on care plan the arrangement used (*e.g.,* meat, 6 o'clock; potatoes, 9 o'clock; vegetables, 12 o'clock)

- Encourage eating of "finger foods" (*e.g.*, bread, bacon, fruit, hot dogs) to promote independence
- Avoid placing food to blind side of person with field cut, until visually accommodated to surroundings; then encourage him to scan entire visual field
3. Specific interventions for people with missing limbs
    - Provide for eating environment that is not embarrassing to individual and allow sufficient time for the task of eating
    - Provide only the amount of supervision and assistance necessary for relearning or adaptation
    - To enhance maximal amount of independence, provide necessary adaptive devices
        Plate guard to avoid pushing food off plate
        Suction device under plate or bowl for stabilization
        Padded handles on utensils for a more secure grip
        Wrist or hand splints with clamp to hold eating utensils
        Bottle with long drinking tube
        Rocker knife for cutting
    - Assist with set-up if needed, opening containers, napkins, condiment packages; cutting meat; buttering bread
    - Arrange food so person has adequate amount of space to perform the task of eating
4. Specific interventions for people with cognitive deficits
    - Provide isolated, quiet atmosphere until person is able to attend to eating and is not easily distracted from the task
    - Supervise feeding program until there is no danger of choking or aspiration
    - Orient person to location and purpose of feeding equipment
    - Avoid external distractions and unnecessary conversation
    - Place person in the most normal eating position he is physically able to assume
    - Encourage person to attend to the task, but be alert for fatigue, frustration, or agitation
    - Provide one food at a time in usual sequence of eating until person is able to eat the entire meal in normal sequence
    - Encourage person to be tidy, to eat in small amounts, and to put food in unaffected side of mouth if paresis or paralysis is present
    - Check for food in cheeks
    - Refer to *Alterations in Nutrition Related to Chewing or Swallowing Difficulties* for additional interventions

## C. Initiate health teaching and referrals as indicated

1. Assess to assure that both person and family understand the reason and purpose of all interventions
2. Proceed with teaching as needed
    - Maintain safe eating methods
    - Prevent aspiration
    - Use appropriate eating utensils (avoid sharp instruments)
    - Test temperature of hot liquids and wear protective clothing (*e.g.*, towel)
    - Teach use of adaptive devices

# Self-Care Deficit
## Related to Inability to Bathe Self

### Assessment

Objective data
>   Impaired visual acuity
>   Impaired hearing acuity
>   Impaired upper limb movement
>   Inability to use hands
>   Uncoordinated movements or spasticity
>   Presence of restrictive devices (splints, casts, braces, traction equipment)
>   Decreased mental alertness

Subjective data

The person states
>   "I can't wash myself"
>   "I don't want (need) a bath"
>   "I'm too tired (weak) to wash myself"
>   "It hurts"

---

**Outcome Criteria**

The person will
  · Perform bathing activity at expected optimal level *or*
  · Demonstrate satisfaction with accomplishments despite limitations
  · Relate feeling of comfort and satisfaction with body cleanliness
  · Demonstrate ability to use adaptive devices
  · Describe causative factors of bathing deficit
  · Relate rationale and procedures for treatment

---

### Interventions

A. Assess causative factors
>   Visual deficits (blindness, field cuts, poor depth perception)
>   Affected or missing limbs (casts, amputations, paresis, paralysis, arthritis)
>   Cognitive deficits (aging, trauma, CVA)

B. Provide opportunities to relearn or adapt to activity
  1. General nursing interventions for inability to bathe
     · Bathing time and routine should be consistent to encourage greatest amount of independence
     · Encourage person to wear prescribed corrective lenses or hearing aid
     · Keep bathroom temperature warm; ascertain individual's preferred water temperature

- Provide for privacy during bathing routine
- Observe skin condition during bathing
- Provide all bathing equipment within easy reach
- Provide for safety in the bathroom (rubber mats, grab bars)
- When person is physically able, encourage use of either tub or shower stall, depending upon which facility is at home (the person should practice in the hospital in preparation for going home)
- Provide for adaptive equipment as needed
  a. Chair or stool in bathtub or shower
  b. Long-handled sponge to reach back or lower extremities
  c. Grab bars on bathroom walls where needed to assist in mobility
  d. Bath board for transferring to tub chair or stool
  e. Safety treads or nonslip mat on floor of bathroom, tub, and shower
  f. Washing mitts with pocket for soap
  g. Adapted toothbrushes
  h. Shaver holders
  i. Hand-held shower spray
- Provide for relief of pain that may affect ability to bathe self*
2. Specific interventions for bathing for people with visual deficits
  - Place bathing equipment in location most suitable to individual
  - Avoid placing bathing equipment to blind side if person has a field cut and is not visually accommodated to surroundings
  - Keep call bell within reach if person is to bathe alone
  - Give the visually impaired individual the same degree of privacy and dignity as any other person
  - Verbally announce yourself before entering or leaving the bathing area
  - Observe the person's ability to locate all bathing utensils
  - Observe the person's ability to perform mouth care, hair combing, and shaving tasks
  - Provide place for clean clothing within easy reach
3. Specific interventions for bathing for people with affected or missing limbs
  - Bathe early in morning or before bed at night to avoid unnecessary dressing and undressing
  - Encourage person to use a mirror during bathing to inspect the skin of paralyzed areas
  - Encourage the person with amputation to inspect remaining foot or stump for good skin integrity
  - For limb amputations, bathe stump twice a day and be sure it is dry before wrapping or applying prosthesis
  - Provide only the amount of supervision or assistance necessary for relearning the use of extremity or adaptation to the handicap
  - For lack of sensation, encourage use of the affected area in the bathing process (an individual tends to forget the existence of body parts in which there is no sensation)
4. Specific interventions for bathing people with cognitive deficits
  - Provide a consistent time for the bathing routine as part of a structured program to help decrease confusion

*May require a physician's order.

- Keep instructions simple and avoid distractions; orient to purpose of bathing equipment
- If person is unable to bathe the entire body, have him bathe one part until he does it correctly; give positive reinforcement for success
- Supervise activity until person can safely perform the task unassisted
- Encourage attention to the task, but be alert for fatigue that may increase confusion
- Apply firm pressure to the skin when bathing; it is less likely to be misinterpreted than a gentle touch
- Use a warm shower or bath to help a confused or agitated person to relax

### C. Initiate health teaching and referrals as indicated

- Communicate to staff and family the person's ability and willingness to learn
- Teach use of adaptive devices
- Ascertain bathing facilities at home and assist in determining if there is any need to make adaptations; refer to occupational therapy or social service for help in obtaining needed home equipment
- Teach to use tub or shower stall, depending on type of facility at home
- If person is paralyzed, instruct him or his family to demonstrate complete skin check on key areas for redness (buttocks, bony prominences)
- Teach to maintain a safe bathing environment

# Self-Care Deficit
## Related to Inability to Dress Self

### Assessment

#### Subjective data

The person reports
"I can't dress myself"
"I don't want to get dressed"
"It hurts to dress myself"
"I'm too tired to get dressed"

#### Objective data

Impaired visual acuity
Inability to use hands
Spasticity, weakness, lack of coordination
Presence of restrictive devices (traction, casts, splints, braces)
Disheveled appearance or inappropriate dress
Decreased mental alertness
Inability to dress self

**Outcome Criteria**

The person will
- Demonstrate increased ability to dress self *or*
- Demonstrate ability to cope with the necessity of having someone else assist him in performing the task
- Demonstrate ability to learn how to use adaptive devices to facilitate optimal independence in the task of dressing
- Demonstrate increased interest in wearing street clothes
- Describe causative factors for dressing deficit
- Relate rationale and procedures for treatments

## Interventions

### A. Assess causative factors

Visual deficits (blindness, field cuts, poor depth perception)
Affected or missing limbs (casts, amputations, arthritis, paresis, paralysis)
Cognitive deficits (aging, trauma, CVA)

### B. Provide opportunities to relearn or adapt to activity

1. Common nursing interventions for self-dressing
   - Encourage person to wear prescribed corrective lenses or hearing aid
   - Promote independence in dressing through continual and unaided practice
   - Choose clothing that is loose fitting, with wide sleeves and pant legs and front fasteners
   - Allow sufficient time for dressing and undressing, since the task may be tiring, painful, or difficult
   - Plan for person to learn and demonstrate one part of an activity before progressing further
   - Lay clothes out in the order in which they will be needed to dress
   - Provide dressing aids as necessary (some commonly used aids include dressing stick, Swedish reacher, zipper pull, buttonhook, long-handled shoehorn, and shoe fasteners adapted with elastic laces, Velcro closures, or flip-back tongues; all garments with fasteners may be adapted with Velcro closures)
   - Encourage person to wear ordinary or special clothing rather than nightclothes
   - Increase participation in dressing by medicating for pain 30 minutes before it is time to dress or undress, if indicated*
   - Provide for privacy during dressing routine
   - Provide for safety by ensuring easy access to all clothing and by ascertaining individual's performance level
2. Specific interventions for dressing for people with visual deficits
   - Allow person to ascertain the most convenient location for clothing, and adapt the environment to best accomplish the task (*e.g.*, remove unnecessary barriers)
   - Verbally announce yourself before entering or leaving the dressing area

---

*May require a physician's order.

- Avoid placing clothing to the blind side if person has a field cut, until he is visually accommodated to surroundings; then encourage him to turn head to scan entire visual field
- Apply adaptive devices (*e.g.,* hand splints) before dressing activity
- Consult or refer to Physical or Occupational Therapy for teaching application of prosthetics to missing limbs

3. Specific interventions for dressing for people with cognitive deficits
   - Make a consistent dressing routine to provide a structured program to decrease confusion
   - Keep instructions simple and repeat them frequently; avoid distractions
   - Introduce one article of clothing at a time
   - Encourage attention to the task; be alert for fatigue, which may increase confusion

## C. Initiate health teaching and referrals as indicated

1. Assess understanding and knowledge of individual and family for above instructions and rationale
2. Proceed with teaching as needed
   - Communicate the individual's ability and willingness to learn to staff and family members
   - Teach use of adaptive devices and techniques that are specific to each disability
   - Teach to maintain a safe dressing environment
   - Attempt to be noncritical in correcting errors

# Self-Care Deficit
## Related to Inability to Toilet Self

### Assessment

#### Subjective data

The person states
> "I can't go to the toilet"
> "It hurts"
> "I can't get out of bed (walk, move)"
> "I can't get to the bathroom in time"
> "I wet myself"
> "I can't control my bowels"

#### Objective data

Impaired visual acuity
Decreased mental alertness
Weakness, lack of coordination
Spasticity
Presence of restrictive devices (traction, casts, splints, braces)
Immobility

**Outcome Criteria**

The person will
- Demonstrate increased ability to toilet self *or*
- Demonstrate that he is coping with inability to toilet self
- Relate positive feelings because of continency
- Demonstrate ability to make use of adaptive devices to facilitate toileting
- Describe causative factors for toileting deficit
- Relate rationale and procedures for treatment

## Interventions

### A. Assess causative factors

Visual deficits (blindness, field cuts, poor depth perception)
Affected or missing limbs (casts, amputations, paresis, paralysis)
Cognitive deficits (aging, trauma, CVA)

### B. Provide opportunities to relearn or adapt to activity

1. Common nursing interventions for toileting difficulties
   - Encourage person to wear prescribed corrective lenses or hearing aid
   - Obtain bladder and bowel history from individual or significant other (see *Alterations in Bowel Elimination* or *Alteration in Patterns of Urinary Elimination*)
   - Ascertain communication system person uses to express the need to toilet
   - Maintain bladder and bowel record to determine toileting patterns
   - Provide for adequate fluid intake and balanced diet to promote adequate urinary output and normal bowel evacuation
   - Promote normal elimination by encouraging activity and exercise within the person's capabilities
   - Avoid development of "bowel fixation" by less frequent discussion and inquiries about bowel movements
   - Be alert to possibility of falls when toileting person (be prepared to ease him to floor without causing injury to either of you)
   - Achieve independence in toileting by continual and unaided practice
   - Allow sufficient time for the task of toileting to avoid fatigue (lack of sufficient time to toilet may cause incontinence or constipation)
   - Avoid use of indwelling catheters and condom catheters to expedite bladder continence (if possible)
2. Specific interventions for toileting for people with visual deficits
   - Keep call bell easily accessible so person can quickly obtain help to toilet; answer call bell promptly to decrease anxiety
   - If bedpan or urinal is necessary for toileting, be sure it is within person's reach
   - Avoid placing toileting equipment to the blind side of an individual with field cut (when he is visually accommodated to surroundings, you may suggest he search entire visual field for equipment)
   - Verbally announce yourself before entering or leaving toileting area
   - Observe person's ability to obtain equipment or get to the toilet unassisted
   - Provide for a safe and clear pathway to toilet area

3. Specific interventions for toileting for people with affected or missing limbs
   - Provide only the amount of supervision and assistance necessary for relearning or adapting to the prosthesis
   - Encourage person to look at affected area or limb and use it during toileting tasks
   - Encourage use of transfer techniques taught by Occupational or Physical Therapy (the nurse should familiarize herself with planned mode of transfer)
   - Provide the necessary adaptive devices to enhance the maximum amount of independence and safety (commode chairs, spill-proof urinals, fracture bedpans, raised toilet seats, support side rails for toilets)
   - Provide for a safe and clear pathway to toilet area
4. Specific interventions for toileting for people with cognitive deficits
   - Offer toileting reminders every two hours, after meals, and before bedtime
   - When person is able to indicate the need to toilet, begin toileting at two-hour intervals, after meals, and before bedtime
   - Answer call bell immediately to avoid frustration and failure to be continent
   - Encourage wearing ordinary clothes (many confused individuals are continent while wearing regular clothing)
   - Avoid the use of bedpans and urinals; if physically possible, provide a normal atmosphere of elimination in bathroom (the toilet used should remain constant to promote familiarity)
   - Give verbal cues as to what is expected of the individual, and give positive reinforcement for success
   - Work to achieve daytime continency before expecting nighttime continency (nighttime incontinence may continue after daytime continency has returned)
   - See *Alteration in Patterns of Urinary Elimination* for additional information on incontinence

## C. Initiate health teaching and referrals as indicated

1. Assess the understanding and knowledge of the individual and significant others of foregoing interventions and rationale
2. Proceed with teaching as needed
   - Communicate person's ability and willingness to learn to staff and family
   - Maintain a safe toileting environment
   - Reinforce knowledge of transferring techniques
   - Teach use of adaptive devices
   - Ascertain home toileting needs and refer to Occupational Therapy or Social Services for help in obtaining necessary equipment

## Bibliography

### Books

American Nurses Association Division on Medical-Surgical Nursing Practice and the Association of Rehabilitation Practice: Standards of Rehabilitation Nursing Practice. Kansas City, American Nurses Association, 1977

Beyers M, Dudas S: The Clinical Practice of Medical-Surgical Nursing. Boston, Little, Brown, 1977

Christopherson VA, Colter PP, Wolanin MP: Rehabilitation Nursing: Perspective and Applications. New York, McGraw-Hill, 1974

Guidelines for Stroke Care. Public Health Service Publ. No. 76-14017. Washington, DC, U.S. Department of Health Education and Welfare, 1976

Hirschberg GG, Lewis L, Vaughan P: Rehabilitation, 2nd ed. Philadelphia, JB Lippincott, 1976
Palmer M, Toms J: Manual for Functional Training. Philadelphia, FA Davis, 1980

## Articles

### Aged

Barton EM: Etiology of dependence in older nursing home residents during morning care: The role of staff behavior. J Pers Soc Psychol 10(3):423–431, 1980
Garvan P, Lee M, Lloyd K et al: Self-care applied to the aged. New Jersey Nurse 10(1):3–6, 1980
Leering C: A structural model of functional capacity in the aged. J Am Geriatr Soc 27(7):314–316, 1979

### General

Ciuca R, Bradish J, Trombly SM: Active range of motion exercises: A handbook. Nursing 8(8):45–49, 1978
Gardiner R: Getting the right piece in the right place: Home aids. Community Outlook 10(2):39–42, 1979
Hailsburg JC: Teaching patients self-care. Nurs Clin North Am 5:223–225, 1970
Kegel B, Carpenter M, Burgess E: Functional capabilities of lower extremity amputees. Arch Phys Med Rehabil 59(3):109–120, 1978
Levin LS: Patient education and self-care: How do they differ? Nurs Outlook 26(3):170–175, 1978
Meissner SE: Evaluate your patient's level of independence. Nursing 10(9):72–73, 1980
Newton A: Clothing: A positive part of the rehabilitation process. J Rehabil 42(4):18–22, 1976
Staff PH: ADL assessment. Scand J Rehab Med (Suppl) 31:153–157, 1980
Sullivan IJ: Self-care model for nursing. ANA Pub. No. G-147, 57–68, 1980
Walter KM: Techniques and concepts: Independent living. Perceptions by professionals in rehabilitation. J Rehabil 46(3):57–63, 1980
Yep JO: Tools for aiding physically disabled individuals increase independence in dressing. J Rehabil 43(5):39–41, 1977
Ziegler JC: Physical reconditioning—Treatment for the convalescent patient. Nursing 10(8):67–69, 1980

### Spinal cord injury

Panchal PD: Rehabilitation of the patient with spinal cord injury. Curr Probl Surg 17(4):254–262, 1980
Rogers JC, Figone JJ: Traumatic quadriplegia: Follow-up study of self-care skills. Arch Phys Med Rehabil 61(7):316–321, 1980
Stauffer S: A master plan for teaching the patient with spinal cord injury. RN 42(7):55–60, 1979
Turgeon E, Nuestadter SB: Helping paralyzed patients regain their independence. Nursing 4(7):83–84, 1974

### Stroke

Adler MK: Stroke rehabilitation: Is age a determinant? J Am Geriatr Soc 28(11):499–503, 1980
Andrews K, Stewart J: Stroke recovery: He can but does he? Rheumatol Rehabil 18(2):43–48, 1979
Dzau RE, Bochme AR: Stroke rehabilitation: A family–team education approach. Arch Phys Med Rehab: 59(5):236–239, 1978
Kavcwak–Keyes MA: Comeback from disaster: Helping the stroke patient learn to help himself. Nursing 9(1):32–35, 1979
Rogers EJ: Goals in hemiplegia care. J Am Geriatr Soc 28(11):497–498, 1980
Stonington HH: Rehabilitation in cerebrovascular diseases. Primary Care 7(3):87–106, 1980

# Self-Concept, Disturbance in

## Definition
Disturbance in self-concept: The state in which the individual experiences or is at risk of experiencing a negative state of change about the way he feels, thinks, or views himself. It may include a change in body image, self-esteem, role performance, or personal identity.

## Etiological and Contributing Factors
A disturbance in self-concept can occur as a response to a variety of health problems, situations and conflicts. Some common sources follow.

### Pathophysiological
Loss of body part(s)
Loss of body function(s)
Severe trauma

### Situational
Divorce, separation from or death of a significant other
Loss of job or ability to work
Hospitalization; chronic or terminal illness
Pain
Surgery
Obesity
Pregnancy
Immobility or loss of function
Need for nursing home placement

### Maturational
Infant and pre-school: Deprivation
Young adult: Peer pressure, puberty
Middle aged: Signs of aging (graying or loss of hair), reduced hormonal levels (menopause)
Elderly: Losses (people, function, financial, retirement)

### Other
Women's movement
Sexual revolution

## Defining Characteristics
Since a disturbance in self-concept may include a change in any one or combination of its four component parts (body image, self-esteem, role performance, personal identity), and since the nature of the change causing the alteration can be so varied, there is no "typical" response to this diagnosis. Reactions may include

Refusal to touch or look at a body part
Refusal to look into a mirror
Unwillingness to discuss a limitation, deformity, or disfigurement
Refusal to accept rehabilitation efforts
Inappropriate attempts to direct own treatment
Denial of the existence of a deformity or disfigurement
Increasing dependence on others
Signs of grieving: weeping, despair, anger
Refusal to participate in own care or take responsibility for self-care (self-neglect)
Self-destructive behavior (alcohol, drug abuse)
Displaying hostility toward the healthy
Withdrawal from social contacts
Changing usual patterns of responsibility
Showing change in ability to estimate relationship of body to environment

## Focus Assessment Criteria

Disturbance in self-concept is manifested in a variety of ways. An individual may respond with an alteration in another life process (see *Spiritual Distress, Fear, Ineffective Individual Coping*). The nurse should be aware of this and utilize the assessment data to ascertain the dimensions affected.

It may be difficult for the nurse to identify the cues and make the inferences necessary to diagnose an alteration in self-concept. Each individual reacts differently to loss, pain, disability, and disfigurement. Therefore, the nurse should determine an individual's usual reactions to problems and feelings about himself before attempting to diagnose a change.

### Subjective data

1. Previous health problems and attitude toward them
    "Tell me about your health in the past; have you ever been sick before?"
    "How did you feel about being sick?"
    "Do you usually view illness as something that happens to everyone or something that happens only to the weak?"
    "In the past, have you had any experiences with hospitals? What were these experiences like?"
    "How do you feel about being in the hospital now?" (if hospitalized)
2. How the client viewed himself in the past and how he views himself now
    "How would you describe yourself?"
    "Has being ill made you feel differently about yourself? About your family?"
3. Pre-illness coping behavior
    "When you have a problem, how do you usually deal with it?"
    "To whom do you usually go for help when you have a problem?"
4. Role responsibilities
    "What do you do for a living? What does the job entail?"
    "Do you think you will be able to return to your job in the future?"
    "What are your major responsibilities at home?"
    "Do you think you will be able to reassume these responsibilities in the future?"
    "Do you anticipate a change in your sexual functioning as a result of this illness?"

5. The significance of an altered body structure or function

"Before you were sick, how did you feel about people who were sick or disabled?"

"How would you feel if your illness resulted in some permanent disability?" (meaning of loss; see Principles for Nursing Care)

6. Current knowledge of the severity of illness

"What events led up to your hospitalization?"

"What do you understand to be your health problem?"

"How serious do you think your illness is?"

"What limitations do you think will result from this illness?"

"How do you feel about this limitation (disability)?" (if expressed)

7. Reaction of significant others to present illness

"Have you discussed your illness with your family?"

"Does your family regularly discuss problems that confront family members?"

"How does your family feel about your illness?"

"Do you think your family really understands what your illness is all about?"

8. What help is available to the individual and his family

"Have you ever used community resources before?" (questions would be based on the nature of the health problems and assistance required)

## Objective data

Assess for the presence of

1. Decision-making ability
   a. Adaptive responses*
      Asks appropriate questions
      Participates in self-care
      Seeks help when necessary
      Is able to make decisions regarding changing jobs and financial arrangements
   b. Maladaptive responses†
      Is unable to make simple decision about self-care
      Refuses to return to work or make decisions regarding work or financial arrangements
2. Response to limitations or deformity
   a. Adaptive responses
      Shows signs of grief and mourning—weeping, despair, anger (helps in acknowledging loss)
      Demonstrates some early denial
      Is preoccupied with limitation or disability
   b. Maladaptive responses
      Denies existence of deformity or disfigurement
      Refuses to touch or look at body part
      Refuses to look in mirror
      Refuses to discuss limitation, deformity, or disfigurement
      Engages in self-destructive behavior
      Refuses to use prosthetic device
      Talks about feelings of worthlessness or insecurity
      Shows a change in ability to estimate relationship of body to environment

---

*An *adaptive response* demonstrates a working through and gradual acceptance of a change or loss.

†A *maladaptive response* shows an inability to accept the change.

3. Independence–dependence patterns
   a. Adaptive responses
      Participates in own care and takes responsibility for self-care
      Uses prosthetic device prescribed
      Allows mutual support between self and family
      Utilizes available resources
   b. Maladaptive responses
      Refuses to participate in self-care (self-neglect)
      Becomes increasingly dependent on others
      Changes usual pattern of responsibility
      Intellectualizes situation; exaggerates independence
4. Socialization and communication
   a. Adaptive responses
      Willingly discusses problems
      Accepts offers of help
      Continues pre-existing socialization patterns
   b. Maladaptive responses
      Withdraws from social contacts (aloofness)
      Exhibits superficial self-confidence or inappropriate laughter
      Is hostile toward the healthy (projection of hostile feelings)
      Does not resume sexual functioning

## Principles and Rationale for Nursing Care

### General

1. Both the client and the nurse have their own personal self-concept. To deal effectively with others, the nurse must be aware of her own behavior, feelings, attitudes, and responses.
2. Self-concept involves a person's feelings, attitudes, and values and affects his reactions to all experiences.
3. Self-concept is learned. A child's concept of self, for example, emerges as a result of changes occurring during earlier developmental stages.
4. The concept of self includes components of body image, self-esteem, role performance, and personal identity.
5. Body image is the mental idea a person has of his body. It is based on past as well as present experience. It is composed of the interrelated phenomena of body surface and depth and the attitudes, emotions, and personality reactions of the individual to his body. It is flexible and subject to change.
6. Self-esteem is a person's personal, subjective judgment of his worthiness. It results from self-evaluation in areas of competence and social acceptance.
7. Alterations in the components of self-concept are described as follows:
   *Body image*: Viewing oneself differently as a result of actual or perceived changes in body structure or function
   *Self-esteem*: Lack of confidence in ability to accomplish that which is desired
   *Role performance*: Inability to perform those functions and activities expected of a particular role in a given society
   *Personal identity*: Disturbance in perception of self ("Who am I?")
8. A nurse's attitude can hinder or facilitate the individual's adaptation to an alteration in self-concept.
9. Intrusive procedures can threaten an individual's sense of wholeness. The nurse should provide a great deal of emotional support during procedures that increase a person's sense of vulnerability.

10. Body image changes constantly. There is often a time lag between the actual body change and the change in body image. The nurse must be aware that during this lag the individual may reject both the diagnosis and the education and treatment prescribed.
11. Body image is influenced during pregnancy in relation to biologic, psychological, and role changes.

## Children

1. The child's development of body image is based on his own body, which is influenced by present and past perceptions of his body, his physiological functioning, his developmental maturation, and the response of others to him.
2. The child strives to master conflicts, and his success or lack of success will influence his pattern for coping throughout his life.
3. The child has periods of decreased self-esteem during the primary grades and again during adolescence.
4. The process of acquiring autonomy, independence, and individuality requires that the child have periods of separation from family even though they may cause anxiety.
5. In order to develop and maintain self-esteem, children need to feel worthwhile, different in some way, and superior and more lovable than any other child.
6. Disturbances in body image are encountered in prepubescent and pubescent children who are either early or late maturing, since children at this age are most comfortable when they are just like their peers.
7. The development of a positive body image by age is charted below.

| Age | Developmental Task |
|---|---|
| Birth to 1 year | Learns to tolerate small frustrations<br>Learns to trust |
| 1 to 3 years | Learns to like body<br>Learns mastery of<br>   Motor skills<br>   Language skills<br>   Bowel training |
| 3 to 6 years | Learns initiative<br>Learns sex typing<br>Identifies with parent models<br>Increases skills (motor language) |
| 6 to 12 years | Develops a sense of industry<br>Has a clear sex role identification<br>Learns peer interaction<br>Develops academic skills |

8. A child learns to see himself the way he is seen by his parents or significant others.
9. The child's personality evolves as the child responds to his changing body and to the environment.

## Loss of body part

1. The loss of a body part or function is followed by a period of grief and mourning. The grief is similar to that following the loss of any valued object.

2. The process of mourning for the loss of a body part or function may include feelings of helplessness, loneliness, sadness, guilt, and anger. The stages of adaptation to loss include shock and disbelief, anger, depression, and eventual acceptance (see *Grieving*).
3. Reorganization of an altered body image is a process: of recognition, acceptance, and resolution.

## Nursing Goals

Through selected interventions the nurse will seek to
- Assist the individual with reconstruction of altered body image
- Enable the individual to achieve or maintain control of body
- Promote self-confidence
- Assist the individual in assuming role-related responsibilities

---

### Outcome Criteria

The person will
- Demonstrate movement toward reconstruction of an altered body image
- Achieve or maintain control of his body
- Begin to assume role-related responsibilities
- Develop confidence in his ability to accomplish what is desired

---

## Interventions

Nursing interventions for the variety of problems that might be associated with a diagnosis of *Disturbance in Self-Concept* are very similar.

### A. Establish a trusting nurse/client relationship

- Encourage person to express his feelings, especially about the way he feels, thinks, or views himself
- Encourage person to ask questions: about his health problem, his treatment, his progress, his prognosis
- Provide reliable information and reinforce information already given
- Clarify any misconceptions the person has about himself, his care, or his caregivers
- Avoid negative criticism
- Provide privacy and a safe environment

### B. Promote social interaction

- Assist person to accept help from others
- Avoid overprotection while still limiting the demands made on the individual
- Encourage movement
- Support family as they adapt

### C. Provide specific interventions in selected situations

1. Pregnancy
    - Encourage the woman to share her concerns
    - Attend to each concern if possible or refer her to others for assistance
    - Discuss the challenges and changes that pregnancy and motherhood bring

- Encourage her to share expectations: her own and those of her significant others
- Assist her to identify sources for love and affection
- Provide anticipatory guidance to both parents-to-be regarding
  a. Fatigue and irritability
  b. Appetite swings
  c. Gastric disturbances (nausea, constipation)
  d. Back and leg aches
  e. Mood swings
  f. Changes in sexual desire
  g. Fear (for self, for unborn baby, of loss of attractiveness, of inadequacy as a mother)
- Encourage the mutual sharing of concerns between spouses

2. Hospitalized child
  a. Prepare child for hospitalization, if possible, with an explanation and a visit to the hospital to meet personnel and examine the environment
  b. Provide child with opportunities to share fears, concerns, anger (see Appendix III for play therapy guidelines)
     - Acknowledge the normalcy of these fears, concerns, anger
     - Correct child's misconceptions (*e.g.*, that he's being punished; that his parents are angry)
     - Encourage family to stay with or visit child, despite the child's crying when they leave; teach them to provide accurate information as to when they will return to reduce fears of abandonment
     - Allow parents to help with care
  c. Assist child to understand his experiences
     - Provide child with an explanation ahead of time, if possible
     - Explain sensations and discomforts of condition, treatments, and medications
     - Encourage crying
  d. Maintain sense of intactness during periods of immobility
     - Encourage movement, no matter how slight
     - During bath, ask child to identify body parts: "Where is your leg?"
     - Allow child access to mirror to provide visualization of body

3. Loss of body part or function
  - Assess the meaning of the loss for the individual and significant others, as related to visibility of loss, function of loss, and emotional investment
  - Expect the individual to respond to the loss with denial, shock, anger, and depression
  - Be aware of the effect of the responses of others to the loss; encourage sharing of feelings between significant others
  - Allow individual to ventilate his feelings and grieve
  - Utilize role-playing to assist with sharing; if person says, "I know my husband will not want to touch me with this colostomy," take the husband's role and discuss her colostomy, then switch roles so she can act out her feelings about her husband's response
  - Explore realistic alternatives and provide encouragement
  - Explore strengths and resources with person
  - Assist with the resolution of a surgically created alteration of body image
    a. Replace the lost body part with prosthesis as soon as possible

    b. Encourage viewing of site

    c. Encourage touching of site

- Begin to incorporate person in care of operative site
- Gradually allow person to assume full self-care responsibility, if feasible
- Refer to *Sexual Dysfunction* for additional information if indicated

## D. Initiate health teaching as indicated

- Teach person what community resources are available, if needed (*e.g.*, mental health centers, such self-help groups as Reach for Recovery, Make Today Count)

## Bibliography

Bille D: The role of body image in patient compliance and education. Heart Lung 6(1):143–147, 1977

Brundage DJ: Altered body image. In Phipps WJ, Long B, Woods N: Medical-Surgical Nursing: Concepts and Clinical Practice. St. Louis, CV Mosby, 1979

Donovan M, Pierce S: Cancer Care Nursing. New York, Appleton-Century-Crofts, 1976

Gruendemann BJ: The impact of surgery on body image. Nurs Clin North Am 10(4):635–643, 1975

McCloskey JC: How to make the most of body image theory in nursing practice. Nursing 6(6):68–72, 1976

McGrory A: A Well Model Approach to Care of the Dying Client. New York, McGraw-Hill, 1978

Murray R: The concept of body image. Nurs Clin North Am 7(4):593–707, 1972

Roberts S: Behavioral Concepts and Nursing Throughout the Life Span. Englewood Cliffs, NJ, Prentice-Hall, 1978

Rubin R: Body image and self-esteem. Nursing Outlook 16(6):20–23, 1968

# Sensory-Perceptual Alterations

*Related to* **Factors Associated with Aging**

*Related to* **Sensory Overload**

## Definition

Sensory-perceptual alterations: A state in which the individual experiences or is at risk of experiencing a change in the amount, pattern, or interpretation of incoming stimuli.*

## Etiological and Contributing Factors

Many factors in an individual's life can contribute to sensory-perceptual alterations. Some common factors are listed below.

### Pathophysiological

Sensory organ alterations (visual, gustatory, hearing, olfactory, and tactile deficits)

Neurological alterations

| | |
|---|---|
| Cerebrovascular accident (CVA) | Neuropathies |
| Encephalitis meningitis | |

Metabolic alterations

| | |
|---|---|
| Fluid and electrolyte imbalance | Acidosis |
| Elevated blood urea nitrogen (BUN) | Alkalosis |

Impaired oxygen transport

| | |
|---|---|
| Cerebral | Respiratory |
| Cardiac | Anemia |

Musculoskeletal changes

| | |
|---|---|
| Paraplegia | Amputation |
| Quadriplegia | |

### Situational

Medications (sedatives, tranquilizers)

Surgery (glaucoma, cataract, detached retina)

Social isolation (terminal or infectious patient)

Physical isolation (reverse isolation, communicable disease, prison)

Radiation therapy

Immobility

Pain

Stress

Environment (noise pollution)

Mobility restrictions (bedrest, traction, casts, Stryker frame, Circoelectric bed)

---

*This diagnostic category differs from the diagnostic category *Alterations in Thought Processes*, which also describes an individual with cognitive alterations, but those alterations are the result of personality and mental disorders, while these are physiological, sensory, motor, or environmental disruptions. This individual is experiencing a change in usual response to stimuli.

Biorhythm alterations (travel, shift-work, hospitalization, special care units—cardiac, trauma, burn)

Substance abuse (alcohol, drugs)

Different culture or language

## Maturational

Infant/child: Maternal deprivation, excessive stimulation

Elderly: Hearing or vision loss, gustatory/olfactory deficits, decreased potential for tactile stimulation, isolation, custodial care

## Defining Characteristics

Disoriented in time or place

Disoriented about people

Altered ability to problem-solve

Altered behavior or communication pattern

Sleep pattern disturbances

Restlessness

Reports auditory or visual hallucinations

Fear

Anxiety

Apathy

## Focus Assessment Criteria

### Subjective data

1. History of symptoms

   The person reports

| | |
|---|---|
| Difficulty concentrating | Fatigue or irritability |
| Anxiety | Unusual sensations |

   Onset and description

| | |
|---|---|
| Precipitated by? | Frequency? |
| Relieved by? | |

2. Assess for presence or history of

| | |
|---|---|
| Recent surgery | Change in biorhythm patterns |
| Recent hospitalization | Mobility restrictions |
| Neurological impairment | Social isolation |
| Sensory organ deficit | Substance abuse (drugs, alcohol) |

### Objective data

1. Assess sensory acuity

   Visual

   Snellen chart

   Newspaper clippings and large lettered index cards

   Aids (contact lenses, glasses)

   Auditory

   Observation of client during normal conversation

   Use of hearing aids

   Tactile

   Thermal sensation

   Sensitivity

   Olfactory/gustatory

2. Assess for the presence of factors that contribute to sensory-perceptual alterations

    Sensory deprivation (isolation, lack of visitors)
    Sensory overload (noise, personnel)
    Physiological alterations
    Medication (side-effects, toxic levels)
    Sleep deprivation
    Fluid, electrolyte, nutritional imbalances
    Crisis, fears, losses

## Nursing Goals

Through selected interventions, the nurse will seek to

- Identify factors that contribute to sensory-perceptual alterations
- Provide sufficient and meaningful sensory input
- Reduce the severity and the incidence of disorientation

## Principles and Rationale for Nursing Care

1. Receiving (reception) and accurately interpreting (perception) incoming stimuli from the environment are essential for survival.
2. People receive information via their five senses. Deficits in one or more senses can alter perception.
3. The five senses can be organized into close (olfactory, gustatory, and tactile) and distant (auditory and visual). When an individual is deprived of a distant sense, he becomes more dependent on the close senses. A blind person will develop a keener sense of touch than a sighted person.
4. Individuals adapt to the stimuli from their internal and external environments. The capacity for this adaptation varies with individuals and also varies at times in the same individual.
5. A disruption in the quality or quantity of incoming stimuli can affect an individual's physiological, emotional, cognitive, and affective domains.
6. Manifestations of sensory deprivation vary with an individual's adaptation ability. Some common manifestations are generalized anxiety, perceptual distortions, inability to think and reason, distortion of time sense, vivid imagery, and illusions and hallucinations.
7. The quality and quantity of sensory input are reduced by immobility or confinement.
8. The elderly are more prone to develop sensory deprivation due to loneliness, physical isolation, and the increased incidence of chronic disabilities experienced during this life stage.
9. An illness state may decrease the efficiency of the sensory organs and thus alter an organism's capacity for adequate reception and perception of information.
10. Sensory overload produces the problem of sensory bombardment and also blocks out meaningful stimuli, thus concurrently producing sensory deprivation.
11. Refer to Principles and Rationale for Nursing Care for *Alterations in Thought Processes* for additional information.

# Sensory-Perceptual Alterations
## Related to Factors Associated with Aging

Factors associated with aging are social isolation, losses (motor, sensory, object, person), attitudes and responses of others, and physiological disorders that can be reduced or eliminated. These factors do not include chronic personality or mental disorders.

## Assessment

### Subjective data

The person expresses
   Fear
   Persecution
   Seeing objects or persons that others cannot see
   Hearing voices that others cannot hear

### Objective data

Change in the person's usual response to stimuli
   Talks to persons not present
   Restless
   Combative
   Withdrawn
   Lack of animation
   Unsmiling
   Rambling
   Shouting

---

**Outcome Criteria**

The person will
   · Demonstrate optimal contact with reality
   · Demonstrate an increase in self-care activities

---

## Interventions

A. Assess for etiological and contributing factors
   1. Physiological factors
         Decreased function (respiratory, renal, endocrine, cerebral, circulatory, sensory — vision, hearing)
         Sleep and rest imbalance
         Fluid and electrolyte imbalance (potassium, sodium; dehydration)
         Nutritional imbalance
         Medication (overdose, side-effects)
   2. Situational factors
         Sensory overload (hospitalization)
         Sensory deprivation (hospitalization, isolation)

Fear of unknown, fear of loss

Actual loss of control, income, significant others, familiar objects and surroundings

Significant others/caregiver factors

Attitude toward aging

Beliefs about confusion

Communication patterns (tone, speed, volume, content)

B. Assess history of the confusion (onset and duration)

Acute or chronic

Sudden or gradual

Continuous or intermittent

Time of day

C. Determine the amount and type of stimuli needed by the individual in the context of his usual life-style

Usual day routine

Work history

Available support systems

Coping patterns

Strengths and limitations

D. Reduce and eliminate reversible physiological factors

1. Monitor physiological functions (electrolytes, circulation, urine output)
2. Maintain optimal physiological functioning
   - Encourage person to remain out of bed as much as possible
   - Teach person to perform isometric and isotonic exercises when in bed
   - Encourage person to change position frequently even if it is just lifting one side off a surface by rolling slightly (see *Activity Intolerance* for specific interventions)
   - To encourage walking, choose a destination or give the walk a purpose (*e.g.*, walk to the lounge for breakfast)
   - Encourage dietary and fluid intake necessary for metabolic requirements (refer to *Alterations in Nutrition* and *Fluid Volume Deficit*)
   - Promote optimal acuity of hearing and vision, *e.g.*, assess adequacy and function of aids (glasses, hearing aids)
   - Provide interventions to ensure adequate periods of sleep
   - Discourage the use of sedatives in older individuals (refer to *Sleep Pattern Disturbance*)
   - Assess person's response to medications
     a. Identify signs and symptoms of overdose
     b. Identify compromised physiological functions that may contribute to such side-effects as toxic levels of medications (*e.g.*, decreased renal function, which may cause certain drugs to accumulate to toxic levels)
     c. Consult pharmacist for possible adverse interactions of two or more drugs
     d. Consult with physician to review present medication regimen and person's response

E. Promote communication that contributes to the person's sense of integrity

1. Examine attitudes about aging (in self, caregivers, significant others)
2. Maintain standards of empathetic, respectful care

- Be an advocate when other caregivers are insensitive to the individual's needs
- Function as a role model with co-workers
- Provide other caregivers with up-to-date information on aging and reality orientation
- Expect empathetic, respectful care and monitor its administration
3. Reduce unessential stimuli, if possible
  - Attempt to assign same caregivers to person
  - Avoid changing rooms
  - Explain procedures and activities prior to event; show equipment
  - Do not move person's belongings; keep them where he can see and use them
4. Attempt to obtain information that will provide useful and meaningful topics for conversations (likes, dislikes; interests, hobbies; work history)
5. Encourage significant others and caregivers to speak slowly and at an average volume (unless hearing deficits are present), as one adult to another, with eye contact, and as if expecting person to understand
6. Provide respect and promote sharing
  - Pay attention to what person is saying
  - Pick out meaningful comments and continue talking
  - Call person by name and introduce yourself each time a contact is made; utilize touch if welcomed
  - Use name the person prefers; avoid Pops or Mom, which can increase confusion and are unacceptable
  - Convey to person that you are concerned and friendly (through smiles, an unhurried pace, humor, and praise; don't argue)

## F. Provide sensory input that is sufficient and meaningful

1. Keep person oriented to time and place
  - Refer to time of day and place each morning
  - Provide person with a clock and calendar large enough to see
  - Provide person with opportunity to see daylight and dark through a window or take person outdoors
  - Single out holidays with cards or pins (*e.g.*, wear a red heart for Valentine's Day)
2. Encourage family to bring in familiar objects from home (photographs, afghan)
  - Ask person to tell you about the picture
  - Focus on familiar topics
3. Discuss current events, seasonal events (snow, water activities); share your interests (travel, crafts)
4. Assess if person can perform an activity with his hands (*e.g.*, latch rugs, wood crafts)
  - Provide reading materials, audio tapes, puzzles (manual, computer, crossword)
  - Encourage person to keep his own records if possible (*e.g.*, intake and output)
  - Provide tasks to perform (addressing envelopes, occupational therapy)
5. If hallucinations and delusions persist, refer to *Alterations in Thought Processes Related to Inability to Evaluate Reality*
6. In teaching a task or activity—for example, eating—break it into small, brief steps by giving only one instruction at a time
  - Remove covers from food plate and cups
  - Locate napkin and utensils

- Add sugar and milk to coffee
- Add condiments to food (sugar, salt, pepper)
- Cut foods
- Proceed with eating
7. Explain all activities
   - Offer simple explanations of tasks
   - Allow individuals to handle equipment related to each task
   - Allow individual to participate in task, such as washing his face
   - Acknowledge that you are leaving and say when you will return

## G. Increase person's self-esteem

- Allow former habits (*e.g.*, reading in the bathroom)
- Encourage the wearing of dentures
- Assist with removal of facial hair
- Ask family to provide spending money
- Ask person his usual grooming routine and encourage him to follow it
- Provide privacy at all times; when it is necessary to expose a body surface, take precautions to cover all other areas (*e.g.*, if washing a back, use towels or blankets to cover legs and front torso)
- Provide for personal hygiene according to person's preferences (hair grooming, showers or bath, nail care, cosmetics, deodorants and fragrances)

## H. Promote a well role

- Discourage the use of nightclothes during the day; have person wear shoes, not slippers
- Encourage self-care and grooming activities
- Have person eat meals out of bed, unless contraindicated
- Promote socialization during meals (*e.g.*, set up lunch for four individuals in lounge)
- Plan an activity each day to look forward to (*e.g.*, bingo, ice-cream-sundae gathering)

## I. Do not endorse confusion

- Never agree with confused statements
- Direct person back to reality; do not allow him to ramble
- Adhere to the schedule; if changes are necessary, advise person of them
- Avoid talking to co-workers about other topics in person's presence
- Provide simple explanations that cannot be misinterpreted
- Remember to acknowledge your entrance with a greeting and your exit with a closure ("I will be back in ten minutes")

## J. Utilize various modalities to provide stimulation for the individual

1. Music therapy
   - Provide soft, familiar music during meals
   - Arrange group song fests
   - Play music during other therapies (physical, occupational)
   - Have person exercise to music
   - Encourage construction of simple instruments and have individuals play them in a rhythm band
   - Organize guest entertainment
   - Use client-developed songbooks (large print and decorative covers)

2. Recreation therapy
   - Encourage arts and crafts (knitting and crocheting)
   - Suggest creative writing
   - Provide puzzles
   - Organize group games
3. Remotivation therapy
   - Use associations and analogies
     "If ice is cold, then fire is ———?"
     "If day is light, then night is ———?"
   - Organize group discussions of current events, interests, activities; involve family, if possible
4. Sensory training
   - Stimulate vision (with mirrors, brightly colored items of different shape, pictures, colored decorations, kaleidoscopes)
   - Stimulate smell (with flowers, coffee, cologne)
   - Stimulate hearing (ring a bell, play records)
   - Stimulate touch (sandpaper, velvet, steel wool pads, silk, stuffed animals)
   - Stimulate taste (spices, salt, sugar, sour substances)

## K. Prevent injury to the individual

1. Discourage the use of restraints; explore other alternatives
   - Put person in a room with others who can help watch him
   - Enlist aid of family or friends to watch person during confused periods
   - If person is pulling out tubes, use mitts instead of wrist restraints
2. Refer to *Potential for Injury* for strategies for assessing and manipulating the environment for hazards

# Sensory-Perceptual Alterations
Related to Sensory Overload

## Assessment

### Subjective data

The person reports
   Visual imagery
   Nightmares
   Difficulty concentrating
   Color perception changes
   Alteration in the size and contour of objects
   Hallucinations

### Objective data

(Occurs in an environment with excessive stimuli)
   Mood alterations
   Sleep pattern disturbances
   Poor appetite

Evidence of lack of self-care
Delusions

---

**Outcome Criteria**

The person will
- Experience decreased symptoms of sensory overload
- Identify and eliminate the potential risk factors if possible
- Describe the rationale for the treatment modality

---

## Interventions

A. Assess causative and contributing factors

Altered sleep and rest pattern (refer to *Sleep Pattern Disturbance*)
Pain (refer to *Alterations in Comfort*)
Excessive noise or light
Critical care unit activity
Health care facility routines
Unfamiliar environment (different culture or language)

B. Reduce or eliminate causative and contributing factors where possible

1. Excessive noise or light
   - Cover nonessential blinking lights at bedside with tape
   - Dim lights at night
   - Encourage use of blindfolds
   - Decrease noise input
     a. Shut off nonessential alarms
     b. Encourage use of earplugs
     c. If possible, limit the use of flasher, etc., during sleep hours
     d. Turn off unnecessary equipment
     e. Position person away from direct source of noise if possible
     f. Curtail nonessential personnel conversation
     g. Avoid loud noises
     h. Discourage TV after 10 p.m.
   - Share with person the source of the noise
   - Discuss the use of a radio with earplugs to provide soft relaxing music
   - Share with personnel the need to reduce noise and provide individuals with uninterrupted sleep for at least 2–4 hours' duration
2. Unfamiliar environment
   - Attempt to reduce fears and concerns by explaining equipment, its purpose and noises
   - Encourage person to share his perceptions of noises
   - Enlist the aid of an interpreter to explain the environment to person who does not speak English

C. Promote reorientation

1. Orient to all three spheres (person, place, time)
   - Address person by name
   - Introduce yourself frequently

- Identify the place
- Identify the time

   "Good morning Mr. Jones. I am Mary Smith. I will be your nurse today."

   "Where are you Mr. Jones? You are in the hospital."

   "Today is May sixth and it is eight thirty in the morning."

2. Explain all activities
   - Offer simple explanations of each task
   - Allow person to handle equipment related to the task
   - Allow him to participate in task, such as washing his face
   - Acknowledge when you leave and when you will return

### D. Promote movement

- Encourage person to remain out of bed as much as possible (eat meals in chair)
- Teach person to perform isometric and isotonic exercises when in bed
- Encourage person to change his position frequently, even if it is just lifting one side off a surface by rolling slightly
- To encourage walking, choose a destination to reach or give the walk a purpose. (walking to the lounge for breakfast)

### E. Utilize measures to prevent injury

- Keep side rails in place and bed in lowest position
- Place call bell in convenient location
- Refer to *Potential for Injury* for additional interventions

### F. Assist person to differentiate reality from fantasy

- Refer to *Alterations in Thought Processes Related to Inability to Evaluate Reality* for additional interventions

### Bibliography

Bolin, RH: Sensory deprivation: An overview. Nurs Forum 13(3):240–258, 1974

Burnside I: Nursing and the Aged. New York, McGraw-Hill, 1981

Chodil J, Williams B: The concept of sensory deprivation. Nurs Clin North Am 5(3):453–465, 1970

Dodd MJ: Assessing mental states. Am J Nurs 78:1501–1503, 1978

Downs F: Bed rest and sensory deprivation. Am J Nurs 74:434–438, 1974

Drummond LK, Scarbrough D: A practical guide to reality orientation: A treatment approach for confusion and disorientation. Gerontologist 18(12):568–573, 1978

Gimbel P: The pathology of boredom and sensory deprivation. Psychiatric Nursing 16(5):12–13, 1975

Kintzel KC: Advanced Concepts in Clinical Nursing, 2nd ed. Philadelphia, JB Lippincott, 1977

Murray R, Huelskoetter M, O'Driscoll D: The Nursing Process in Later Maturity. Englewood Cliffs, NJ, Prentice-Hall, 1980

Nowakowski L: Disorientation—signal or diagnosis? Journal of Gerontological Nursing 6(4):197–202, 1980

Schultz P: Sensory Restriction: Effects on Behavior. New York, Academic Press, 1965

Severtsen B: Sensory impairment: Its effects on the family. In Hymovich D, Barnard M (eds): Family Health Care, pp. 293–304. New York, McGraw-Hill, 1979

Shelby S: Sensory deprivation. Image 10(2):49–55, 1978

Solomon L: Sensory Deprivation. Cambridge, MA, Harvard University Press, 1961

Trockman G: Caring for the confused or delirious patient. Am J Nurs 78:1495–1499, 1978

Zubek S: Sensory Deprivation: Fifteen Years of Research. New York, Appleton-Century-Crofts, 1969

# Sexual Dysfunction

*Related to* **Impotence**

*Related to* **Ineffective Coping**

*Related to* **Lack of Knowledge**

*Related to* **Change or Loss of Body Part**

*Related to* **Physiological Limitations**

## Definition

Sexual dysfunction: The state in which an individual experiences or is at risk of experiencing a change in sexual health or sexual function that is viewed as unrewarding or inadequate.

## Etiological and Contributing Factors

An alteration in sexual patterns can occur as a response to a variety of health problems, situations, and conflicts. Some common sources are indicated below.

### Pathophysiological

Endocrine
  Diabetes mellitus
  Decreased hormone production
  Myxedema
Genitourinary
  Chronic renal failure
  Premature or retarded ejaculation
  Priapism
  Chronic vaginal infection
Neuromuscular and skeletal
  Arthritis
  Multiple sclerosis
  Amyotropic lateral sclerosis
Cardiorespiratory
  Myocardial infarction
  Congestive heart failure
Cancer
Liver disease

Hyperthyroidism
Addison's disease
Acromegaly

Decreased vaginal lubrication
Vaginismus
Altered structures
Venereal disease

Disturbances of nerve supply to brain, spinal cord, sensory nerves, and autonomic nerves

Peripheral vascular disorders
Chronic respiratory disorders

### Psychological

Fear of failure
Fear of pregnancy
Depression

Anxiety
Guilt
Vulnerability

## Situational

Partner
>>> Unwilling
>>> Uninformed
>>> Abusive

Not available
Separated
Divorced

Environment
>>> Unfamiliar
>>> No privacy

Hospital

Stressors
>>> Job problems
>>> Financial worries

Conflicting values
Religious conflict

Lack of knowledge
Fatigue
Obesity
Pain
Alcohol ingestion
Medications
Radiation treatment
Altered self-concept from change in appearance (trauma, radical surgery)

## Maturational

Ineffective role models
Negative sexual teaching
Absence of sexual teaching
Aging (separation, isolation)

## Defining Characteristics

Verbalization of problem
Dissatisfaction with sex role (perceived or actual)
Reports limitations on sexual performance imposed by disease or therapy
Fears future limitations on sexual performance
Misinformed about sexuality
Lacks knowledge about sexuality and sexual function
Value conflicts involving sexual expression (cultural, religious)
Reports sexual dissatisfaction or decreased libido
Altered relationship with significant other

## Focus Assessment Criteria

### Guidelines in taking a sexual history

Take sexual history in a private, relaxed setting to ensure confidentiality
Do not judge the individual by your own norms
Permit the individual to refuse to answer
Clarify vocabulary
Strive to be open, warm, objective, unembarrassed, and reassuring
Assume the individual has had some form of sexual experience
Several interviews may be necessary to complete the history

### Subjective data

1. General
>> Age, sex, marital status
>> Quality of relationship with significant other
>> Number of children and siblings

Religious and cultural background

Job and financial status

Medical and surgical history

Drug therapy (present and past—type, dosage, frequency)

2. Sexual knowledge and attitudes

Source of sexual information

Knowledge of anatomy and physiology

Childhood sexual experiences (parental influence, religious influence, masturbation)

Attitudes concerning sexual variations

Myths and taboos

Menstruation

Birth control methods

3. Sexual function

Usual pattern

Present pattern

Satisfaction (individual, partner)

Erection problems for male (attaining, sustaining)

Ejaculation problems for male (premature)

4. Sexual problem

Description

Onset (when, gradual, sudden)

Pattern over time ($\uparrow$, $\downarrow$, unchanged)

Person's concept of cause

Knowledge of problem by others (physician, support system)

Past diagnostic studies and treatments

Expectations

5. School-age child*

Knowledge

"What is the difference between boys and girls?"

"What do you know about having babies?"

"Who taught you? At what age?"

Body changes

"Is your body changing in any way? How? Why?"

"How do you feel about these changes?"

Masturbation

"Almost everyone touches their body; how do you feel about this?"

6. Adolescent

Knowledge and attitudes

"What were your parent's attitudes toward sex, nudity, and touching?"

"Were these subjects discussed in your home?"

"How are babies made?"

"What are some methods of birth control?"

Body changes

"Is your body changing in any way? How? Why?"

"How do you feel about these changes?"

Sexual activity

"Some young people are sexually active; how do you feel about that?"

*Data that relate to children or adolescents may be more appropriately labeled *Disturbance in Self-Concept* or *Knowledge Deficit*

## Nursing Goals

Through selected interventions, the nurse will seek to
- Assess the sexual health of the individual
- Identify factors that compromise sexual health
- Assist the individual to reach optimal sexual health

## Principles and Rationale for Nursing Care

### General

1. All humans are sexual beings. Sexuality is an integral part of one's identity.
2. Sexuality encompasses how one feels about oneself and how one interacts with others. Sexual function is the choice an individual makes in the manner or form of how one will express sexuality. Sexuality and sexual function are influenced by age, marital status, value system, knowledge, sexual patterns, resources (social, economic, geographic), culture, physical health, and emotional health.
3. Sexual health care is often given low priority by nurses. In promoting sexual health the nurse generalist can:
   Assess individuals for sexual problems
   Provide accurate information
   Make referrals for individuals with complex sexual problems
4. The nurse must educate herself regarding sexuality and sexual health through the life span. She must examine her own beliefs and feelings regarding sexuality and sexual function and what is considered to be sexually normal and abnormal.
5. Sexuality and sexual function are not restricted solely to the young and healthy.
6. Sexual gratification is an individual matter. It encompasses self-pleasure and giving pleasure to others.
7. Sexual expression is not limited to intercourse. It includes closeness, touching, and one's approach to others.
8. Satisfaction and gratification can be experienced from responses to interactions other than sexual organ interaction.
9. Sexual preferences are an individual matter. Homosexuality is not a diagnosis unless the person sees it as a problem. In such a situation another nursing diagnosis might be more appropriate: for example, *Disturbance in Self-Concept.*
10. Sexual expression is essential for complete well-being and should be nurtured in all age groups.
11. Masturbation may be a necessary outlet for sexual release.
12. Individuals must have the opportunity to make their own decisions regarding sexual function.
13. Individuals decide what is normal for them. Mutually satisfying acts between consenting adults is considered normal.
14. As stress increases, there is a negative influence on sexual performances that conversely increases stress.
15. Sexual options available to the cord-injured person are influenced (Woods) by sexual value system, previous sexual function, upper-extremity muscle strength, presence of hip flexors and extensors, presence of appliances (casts, catheters), and availability of a caring partner.
16. Cord injuries do not usually affect fertility. Paraplegic females can become pregnant and deliver vaginally.

### Aging and sexuality

1. Aging influences sexual anatomy and physiology, but the elderly person is physically able to engage in sexual activity.

Table II–10. **Effects on Intercourse of Normal Aging Changes**

| Hormonal Change | Phase of Intercourse | | | |
| --- | --- | --- | --- | --- |
| | Excitement | Plateau | Orgasm | Resolution |
| Female ↓ Estrogen | ↑ Lubrication time | Little change | ↓↑ Uterine contractions | Quick return to preintercourse state |
| Male ↓ Testosterone | ↓ Sex flush, erection delay | Longer, ↑ penile circumference | Shorter duration | Refractory period from 10–24 hr, loss of erection in seconds/minutes |

2. The normal aging changes in the reproductive system are indicated in Table II–10.
3. Decreased levels of hormones influence tissue elasticity. Females have decreased tone in breasts, thinning and loss of elasticity of the vaginal wall, and shortening of its length. Males experience decreased production of spermatozoa, decreased ejaculation force, and smaller, less firm testicles.
4. The need for intimacy and love may be more critical for the elderly who are experiencing diminishing meaningful relationships.
5. Past sexual function (enjoyment, interest, frequency) are predicators of sexual activity for the aging.

## Drugs and sexuality

1. Drugs can influence sexual function positively and negatively. Table II–11 illustrates their effects.

Table II–11. **Drugs That Alter Sexual Behavior**

| Drug | Probable Effects |
| --- | --- |
| **Antihypertensives** | Produce vasodilation and decreased cardiac output; depress CNS |
| Guanethidine (Esimil) | |
| Reserpine (Serpasil) | Cause impotence in men and decreased vaginal lubrication in women |
| Mecamylamine (Inversine) | |
| Trimethaphan (Arfonad) | |
| Spironolactone (Aldactone) | |
| Methyldopa (Aldomet) | |
| Phenoxybenzamine (Dibenzyline) | |
| Clonidine (Catapres) | |
| Propranolol (Inderal) | |
| Pargyline (Eutonyl) | |
| **Antidepressants** | Peripheral blockage of nervous innervation of sex glands |
| Imipramine (Tofranil) | |
| Desipramine (Norpramin, Pertofrane) | May have positive effect, since they decrease depression |
| Amitryptyline (Elavil) | |

*(continued)*

Table II–11. **Drugs That Alter Sexual Behavior** (*continued*)

| Drug | Probable Effects |
| --- | --- |
| **Antidepressants** (*continued*) | |
| Nortriptyline (Aventyl) | |
| Protriptyline (Vivactil) | |
| Phenelzine sulfate (Nardil) | |
| Tranylcypromine sulfate (Parnate) | |
| **Antihistamines** | Block parasympathetic nervous innervation of sex glands |
| Diphenhydramine (Benadryl) | |
| Promethazine (Phenergan) | |
| Chlorpheniramine (Chlor-Trimeton) | |
| **Antispasmodics/Anticholinergics** | Inhibit parasympathetic innervation of sex glands |
| Methantheline (Banthine) | |
| Glycoyrrolate (Robinul) | |
| Hexocyclium (Tral) | |
| Poldine (Nacton) | |
| Diphenoxylate hydrochloride with atropine (Lomotil) | |
| **Sedatives and Tranquilizers** | Block autonomic innervation of sex glands |
| Chlorpromazine (Thorazine) | May have positive effect because they produce tranquilization and relaxation |
| Prochlorperazine (Compazine) | |
| Thioridazine (Mellaril) | May have negative effect influencing libido |
| Mesoridazine (Serentil) | |
| Chlordiazepoxide (Librium) | |
| Diazepam (Valium) | |
| Phenoxybenzamine (Dibenzyline) | |
| Chlorprothixene (Taractan) | |
| Haloperidol (Haldol) | |
| **Oral Contraceptives** | Remove fear of pregnancy |
| **Alcohol** | In small amounts, may increase libido |
| | In large amounts, impairs neural reflexes involved in erection and ejaculation |
| | Chronic use may cause impotence |
| **Narcotics** | Central sedation causes impotence in chronic users |
| **Cancer chemotherapy agents** | Possible temporary sterility or neurotoxicity in males, causing impotence |
| **Estrogen** | Suppresses sexual function in males |
| **Diuretics** | Chronic use may cause impotence |
| Ethacrynic acid (Edecrin) | |
| Furosemide (Lasix) | |

# Sexual Dysfunction
## Related to Impotence

Impotence is the inability to achieve or sustain an erection for satisfying intercourse.

### Assessment

Subjective data

The person states he is unable to have or sustain an erection

Objective data

Monitoring of nocturnal penile tumescence to determine if erection occurs during REM sleep

---

**Outcome Criteria**

The person will
  · Relate satisfying sexual relationships

---

### Interventions

A. Assess causative or contributing factors

Degenerative physiological factors
  Neurological (diabetes mellitus, multiple sclerosis)
  Circulatory (severe anemia, arteriosclerosis)
Trauma (surgical injury)
  Spinal cord injury or lesion
  Prostatectomy
  Arteriofemoral bypass
  Sympathectomy
  Abdominal-perineal resection
Chemical influences
  Alcohol
  Drugs (see Table II–11)
Psychogenic influences
  Almost any stressor

B. Discuss with individual and significant other the varied etiologies of temporary impotence
  · Convey the normalcy of the situation
  · Relate the interrelationship of stress and the ability to perform sexually
  · Review with individual any changes that may have occurred in his life (*e.g.,* financial, career, significant other, health)
  · Assist with constructive problem-solving (see Appendix *VI*)
  · Identify stress reduction techniques that can be incorporated into his life (see Appendix *IV*)
  · Assist individual or couple to examine their relationships
    What are the benefits of the relationship?

How can each person improve the relationship?
How does the couple handle conflicts?
- Refer individuals or couples to professional counseling when indicated
- See *Sexual Dysfunction Related to Ineffective Coping* for additional interventions

## C. Facilitate or enhance sexual expression in individuals with irreversible impotence

- Explain the cause of the impotence, if known
- Discuss alternate means for sexual satisfaction for self and partner (vibrator, touching, oral-genital techniques, body massage); consider past sexual experiences prior to giving specific techniques
- Refer to pertinent literature in bibliography for specific information
- Explain penile implants, function, limitations, surgical procedure, and cost
- Refer to a urologist for further details

## D. Initiate health teaching and referrals when appropriate (sex therapy, psychotherapy)

# Sexual Dysfunction
## Related to Ineffective Coping

Ineffective coping (associated with sexual dysfunction) is the difficulty or inability to adapt to stressors or changes in life-style that negatively influence sexual function.

## Assessment

### Subjective data

The person reports
  Multiple stressors that are accompanied by altered sexual function
    Job-related stress                Death of partner or significant
    Financial worries                   other
    Relocation                        Job change
    Divorce                           Disability of spouse
    Separation from partner
  Feelings
    Depression                        Frustration
    Anxiety                           Impaired or absent libido
    Severe fatigue

---

**Outcome Criteria**

The person will
- Identify stressors in life
- Identify constructive coping patterns
- Resume previous sexual activity

---

## Interventions

A. Assess for causative factors

Job change or problems
Financial worries
Relocation
Divorce or separation from partner
Death of significant other
Severe fatigue
Depression
Disability of spouse

B. Assist person in modifying life-style to reduce stress

· Encourage identification of present stressors in life; group as those he can control and those he cannot

| Can Control | Can't Control |
|---|---|
| Personal lateness | Report due |
| Involvement in community activities | Daughter's illness |

· Assist in analyzing the problem
What is it?
Who or what is responsible?
What are the options?
What are the advantages and disadvantages of each option?

C. Identify alternative methods for dispersing sexual energy when partner is unavailable or unwilling

· Utilize masturbation, if acceptable to individual
· Teach the physical and psychological benefits of regular physical activity (at least 3 times a week for 30 minutes)—yoga, walking or running, exercise (aerobics, dance) (see *Alterations in Health Maintenance*, for an exercise program)
· If partner is deceased, explore opportunities to meet and socialize with others (night school, singles club, community work)
· See Appendix *VI* for problem-solving techniques

D. Initiate health teaching and referrals as indicated

Marriage counselor
Psychiatrist or psychologist
Sex therapist
Social service (for assistance with job, financial, housing, or family problems)

# Sexual Dysfunction
Related to Lack of Knowledge

## Assessment

The person expresses
Anxiety about normal physical development (small breasts; small penis)
Misinformation
"I will get pregnant if I kiss him"
"Babies come from storks"
"I can't get pregnant if I douche after intercourse"

---

### Outcome Criteria

The person will
- Relate valid information regarding sexual structure and function
- Identify those myths or misinformation about sexual matters that he formerly believed

---

## Interventions

A. Assess the adolescent or adult's knowledge and attitudes concerning sexuality and sexual function
Source of sexual information
Knowledge of anatomy and physiology, menstruation
Childhood sexual experiences (religious influence, parental influence, masturbation)
Attitudes concerning sexual variations
Myths and taboos
Feelings about changes in body

B. Eliminate or reduce causative or contributing factors to lack of knowledge
1. Fear of embarrassment or recrimination
   - Allow individual to set limits
   - Provide privacy
   - Be nonjudgmental both verbally and nonverbally
   - Validate normalcy of person's feelings
2. Negative beliefs or attitudes about sexuality
   - Explore sociocultural, religious, and parental influences on person's beliefs
   - Discuss the bio-psychosocial dimensions of sexuality for adults
   - Correct all erroneous information
3. Provide knowledge concerning sexuality appropriate for person's maturational level, or educate parents regarding appropriate information to give child

C. Initiate health teaching if indicated
Refer person (adult, adolescent, parents) to appropriate literature on sexuality and sexual function (see Bibliography)

# Sexual Dysfunction
## Related to Change or Loss of Body Part

## Assessment

### Subjective data
The person reports
 An altered sexual function
 Feelings of undesirability
 Partner unwilling to look at affected part
 Partner's change in usual responses (social, sexual)

### Objective data
 Withdrawn behavior
 Depression
 Unwillingness to acknowledge loss
 Unwillingness to look at affected area

---

**Outcome Criteria**

The person will
- Demonstrate movement toward accepting the altered part
- Resume sexual activity

---

## Interventions

A. Assess causative or contributing factors

 Anatomic disruptions from surgery (mastectomy, hysterectomy, uterostomal surgery, prostatectomy, amputation)
 Pregnancy
 Obesity
 Trauma (burns, scarring)
 Chronic disease

B. Assess the stage of adaptation of the individual and his partner to the loss (denial, depression, anger, resolution; see *Grieving*)

C. Encourage individuals to share concerns
- Explain the normalcy of the foregoing responses to loss
- Explain the need to share concerns with partner
 The imagined response of partner
 The fear of rejection
 Fear of future losses
 Fear of physically hurting partner
- Maintain modesty and privacy
- Help individual realize that his body changes are acceptable by spending time with him

- Encourage the couple to discuss the strengths of their relationship and to assess the influence of the loss on their strengths

D. Encourage person to resume sexual activity as close to previous pattern as possible
  - Suggest that intercourse be resumed as soon as possible*
  - Advise modifying positions because of alteration
  - Teach the use of pillows to provide comfort (mastectomy, amputation)
  - Caution the person against covering the affected body part (delays confronting the actual or perceived fear)
  - Teach techniques to control drainage or odor prior to sexual activity (change colostomy bag or dressing; utilize a light scent such as aftershave or perfume)
  - Encourage the individual or couple to read about various sexual techniques and responses (see Bibliography)
  - Encourage individuals to experiment and enjoy each other

E. Initiate health teaching and referrals as indicated; discuss with individuals or couples the availability of self-help groups
  > Reach for Recovery (post-mastectomy)
  > Encore program (post-mastectomy)
  > United Ostomy Association

# Sexual Dysfunction
## Related to Physiological Limitations

### Assessment

Subjective data
The person reports the following as interfering with sexual function

| | |
|---|---|
| Chest pain | Fatigue |
| Shortness of breath | Decreased vaginal secretions |
| Joint pain | Paralysis |

Objective data
> Dyspnea
> Joint deformities
> Paralysis

*May require a physician's order.

**Outcome Criteria**

The person will
  * Identify practices that conserve energy and oxygen requirements during sexual activity
  * Describe the rationale for interventions
  * Engage in sexual activity that is satisfying

## Interventions

### A. Assess causative or contributing factors

Limited oxygen reserve
Decreased cardiac output
Pain
Inability to assume positions
Inability to experience sensations at genitourinary level

### B. Teach techniques to

1. Reduce oxygen consumption
   * Do not lie flat
   * Use oxygen during sexual activity if indicated
   * Engage in sexual activity after IPPB treatment or postural drainage
   * Plan sexual activities for timeof day person is most rested
   * Utilize positions for intercourse that are comfortable and permit unrestricted breathing (side to side; compromised individual on top)
2. Reduce cardiac workload
   * Cardiac patients should avoid sexual activity
       In extremes of temperature
       Directly after eating or drinking
       When intoxicated
       When tired
       With unfamiliar partner (when other stressors are present, *e.g.,* alcohol, fatigue)
       In unfamiliar environment
   * Rest before engaging in sexual activity (mornings are best)
   * Cardiac patients should terminate sexual activity if chest discomfort or dyspnea occurs
3. Reduce or eliminate pain
   * If vaginal lubrication is decreased, use a water-soluble lubricant
   * Refer person with vaginismus to gynecologist
   * Take medication for pain before beginning sexual activity
   * Use whatever relaxes individual before beginning sexual activity (hot packs, hot showers)
4. Teach techniques for intercourse for individuals with specific alterations
   a. Inability to abduct hip joints (woman)
       * Posterior vaginal entry
       * Woman supine with hips abducted and pillow under thigh and knee

- Woman supine with knees flexed
- Woman kneeling with posterior vaginal entry by partner
- Woman standing with posterior vaginal entry by partner

b. Spinal cord injury
- Consider that the sexual options available are dependent on the values and extent of injury
- Modify positions if necessary (quadriplegic, partner on top; paraplegic can assume most positions)
- If partner must initiate all pelvic thrusting then partner must assume the top position
- Water beds amplify pelvic movements
- Individuals with chronic urinary tract infections should be taught to wash well and empty the bladder completely before sexual activity to prevent infecting partner
- Individuals with Foley catheters can lubricate with a water-soluble jelly and tape catheter to their penis or leg. It is, however, better to remove the catheter if possible

c. Pregnant woman
- Discuss the effects of stress, fatigue, and the other changes that pregnancy and motherhood bring on libido and sexual function
- Allow her to verbalize her concerns and beliefs about pregnancy and coitus
- Advise that coital positions may need to be varied according to the woman's contour (side-lying during 8th and 9th months)
- Orgasms from intercourse or masturbation should be discouraged if spotting or bleeding occurs, fetal membranes rupture prematurely, or there is a repeated history of miscarriage
- Vaginal discomfort during coitus can be reduced with the use of a water-soluble lubricant
- Intercourse can usually be resumed after delivery when the woman is comfortable participating

5. Promote the stimulation of alternate senses and perceptions
- The use of erotic material may help prepare the individual for sexual response
- Encourage techniques to pleasure partner that provide satisfaction for individual (vibrators, touching, oral–genital intercourse, body massaging, anal stimulation)

## C. Provide health teaching and referrals when indicated

- Partner must be included in counseling and teaching to be aware of limitations
- Encourage individual to consult others with similar alterations for an exchange of information
- Refer individual and partner to pertinent literature and organizations (see Bibliography)

## Bibliography

Adams G: The sexual history as an integral part of the patient history. Matern Child Nurs J 1(3):170–175, 1976

Baxter R: Sex counseling and the spinal cord injured patient. Nursing 8(9):46–52, 1978

Calderone M, Johnson E: Family Book About Sexuality. New York, JB Lippincott, 1981

Carey P: Temporary sexual dysfunction in reversible health limitations. Nurs Clin North Am 10(3):575–585, 1975

Comfort A: Sexual Consequences of Disability. Philadelphia, GF Stickley, 1978

Comfort J, Comfort A: The Facts of Love, Living, Loving and Growing Up. New York, Crown Publishers, 1979

Davies H: Sexual dysfunction in diabetes: Psychogenic and physiologic factors. Medical Aspects of Human Sexuality 12:48–53, 1978

Evans R, Halar EM, DiFreece AB et al: Multidisciplinary approach to sex education of spinal cord injured patients. Phys Ther 56:541–545, 1976

Falk G, Falk UA: Sexuality and the aged. Nursing Outlook 10(1):51–55, 1980

Hickman B: All about sex—despite dialysis. Am J Nurs 77:606–609, 1977

Hogan R: Human Sexuality: A Nursing Perspective. New York, Appleton-Century-Crofts, 1980

Kennerly S: What I learned about mastectomy. Am J Nurs 77:1430–1432, 1977

Kolodney RC, Masters WH, Johnson VE et al: Textbook of Human Sexuality for Nurses. Boston, Little, Brown, 1979

Krozy R: Becoming comfortable with sexual assessment. Am J Nurs 78:1036–1038, 1978

Macrae I, Henderson M: Sexuality and irreversible health limitations. Nurs Clin North Am 10(3):587–597, 1975

Masters WH, Johnson VE: Human Sexual Inadequacy. Boston, Little, Brown, 1970

Masters WH, Johnson VE: The Pleasure Bond. Boston, Little, Brown, 1970

Mims FH, Sevenson M: A model to promote sexual health care. Nurs Outlook 26(2):121–125, 1978

Mooney T: Sexual Options for Paraplegics and Quadriplegics. Boston, Little, Brown, 1975

Peach E: Counseling sexually active very young adolescent girls. Matern Child Nurs J 5(3):191–195, 1980

Pettyjohn RD: Health care of the gay individual. Nurs Forum 17:367–371, 1979

Pogoncheff E: The gay patient—what not to do. RN 42:46–48, 1979

Siemens S, Brandzel R: Sexuality: Nursing Assessment and Intervention. Philadelphia, JB Lippincott, 1982

Schiller P: The nurse's role as sex counselor. Nursing Care 10:10–13, 1977

Watts RJ: Sexuality and the middle-aged cardiac patient. Nurs Clin North Am 11(2):349–359, 1976

Wood R, Rose R: Penile implants for potency. Am J Nurs 78:229–231, 1978

Woods NF: Human Sexuality in Health and Illness, 2nd ed. St. Louis, CV Mosby, 1979

## Pertinent Organizations and Literature for the Consumer

"Sex Can Help Arthritis" (pamphlet), available from the Arthritis Foundation (local chapters)

Sex and Spinal Cord Injured, Superintendent of Documents, U.S. Government Printing Office, Washington, DC 20402

Sex Information and Education Council of the United States, 80 Fifth Avenue, New York, NY 10011

Bibliographies for professionals and the general public (e.g., aging, disabilities, children). Planned Parenthood, Publications Section, 810 Seventh Avenue, New York, NY 10019

American Cancer Society, 77 Third Avenue, New York, NY 10017

American Fertility Society, 1608 14th Avenue South, Birmingham, AL 35205

National Clearinghouse for Family Planning Information, P.O. Box 2225, Rockville, MD 20852

United Ostomy Association, 1111 Wilshire Boulevard, Los Angeles, CA 90017

"Sex Education for Adolescents," American Library Association, Order Department, 50 East Huron Street, Chicago, IL 60611

Public Affairs Pamphlets, 381 Park Avenue South, New York, New York 10016 (many inexpensive pamphlets for parents; send for free catalog)

# Skin Integrity, Impairment of

*Related to* **Pruritus**

*Related to* **Immobility: Potential**

*Related to* **Pressure Ulcer**

*Related to* **Stoma Problems**

## Definition

Impairment of skin integrity, actual or potential: A state in which the individual's skin is altered or is at risk of becoming altered.

## Etiological and Contributing Factors

Pathophysiological

Autoimmune alterations
    Lupus erythematosus                Scleroderma
Metabolic and endocrine alterations
    Diabetes mellitus                  Renal failure
    Hepatitis                          Jaundice
    Cirrhosis                          Cancer
Nutritional alterations
    Obesity                            Edema
    Dehydration                        Emaciation
Impaired oxygen transport
    Peripheral vascular alterations    Anemia
    Arteriosclerosis                   Cardiopulmonary disorders
Medications (steroid therapy)
Psoriasis
Infections
  Bacterial (impetigo, folliculitis, cellulitis)
  Viral (herpes zoster [shingles], herpes simplex)
  Fungal (ringworm [dermatophytosis], athlete's foot, vaginitis)

Situational

Chemical
    Radiation                          Excretions
    Hyperthermia                       Secretions
Environmental
    Humidity                           Contact dermatitis
    Parasites                            (poison plants—ivy, sumac)
    Bites (insect, animal)
Immobility
  Imposed

Related to pain, fatigue, motivation, sedation
Stress
Pregnancy
Allergy (drug, food)
Surgery

## Maturational

Infants and children: Diaper rash, childhood diseases (chicken pox)
Elderly: Dryness, thin skin

## Defining Characteristics

Denuded skin
Erythema
Lesions (primary, secondary)
Pruritus
Disruptions of skin layer (incision, pressure sores, stomas, fistulas, burns)

## Nursing Goals

Through selected interventions, the nurse will seek to
  • Prevent damage to healthy skin
  • Prevent secondary infection
  • Reverse the inflammatory process and relieve symptoms

## Focus Assessment Criteria

### Subjective data

1. History of symptoms
    Onset
    Precipitated by what?            Frequency?
    Effects on life-style            Relieved by what?
        Occupation                    Role functions
        Financial                     Social/sexual
2. History of exposure (if allergy is suspected)
    Carrier of contagious disease
    Chemicals, paints, cleaning agents, plants
    Heat or cold
3. Medical/surgical history
4. Current drug therapy
    What drugs? How often? When was last dose taken?
    Effect on symptoms
5. Factors contributing to the development or extension of pressure ulcers (assess
   for)
    Skin deficits
        Dryness                       Thinness
        Edema                         Excessive perspiration
        Obesity
    Impaired oxygen transport
        Edema                         Arteriosclerosis
        Anemia                        Cardiopulmonary disorders
        Peripheral vascular disorders

Chemical/mechanical irritants
  Radiation     Casts, splints, braces
  Incontinence (feces, urine)     Spasms
Nutritional deficits
  Protein deficiencies     Mineral deficiencies
  Vitamin deficiencies     Dehydration
Systemic disorders
  Infection     Cancer
  Diabetes mellitus     Hepatic or renal disorders
Sensory deficits
  Neuropathy     Comatose
  Confusion     Cord injury
Immobility

## Objective data*

1. Skin characteristics

| Color | Texture | Turgor | Vascularity | Moisture | Temperature |
|-------|---------|--------|-------------|----------|-------------|
| Pigment | Coarse | Good | Bruising | Dry | Cool, <98.6° |
| Pallor | Thick | Poor | Bleeding | Moist | Warm, >98.6° |
| Cyanosis | Thin | | Angioma | Normal | Normal |
| Jaundice | | | Petechiae | | |
| Flushed | | | Purpura | | |
| | | | Telangiectasis | | |

2. Lesions (primary, secondary; see Table II-12)
       Type         Shape
       Location       Size
       Distribution   Drainage
       Color
3. Circulation
       Is erythema present?
       Does the skin blanch when pressure is applied?
       Does erythema subside within 30 minutes after pressure is removed?
4. Edema
       Note degree and location
       Palpate over bony prominences for sponginess (indicates edema)

## Principles and Rationale for Nursing Care

### Physiology

1. Skin consists of two layers: the outer (epidermis) and the deeper (dermis).
2. The epidermis (outer layer) functions as a barrier to protect inner tissues (from injury, chemicals, organisms); as a receptor for a range of sensations (touch, pain, heat, cold); as a regulator of body temperature through radiation (giving off heat), conduction (transfer of heat), and convection (movement of warm air

---

*Dark or black skin should be assessed in good light (daytime preferred). Palpation is usually more beneficial than observation. Borders of rashes can be felt and also the skin surface can indicate increased warmth (inflammation) and tautness (edema) when felt.

Table II–12. **Primary and Secondary Lesions**

| *Primary* | *Secondary* |
|---|---|
| **Macules** | **Scales** |
| Circumscribed, flat discolorations of the skin<br>*Examples*: Freckles, flat nevi | Abnormal epidermal cells that thicken and flake off<br>*Examples*: Dandruff, psoriasis |
| **Papules** | **Crusts** |
| Smaller-than-1-cm circumscribed, elevated, superficial, solid lesions<br>*Examples*: Elevated nevi, warts | Dried-up serum on the surface of the skin produced when skin is damaged<br>*Examples*: Impetigo, infected dermatitis |
| **Nodules** | **Fissures** |
| Solid elevation, usually greater than 1 cm in diameter; extend deeper into dermis than papules<br>*Example*: Epitheliomas | Linear breaks in the skin, sharply defined, with abrupt walls<br>*Examples*: Congenital syphilis, athlete's foot |
| **Tumors** | **Erosion** |
| Larger-than-1-cm solid lesions with depth; they may be above, level with, or beneath the skin<br>*Example*: Tumor stage of mycosis fungoides | Loss of epidermis that does not extend into the dermis<br>*Example*: Abrasion |
| **Plaques** | **Ulcers** |
| Larger-than-1-cm circumscribed, elevated, superficial, solid lesions<br>*Examples*: Localized mycosis fungoides, neurodermatitis | Irregularly sized and shaped excavations in the skin extending into the dermis or below<br>*Examples*: Stasis ulcers of the legs, tertiary syphilis |
| **Wheals** | **Scars** |
| Types of plaques; result is transient edema in dermis | Formations of connective tissue replacing tissue loss through injury or disease<br>*Example*: Keloids |
| **Vesicles** | **Atrophy** |
| Up-to-1-cm circumscribed elevations of the skin, containing serous fluid<br>*Examples*: Early chickenpox, contact dermatitis | Decrease in the volume of dermis<br>*Example*: Striae |
| **Bullae** | |
| Larger-than-1-cm circumscribed elevations containing serous fluid<br>*Examples*: Pemphigus, second-degree burns | |

     molecules away from body); as a regulator of water balance by preventing water and electrolyte loss; and as a receptor for Vitamin D from the sun.

3. The balance (homeostasis) of the skin surface is dependent on the equilibrium between cell production and renewal and cell destruction or loss.

4. Chalone is a hormone that is thought to inhibit the mitotic rate and the maturation rate of the epidermis. High chalone levels depress epidermis

regeneration. Chalone levels are high during daytime stress and activity and lower during sleep. Healing is therefore promoted during rest and sleep.

5. The skin's responses to antigens are capillary dilation (erythema), arteriole dilation (flare), and increased capillary permeability (wheal), which all contribute to the localized edema, spasms, and pruritus.

6. Application of heat causes local vasodilation, which promotes healing but increases pruritus and edema.

7. Application of cold causes local vasoconstriction, which decreases edema and pruritus but retards healing.

8. Skin lesions can be described as primary or secondary. *Primary lesions* are the initial responses of the skin to an irritant. *Secondary lesions* result from changes that take place in primary lesions (see Table II-12).

## Pruritus

1. Pruritus (itching) is the most common skin alteration. It can be a response of the skin to an allergen or it can be a sign or symptom of a systemic disease, as cancer, liver or renal dysfunction, or diabetes mellitus.

2. Pruritus is aggravated by excessive warmth, excessive dryness, rough fabrics, fatigue or stress, and monotony (lack of distractions).

## Wound healing (surgical, trauma, pressure ulcers)

1. Wound healing is delayed by wound infection, factors that impair cell production, factors that increase cell destruction, and inadequate nutrition.

2. Cell production is impaired by hypovolemia (*e.g.*, dehydration), stress (↑ chalone levels), activity (↑ chalone levels), and loss of sleep. It is also impaired by nutritional deficiencies (Vitamin C, protein) and by conditions that contribute to nutritional deficiencies (*e.g.*, liver disease, cancer, renal disease). Other factors affecting cell production are a compromised blood supply/stasis as in obesity, diabetes mellitus, the elderly, and the anemic; as well as radiation and certain medications—steroids, antimetabolites, and smooth-muscle relaxants.

3. Wound healing requires the following nutritional considerations (Constantian):

   Increased protein-carbohydrate intake sufficient to prevent negative nitrogen balance, hypoalbuminemia, and weight loss

   Increased daily intake of vitamins and minerals

   Vitamin A, 10,000 IU to 50,000 IU

   Vitamin B, 0.5 mg to 1.0 mg per 1,000 diet calories

   Vitamin $B_2$, 0.25 mg per 1,000 diet calories

   Vitamin $B_6$, 2 mg

   Niacin, 15 to 20 mg

   Vitamin $B_{12}$, 400 mg

   Vitamin C, 75 mg to 300 mg

   Vitamin D, 400 mg

   Vitamin E, 10 IU to 15 IU

   Traces of zinc, magnesium, calcium, copper

   Adequate oxygen supply and the blood volume and ability to transport it

4. Pressure ulcers (decubitus ulcers) are localized areas of necrosis resulting when the blood supply to that area falls below that required for survival. Destruction of the skin surface and underlying tissues is caused by tissue anoxia and the subsequent breakdown of the skin.

5. The nurse can prevent or reduce the development of pressure ulcers by intervening in reducing the amount of pressure, the time, and its repetition and by promoting optimal tissue condition.

## Ostomy-related

1. Skin irritations at the stoma site are usually caused by mechanical or chemical irritants, infections and inflammations, or an allergic reaction. *Mechanical irritants* include the frequent removal of tape, tight clothes, and prolonged or frequent bending or sitting. *Chemical irritations* result from exposure to urinary or gastric juices resulting from use of too large an appliance opening and from soap. *Infections and inflammations* are caused by the excessive stripping of skin, prolonged antibiotic therapy, overzealous cleaning, and occlusive appliances. *Allergic responses* are produced by adhesives and barriers.
2. A well-fitted appliance is one that protects all the surrounding skin surface from drainage.
3. The repeated removal and reapplication of adhesive-held appliances removes the epidermis, the protective layer of the skin.
4. The use of a belt-held appliance is an individual choice. Their use is usually discouraged because they can impair circulation and cause irritations by shifting during body motions.
5. Various skin products (barriers, adhesives), are available for ostomy appliances. Table II–13 illustrates the uses and limitations of selected products.

(*text continues on page 430*)

Table II–13. **Comparative Strengths of Ostomy Adhesives**

| Product | Consistency | | | | | Sensitivities | Normal Skin | Moist Skin | Excoriated Skin | Special Considerations |
| --- | --- | --- | --- | --- | --- | --- | --- | --- | --- | --- |
| | Paste | Solid | Powder | Liquid | Film | | | | | |
| Colly-Seal | | √ | | | | Rare | + | + | + | Lasts longer than Karaya (not a true adhesive); needs to be worn with belted appliance |
| Crixiline | | √ | | | | Rare | + | + | + | Melts readily, difficult to remove (use mineral oil) |
| Holli-Hesive | | √ | | | | Rare | + | + | + | Does not melt easily |
| Holliseal | | √ | | | | Rare | + | + | + | More effective in the presence of urine |
| Karaya | | | √ | | | Occasional | − | + | + | All consistencies produce burning, stinging when applied to irritated skin |
| | √ | | | | | Common | + | − | − | |
| | | | √ | | | Occasional | + | + | − | |
| Op Site | | | | | Film | | + | − | − | May be used over isolated denuded areas if sealed around them |

+ = Will adhere
− = Won't adhere

| Product | | | | + / − | + / − | + / − | Comments |
|---|---|---|---|---|---|---|---|
| Relia Seal | √ | | Rare | + | − | − | Effective in the presence of urine; also used for colostomy care |
| Skin Gel | √ | | Rare | + | Intact only | − | Always allow to dry before placing appliance over it |
| Skin Prep | √ | | Rare | + | Intact only | − | Same as Skin Gel |
| Stomahesive | √ | | Rare | + | + | + | May be used on excoriated skin and left on 3 days for healing to take place |
| | | √ | Rare | + | + | + | May sting momentarily due to alcohol base |
| | | √ | Rare | + | + | + | Use as filler for depressed areas; forms gel when moist |
| Surgical cement | √ | | Common | + | − | − | Must be allowed to dry before using appliance |
| Tincture of benzoin compound | √ | | Common | + | − | − | Not recommended, due to sensitivities |
| Tincture of benzoin (plain) | √ | | Rare | + | | + | Used as tactifier and barrier under adhesive |

+ = Will adhere
− = Won't adhere

# Impairment of Skin Integrity
## Related to Pruritus

Pruritus is an unpleasant, irritating, cutaneous sensation of itching that causes a desire to scratch.

### Assessment

Subjective data
The person reports itching sensations

Objective data
Scratch marks/redness (erythema)
Restlessness, irritability
Rash or lesions

---

**Outcome Criteria**

The person will
- Experience decreased pruritus
- Describe causative factors when known
- Describe rationale and procedure for treatment

---

### Interventions

A. Assess causative and contributing factors

Exposure to a contagious disease (rubella, fungus)
Exposure to chemical irritant (paints, oils, cleaning agents, cosmetics)
Systemic disease (liver disease, diabetes, collagen disease, renal disease, leukemia, Hodgkin's)
Parasites
Dry skin
Hypersensitivity to drug, food, insect bite
Psychogenic stress (acute or chronic)

B. Reduce or eliminate causative and contributing factors if possible

1. Maintain hygiene without producing dryness
   - Baths should be given infrequently
   - Use cool water when acceptable
   - Use mild soap (Castile, lanolin) or a soap substitute
   - Blot skin dry; do not rub
   - Apply cornstarch or powder lightly to skin folds by sprinkling on hand to avoid caking of powder; in bacterial or fungal conditions, use antifungal or anti-yeast powder preparations
2. Prevent excessive dryness
   - Lubricate skin with baby oil or lotion unless contraindicated; pat on by hand or with gauze

- Apply lubrication after bath to help moisture retention
- Apply wet dressings continuously or intermittently to relieve itching and remove crusts and exudate
- Provide for tub soaks for 20 to 30 minutes with temperature of 32° to 38° C; water can contain oatmeal powder, potassium permanganate, cornstarch, or sulfur*
3. Promote comfort and prevent further injury
   - Advise against scratching; explain the scratch-itch-scratch cycle
   - Secure an antihistamine order if itching is unrelieved
   - Utilize mitts (or cotton socks) if necessary on children and confused adults
   - Maintain trimmed nails to prevent injury; file after trimming
   - Remove particles from bed (food, caked powder)
   - Use old soft sheets and avoid wrinkles in bed; if incontinent pads are used, place draw sheet over them to elminate direct contact with skin
   - Avoid using perfumes and scented lotions
   - Wash clothes in a mild detergent and put through a second rinse cycle to reduce residue
   - Prevent excessive warmth, by use of cool room temperatures and low humidity, light covers with bed cradle; avoid overdressing
   - Apply ointments with gloved or bare hand, depending on type, to lightly cover skin; rub creams in entirely
   - Utilize frequent thin applications of ointment rather than one thick application
4. In children
   - Explain to child why he can't scratch
   - Dress child in long sleeves, long pants, or a one-piece outfit to prevent scratching
   - Avoid overdressing child, which will increase warmth
   - Before bedtime, give child a tepid bath with two cups of cornstarch
   - Use cotton blankets or sheets next to skin
   - Remove furry toys that may increase lint and pruritus
   - Teach child to press area that itches but not to scratch, or to put a cool cloth on the area if permitted

## C. Proceed with health teaching when indicated

- Explain causes of pruritus and their possible avoidance to person and significant other
- Explain interventions that relieve symptoms
- Explain factors that increase symptoms
- Teach person to avoid fabrics that irritate skin (wool, coarse textures)
- Refer to allergy-testing if indicated
- For further interventions refer to *Ineffective Individual Coping* if pruritus is stress-related

*May require a physician's order.

# Potential Impairment of Skin Integrity
Related to Immobility

## Assessment

Subjective data

The person reports fatigue; inability to move or turn

Objective data

Prescribed bedrest or immobility
Contributing factors

| | |
|---|---|
| Skin deficits | Sensory deficit |
| Impaired oxygen transport | Irritants |
| Nutritional deficit | |

---

**Outcome Criteria**

The person will
- Express willingness to participate in prevention of pressure sores
- Describe causation and prevention measures
- Explain rationale for interventions

---

## Interventions

A. Identify persons who are at risk for developing pressure sores; assess for

Skin deficits

| | |
|---|---|
| Dryness | Thinness |
| Edema | Excessive perspiration |
| Obesity | |

Impaired oxygen transport

| | |
|---|---|
| Edema | Arteriosclerosis |
| Anemia | Cardiopulmonary disorders |
| Peripheral vascular disorders | |

Chemical/mechanical irritants

| | |
|---|---|
| Radiation | Casts, splints, braces |
| Incontinence (feces, urine) | Spasms |

Nutritional deficits

| | |
|---|---|
| Protein deficiencies | Mineral deficiencies |
| Vitamin deficiencies | Dehydration |

Systemic disorders

| | |
|---|---|
| Infection | Cancer |
| Diabetes mellitus | Hepatic or renal disorders |

Sensory deficits

| | |
|---|---|
| Neuropathy | Comatose |
| Confusion | Cord injury |

Immobility

B. Attempt to reduce contributing factors in order to lessen the possibility of development of a pressure ulcer

1. Incontinence of urine or feces
   - Maintain sufficient fluid intake for adequate hydration (approximately 2500 ml daily, unless contraindicated); check mucous membranes in mouth for moisture and urine specific gravity
   - Establish a schedule for emptying bladder (begin with q 2 hours)
   - If person is confused, determine what his incontinent pattern is and intervene before incontinence occurs
   - Alternatives (if above fails) in order of choice
     a. External catheter*
     b. Intermittent catheterization every 4–8 hours, depending on individual*
     c. Continuous Foley catheter with bladder training for eventual removal*
   - Explain problem to individual and secure cooperation for plan
   - When incontinent, wash preferably with a commercial wash for perineal care and apply a protective cream for the perineal region
   - Check person frequently for incontinence when indicated
   - For additional interventions refer to *Alteration in Patterns of Urinary Elimination Related to Incontinence*

2. Immobility
   a. Encourage range-of-motion exercise and weight-bearing mobility when possible to increase blood flow to all areas
   b. Promote optimal circulation when in bed
      - Utilize turning schedule that relieves vulnerable area most often (e.g., if vulnerable area is the back, turning schedule would be left side to back, back to right side, right side to left side, and left side to back)
      - Turn person or instruct him to turn or shift weight every 30 minutes to 2 hours, depending on other causative factors present and the ability of the skin to recover from pressure
      - Frequency of turning schedule should be increased if any reddened areas that appear do not disappear in 1 hour after turning
      - Position person in normal or neutral position with body weight evenly distributed (see Fig. II–4 under *Impaired Physical Mobility*)
      - Keep bed as flat as possible to reduce tissue pressure; limit Fowler's position to only 30 minutes at a time
      - Use foam blocks or pillows to provide a bridging effect to support the body above and below the high risk or ulcered area, so affected area does not touch bed surface
      - Alternate or reduce the pressure on the skin surface with
         Wafer barrier (*e.g.*, Stomahesive, Hollihesive)
         Commercial fat pads over bony prominences
         Moisture-permeable adhesive
         Telfa or ABD dressings
         Alternating mattress
         Sheepskin, egg-crate mattress, foam protectors
         CircOlectric bed

*May require a physician's order.

    Stryker frame
    Flotation devices

  c. Utilize enough personnel to lift person up in bed or chair rather than pull or slide skin surfaces

  d. To reduce shearing forces, support feet with footboard to prevent sliding

  e. Promote optimal circulation when person is sitting
- Limit sitting time for person at high risk for ulcer development
- Instruct person to lift self using chair arms every 10 minutes if possible or assist person in rising up off the chair every 10 to 20 minutes, depending on risk factors present
- Do not elevate legs unless calves are supported to reduce the pressure over the ischia tuberositates
- Pad chair with at least 2 inches of foam rubber padding

  f. Inspect areas at risk to develop ulcers with each position change

| | |
|---|---|
| Ears | Elbows |
| Occiput | Trochanter |
| Heels | Ischia |
| Sacrum | Scapula |
| Scrotum | |

  g. Observe for erythema and blanching and palpate for warm and tissue sponginess with each position change

  h. Massage vulnerable areas with each position change

3. Malnourished state
- Increase protein and carbohydrate intake to maintain a positive nitrogen balance; utilize daily weights and serum albumin level to monitor status
- Ascertain that daily intake of vitamins and minerals is maintained with diet or supplements (See Principles for recommended amounts)
- See *Alterations in Nutrition: Less Than Body Requirements Related to Anorexia* for additional interventions

4. Sensory deficit
- Inspect person's skin every 2 hours, since he will not notice early discomfort
- Teach person or family to inspect skin with mirror

D. Initiate health teaching as indicated
- Instruct person and family in specific techniques to utilize at home to prevent pressure ulcers

# Impairment of Skin Integrity
## Related to Pressure Ulcer

A pressure ulcer is an area of cellular necrosis from tissue hypoxia resulting from pressure.

### Assessment

Subjective data

The person may report no discomfort or may report pain or numbness

## Objective data

The following signs may be noted over a bony prominence (sacrum, heel), or under a cast or brace

| | |
|---|---|
| Elevated skin temperature | Blister |
| Redness | Drainage wound |
| Blanching on pressure | Tissue erosion |

---

### Outcome Criteria

The person will
- Identify causative factors for pressure ulcers
- Identify rationale for prevention and treatment
- Participate in the prescribed treatment plan to promote wound healing

---

## Interventions

1. Identify the stage of pressure sore development

    Stage 1: Transient circulatory disturbance (redness, blanching on pressure) that disappears after pressure is removed

    Stage 2: Reddened or blanched area with no break in skin that does not disappear after pressure is removed

    Stage 3: Erythema and edema with blister or skin break

    Stage 4: Full-thickness lesion extends to subcutaneous fat, may have serosanguinous drainage

    Stage 5: Full-thickness lesion extends to deep fascia, muscle, and bone

2. Reduce or eliminate factors that contribute to the development or extension of pressure ulcers
    - Refer to *Impairment of Skin Integrity Related to Immobility*

3. Promote healing and prevent extension of the ulcer in stages 1, 2, and 3
    a. Wash reddened area gently with a mild soap for 1 to 3 minutes, rinse area thoroughly to remove soap, and pat dry
    b. Massage skin around the affected area to stimulate circulation
    c. Protect the skin surface with one of or a combination of the following
        - Dust area with karaya powder and remove excess
        - Apply a thin coat of Skin Prep or Skin Gel
        - Cover area with moisture-permeable adhesive
        - Cover area with a wafer barrier (*e.g.*, Stomahesive, Holli-Hesive) and secure with 2 strips of 1 inch micropore tape; leave in place for 2 to 3 days unless a whitish area appears
        - Apply a liquid copolymer skin barrier (*e.g.*, Bard)
        - Apply Granulex spray q 8 hours according to manufactor's instructions
        - Apply a commercial fat pad according to manufactor's directions
        - Apply Telfa or ABD dressings if more protection is needed
        - Pad bony prominences with foam protectors or sheepskin
    d. Increase dietary intake to promote wound healing
        - Increase protein and carbohydrate intake to maintain a positive nitrogen balance; utilize daily weights and serum albumin level to monitor status
        - Ascertain that daily intake of vitamins and minerals is maintained with diet or supplements (see Principles for recommended amounts)

• See *Alterations in Nutrition: Less Than Body Requirements Related to Anorexia* for additional interventions
4. Consult with physician for treatment of stage 4 and 5 pressure ulcers
5. Initiate health teaching and referrals as indicated
   • Instruct person and family on care of ulcers
   • Teach the importance of good skin hygiene and optimal nutrition
   • Refer to community nursing agency if additional assistance at home is needed

# Impairment of Skin Integrity
## Related to Stoma Problems

### Assessment

Subjective data

The person reports

| | |
|---|---|
| Itching | Inability to keep appliance on |
| Burning | Inability to apply appliance |

Objective data

| | |
|---|---|
| Erythema | Weeping sore |
| Macule or papule | Vesicle |
| Dry scales | Pustule |
| Excoriation | Abscess |
| Calcium deposits (urostomate) | |

---

**Outcome Criteria**

The person will
• Be free of stoma-related skin problems
• Describe factors that contribute to skin alterations
• Demonstrate correct application of the appliance and related skin care

---

### Interventions

A. Assess causative and contributing factors

Lack of knowledge
Ill-fitting or improper appliance
Difficulty or inability to perform stoma care
Improper location
Sensitivity to appliance material
Infection and inflammation

B. Eliminate or reduce contributing factors

1. Teach causes of skin alteration
   Mechanical irritation (pulling off adhesive; tight clothing or appliance belt)

Chemical irritants (soap; gastric secretions)

Infections (fungal, bacterial)

Excessive stripping of skin

Prolonged antibiotic therapy

Overzealous cleansing

2. Demonstrate method for selecting the right size appliance
   - Inform person that stoma will become smaller as the surgical area heals
   - After a stoma has healed, inform person that its size can vary depending on illness, hormonal levels, weight gain or loss
   - Utilize appliance manufacturer's stoma measuring card if possible
   - If stoma's size or form does not fit manufacturer's size chart to provide optimal skin protection, teach person to make individual pattern for cutting appliance backing
     a. If stoma is oval, using standard measuring guide (width, length), place a piece of clean folded paper over stoma, mark length, refold in opposite direction, and mark width
     b. If stoma is irregular, place a piece of plastic (*e.g.,* plastic wrap or wrapper for skin barriers) and trace with a marking pen; remember to reverse plastic to use as pattern

3. Teach person the proper cleansing of the skin around the stoma
   - Encourage gentle cleansing; use mild soap
   - Rinse the surface area well to remove soap residue
   - Blot skin, do not rub
   - Encourage individuals with dry skin to avoid soap or use it only on alternate days
   - If skin is intact, instruct that it is not necessary (and could cause irritations) to remove Karaya crusts
   - If skin is irritated, Karaya crusts can be removed; moisten the Karaya with water and remove it with a *dry* gauze pad or cloth
   - Use adhesive remover if necessary

4. Demonstrate application of appliance to increase wearing time and decrease skin irritation
   - Apply on a firm, smooth surface; encourage person to lie down or stand while placing the appliance to increase the skin surface's tautness
   - Be aware that some appliances can adhere to wet surfaces while others will not (see Table II–13).
   - When using adhesive or cement, apply to skin surface and appliance surface and allow to dry at least 1 minute before joining them
   - Uneven skin around the stoma (body folds, scars, depressions) can be filled with Karaya paste or Stomahesive paste

5. Teach ways to adjust for improper location
   - An inverted stoma may need a firm convex custom face plate (reusable)
   - A stoma in a body fold may need a flexible face plate with a skin barrier
   - A belt on an appliance may help, but caution against using a belt that is too tight and also instruct person to check to see if the belted appliance shifts during body motions

6. Teach individual to test sensitivity to appliance material by patch test
   - Apply a small patch of a new product or adhesive to any part of the body not near the stoma and leave on for 24 hours; if a rash occurs, discontinue use
   - If person has many sensitivities, he can be instructed to apply a copolymer skin barrier to the skin area before trying another patch test

- Instruct him to request a small supply of a new product from the manufacturer in order to prevent unnecessary expense if the product proves unsatisfactory
3. Infection and inflammation
   - Do not cover infected area with occlusive or nonabsorbent material
   - Use systemic or topical preparations to treat infections, per physician's order
      a. Topical antibiotics for bacterial infections often interfere with appliance adherence
      b. Topical powders for fungal infections can be dusted on lightly and the excess brushed off; appliance adherence is usually unaffected
   - Topical hydrocortisone is often used to treat inflammations; a cream with a non-greasy base is smoothed on sparingly and allowed to dry before appliance adhesive is applied
   - Aerosol products are convenient, but the propellants in them can cause drying and irritation if used over a long period of time
   - Instruct person to expose irritated skin to air for half hour to one hour between appliance changes (a small fan can be used to circulate air over the peristomal skin)
   - A person with an ileostomy or urostomy must control drainage when the appliance is off
      For ileostomy, mop up as it drains
      For urostomy, fill an empty round pill bottle with gauze and hold it over stoma
   - Warn never to use heat in any form (sun lamp, heat lamp) because it contributes to ulcerations resulting from tissue drying
   - With extensive irritation, use barriers such as disks, wafers, or squares, which protect the skin but permit healing
   - Instruct person to consult physician or enterostomal therapist if
      The appliance will not adhere properly
      The irritation gets worse
      The irritation persists for more than a week

## C. Initiate health teaching and referrals as indicated

- Provide an opportunity to demonstrate the procedure for preparing and applying the appliance
- Refer to pertinent literature (see Bibliography)
- Refer to pertinent organizations
   American Cancer Society (local)
   United Ostomy Association (local, state)

## Bibliography

### Books and Articles

Ahmed MC: Op site for decubitus care. Am J Nurs 82:61–64, 1982

Allison JR, Rist T: Skin infections may be outward signs of inner disorders. Geriatrics 30(2):87–95, 1975

Broadwell D, Johnson B: Principles of Ostomy Care. St. Louis, CV Mosby, 1982

Bruno P: Skin problems. In Carnevali D, Patrick M: Nursing Management for the Elderly. Philadelphia, JB Lippincott, 1979, pp 457–478.

Carlson R: Aging skin: Understanding the inevitable. Geriatrics 30(2):51–54, 1975

Constantian M: Pressure Ulcers: Principles and Techniques of Management. Boston, Little, Brown, 1980

Gruis M, Innes B: Assessment: Essential to prevent pressure sores. Am J Nurs 16:1762–1764, 1976

Hill GL: Ileostomy Surgery, Physiology and Management. New York, Grune & Stratton, 1976

Jacobs A: Eruptions in the diaper area. Pediatr Clin North Am 25:209–224, 1978

Jillson OF: The why and how of managing common skin problems. Consultant 19(8):32–34, 1979

King R: Assessment and management of soft tissue pressure. In Martin N, Holt N, Hicks D: Comprehensive Rehabilitative Nursing. New York, McGraw-Hill, 1981

Kretschmer KP: The Intestinal Stoma. Philadelphia, WB Saunders, 1978

Rodriguez DB: Treatment for three ostomy patients with systemic skin disorders. Journal of Enterostomal Therapy 8(5):31–32, 1981

Williams A: A study of factors contributing to skin breakdown. Nurs Res 21:238–243, 1972

## Pertinent Literature for the Consumer

Jetter KF: These Special Children.

Mullen BD, McGinn K: The Ostomy Book. Available from the Bull Publishing Company, P.O. Box 208, Palo Alto, CA 94302.

# Sleep Pattern Disturbance

## Definition

Sleep pattern disturbance: The state in which the individual experiences or is at risk of experiencing a change in the quantity or quality of his rest pattern as related to his biological and emotional needs.

## Etiological and Contributing Factors

Many factors in an individual's life can contribute to sleep pattern disturbances. Some common factors are listed below.

Pathophysiological

Impaired oxygen transport
    Angina      Respiratory disorders
    Peripheral arteriosclerosis      Circulatory disorders
Impaired elimination (bowel or bladder)
    Diarrhea      Retention
    Constipation      Dysuria
    Incontinence      Frequency
Impaired metabolism
    Hyperthyroidism      Hepatic disorders
    Gastric ulcers

Situational

Immobility (imposed by casts, traction)
Lack of exercise
Pain
Anxiety response
Pregnancy
Life-style disruptions
    Occupational      Sexual
    Emotional      Financial
    Social
Environmental changes
    Hospitalization (noise, disturbing      Travel
      roommate, fear)
Medications
    Tranquilizers      Steroids
    Sedatives      Soporifics
    Hypnotics      MAO inhibitors
    Antidepressants      Anesthetics
    Antihypertensives      Barbiturates
    Amphetamines

Maturational

> Neonates: Anoxia
> Infants and children: Nightmares, fears
> Adults: Parenthood
> Elderly: Chronic illness, depression

## Defining Characteristics

### Adults

> Difficulty falling or remaining asleep
> Fatigue on awakening or during the day
> Dozing during the day
> Agitation
> Mood alterations

### Children

Sleep disturbances in children are frequently related to fear, enuresis, or inconsistent responses of parents to child's requests for changes in sleep rules, such as requests to stay up late.

> Reluctance to retire
> Frequent awakening during the night
> Desire to sleep with parents

## Focus Assessment Criteria

### Subjective data

1. History of symptoms
   Complaints of
   - Sleeplessness
   - Anxiety
   - Irritability
   - Depression
   - Fear (nightmares, dark, maturational situations)

   Onset and duration
   Location
   Description
   - Precipitated by what?
   - Aggravated by what?
   - Relieved by what?

2. Sleep requirements
   In order to establish the amount of sleep an individual needs, have him go to bed and sleep until he wakes in the morning (without an alarm clock). This should be done for a few days and the average of the total sleeping hours calculated—with the subtraction of 20 to 30 minutes, which is the time most people need to fall asleep.

3. Sleep patterns (present, past)
   Usual bedtime and arising time
   Difficulty in getting to sleep, staying asleep, awakening
   Reasons for difficulty
   Use of sleep aids or rituals
   - Warm bath
   - Drink or food (milk, wine)
   - Medications
   - Pillows
   - Position
   - Toy, book

   Naps (frequency, length)

Objective data

Physical characteristics
  Drawn appearance (pale, dark circles under eyes, puffy eyes)
  Yawning
  Dozing during the day
  Decreased attention span

## Nursing Goals

Through selected interventions, the nurse will seek to
- Provide comfort measures to induce sleep
- Reduce or prevent discomforts that may interfere with the individual's normal sleep and rest patterns
- Increase the quality and quantity of the individual's rest pattern during periods of added physiological and emotional stress

## Principles and Rationale for Nursing Care

### General

1. The average adult requires approximately 20 minutes to fall asleep.
2. The amount of sleep a person needs varies with life-style, health, and age.
3. The average amount of sleep needed according to age follows (William).

| Age | Hours of Sleep |
|---|---|
| Newborn | 10.5 to 23 |
| 6 months | 12 to 16 |
| Over 6 months to 4 years | 12 to 13 |
| 5 to 13 years | 7 to 8.5 |
| 13 to 21 years | 7 to 8.75 |
| Adults under 60 | 6 to 9 |
| Adults over 60 | 7 to 8 |

4. The quality of sleep and the ability to fall asleep and remain asleep for a sufficient period are a direct measurement of the physiological, psychological, and spiritual health of the individual.
5. Age affects the amount of time spent in each stage of sleep as well as the amount of time one needs to engage in sleep in order to replenish body energies. The neonate spends the greatest amount of time sleeping, and spends the most time in REM sleep (see numbers 5 and 6 in next section).
6. Older adults require the same or slightly less sleep than younger adults but can experience a decreased intensity of sleep related to nighttime wakenings.
7. Moderate sleep deprivation can produce behaviors of withdrawal, depression, memory lapses, apathy, irritability, confusion, and even hallucinations.
8. Fear (of recurrent nightmares, the dark) may interfere with sleep or create a reluctance to go to sleep.
9. Depression usually influences sleep in the form of initial insomnia (difficulty getting asleep). Depressed individuals may then increase their sleeping hours (daytime and nighttime).
10. The use of sedatives to induce sleep will also inhibit other mental and physical activities (respiration, cognition, circulation, digestion, elimination).
11. Chronic insomnia and chronic use of hypnotics reflect ineffective individual coping and require intensive therapeutic interventions.

12. Use of hypnotics by the elderly is usually contraindicated because of decreased renal function, which increases the toxicity of the drug. If sedatives are required, antihistamines will provide the needed sedation with fewer adverse side-effects.

## Physiological

1. Sleep is a restorative and recuperative process that facilitates cellular growth and the repair of damaged and aging body tissues.
2. The sleep process is hypothesized to be dependent on the action of the reticular activating system. Impulses are transported to the reticular activating system where epinephrine is secreted. Brain stem activity is therefore increased. It is speculated that after a period of time the impulses become fatigued, decreasing their output, and sleep spreads throughout the body.
3. There are different levels of sleep at which the various body tissues relax and rejuvenate. Each level has its own structure and function.

   Stage I: The individual becomes very drowsy and his musculature relaxes

   Stage II: Progressive muscular relaxation occurs, with decreasing cerebral activity

   Stage III: Physiological alterations become evident—vital signs become depressed, gastrointestinal function accelerates to facilitate cellular metabolism, and venous dilation occurs to accelerate the exchange of cellular metabolites

   Stage IV: The individual is in a deep sleep pattern; body functions decrease to an extremely depressed level of functioning

4. The entire sleep cycle is completed in an interval of 70 to 100 minutes and repeats itself frequently during the course of the sleep pattern. During stages 1 and 2 the sleeper can be awakened by relevant stimuli, but in stages 3 and 4 the stimuli must be louder and stronger to awaken the sleeper.
5. Sleep can be divided into two major kinds: rapid eye movement (REM) and non-rapid eye movement.
6. REM is the active phase of the sleep cycle that appears at the end of stage I. This phase is characterized by increased irregular vital signs, penile erections, flaccid musculature, and the release of adrenal hormones. REM sleep occurs approximately four to five times a night and is essential to one's sense of well-being.
7. During sleep the basal metabolic rate and the volume of urine production is decreased, but the secretion of sweat and gastric juice is increased.

## Pregnancy

1. Pregnant women require increased periods of sleep because of physical and emotional stressors.
2. Insomnia during pregnancy is influenced by conflicts and anxieties of pregnancy and impending motherhood, fetal activity, musculoskeletal discomforts, and abdominal pressure.

---

**Outcome Criteria**

The person will
- Describe factors that prevent or inhibit sleep
- Identify techniques to induce sleep
- Demonstrate an optimal balance of rest and activity

## Interventions

Since a variety of factors can disrupt sleep patterns, the nurse should consult the index for specific interventions to reduce certain factors (*e.g.*, pain, anxiety, fear). The following suggests general interventions for promoting sleep and specific interventions for selected clinical situations.

### A. Identify causative contributing factors

Pain (see *Alterations in Comfort: Pain*)
Fear (see *Fear*)
Stress or anxiety (see *Anxiety*)
Immobility or decreased activity
Pregnancy
Urinary frequency or incontinence (see *Alterations in Patterns of Urinary Elimination*)
Unfamiliar or noisy environment

### B. Reduce or eliminate evironmental distractions and sleep interruptions

1. Noise
   - Close door to room
   - Pull curtains
   - Unplug telephone
   - Provide soft music (*e.g.*, a radio with earplugs)
   - Eliminate 24-hour lighting
   - Provide night lights
   - Decrease the amount and kind of incoming stimuli (*e.g.*, staff conversations)
   - Cover blinking lights with tape
   - Reduce the volume of alarms and TVs
   - Place with compatible roommate if possible
2. Interruptions
   - Organize procedures to provide the fewest number of disturbances during sleep period (*e.g.*, when individual awakens for medication also administer treatments and obtain vital signs)
   - Avoid unnecessary procedures during sleep period
   - Limit visitors during optimal rest periods (*e.g.*, after meals)
   - If voiding during the night is disruptive, have person limit his nightime fluids and void before retiring

### C. Increase daytime activities as indicated

- Establish with person a schedule for a daytime program of activity (walking, physical therapy)
- Limit amount and length of daytime sleeping
- Provide others to communicate with person and stimulate wakefulness

### D. Provide comfort measures to induce sleep

- Assess with person, family, or parents the usual bedtime routine—time, hygiene practices, rituals (reading, toy)—and adhere to it as closely as possible
- Encourage or provide p.m. care
  Bathroom or bedpan
  Personal hygiene (mouth care, bath, shower, partial bath)
  Clean linen and bedclothes (freshly made bed, sufficient blankets)

- Utilize sleep aids
    Desired bedtime snack (avoid highly seasoned and high-roughage foods)
    Reading material
    Back rub or massage
    Soft music or tape-recorded story
- Utilize pillows for support (painful limb, pregnant or obese abdomen, back)

## E. Reduce the potential for injury during sleep
- Utilize side rails if needed
- Place bed in low position
- Provide adequate supervision
- Provide night lights
- Place call bell within reach
- Ensure that an adequate length of tubing is available for turning (IV tubing, levin tube)

## F. Provide health teaching and referrals as indicated
- Teach the importance of regular exercise for at least ½ hour three times a week (if not contraindicated) to reduce stress and promote sleep (walking, running, areobic dance and exercise)
- Teach the pregnant woman
    Not to stand when she can sit
    To elevate feet when sitting
    Not to sit when she can lie down
    To adjust her schedule to provide for an afternoon rest (*e.g.*, upon returning home from work)
- Explain to person and significant others the causes of sleep/rest disturbance and possible ways to avoid them
- Explain interventions that relieve symptoms

## Bibliography

Fass G: Sleep, drugs and dreams. Am J Nurs 71:2316–2320, 1971

Grant DA, Klell C: For goodness' sake—let your patient sleep! Nursing 4:54–57, 1974

Hayter J: The rhythm of sleep. Am J Nurs 80:457–461, 1980

Hilton BA: Quality and quantity of patient's sleep and sleep disturbing factors in a respiratory intensive care unit. J Adv Nurs 1:453–468, 1976

Kleitman N: Sleep and Wakefulness. Chicago, University of Chicago Press, 1963

William D: Sleep and disease. Am J Nurs 71:2321–2324, 1971

Woods N: Patterns of sleep in post-cardiotomy patients. Nurs Res 2(4):437–452, 1972

Zelechowski G: Helping your patient sleep: Planning instead of pills. Nursing 7:63–65, 1977

Zelechowski G: Sleep and the critically ill. Critical Care Update 6(2):5–13, 1979

Zwillich CW: Uncovering the mysteries of sleep. Arch Intern Med 138(2):195, 1978

# Social Isolation

## Definition
Social isolation: The state in which the individual experiences a need or desire for contact with others but is unable to make that contact.*

## Etiological and Contributing Factors
A state of social isolation can result from a variety of situations and health problems that are related to a loss of established relationships or to a failure to generate these relationships. Some common sources follow.

### Situational
Death of a significant other
Divorce
Extreme poverty
Hospitalization or terminal illness (dying process)
Moving to another culture (*e.g.*, unfamiliar language)
Drug or alcohol addiction
Obesity
Cancer (disfiguring surgery of head or neck, superstitions of others)
Physical handicaps (paraplegia, amputation, arthritis, hemiplegia)
Emotional handicaps (extreme anxiety, depression, paranoia, phobias)
Homosexuality
Loss of usual means of transportation
Incontinence (embarrassment, odor)

### Maturational
Elderly: Sensory losses, motor losses, loss of significant others

## Defining Characteristics
Since social isolation is a subjective state, all inferences made regarding a person's feelings of aloneness must be validated. Because the causes vary and people show their aloneness in different ways, there are no absolute cues to this diagnosis.

### Possible subjective reactions
Expressed feelings of unexplained dread or abandonment
Desire for more family or nurse contact
Time passing slowly ("Mondays are so long for me")

*Social isolation is a negative state of aloneness. It is a subjective state that exists whenever a person says it does and is perceived as imposed by others. Social isolation is *not* the voluntary solitude that is necessary for personal renewal, nor is it the creative aloneness of the artist or the loneliness—and possible suffering—one may experience as a result of seeking individualism and independence (*e.g.*, moving to a new city, going away to college).

## Associated characteristics

Inability to concentrate and make decisions
Feelings of uselessness
Doubts about ability to survive

## Behavior changes

Increased irritability or restlessness
Underactivity (physical or verbal)
Inability to make decisions
Increased signs and symptoms of illness (a change from previous state of good health)
Appearing depressed, anxious, or angry
Postponing important decision-making
Failure to interact with others nearby
Sleep disturbance (too much or insomnia)
Change in eating habits (overeating or anorexia)

Social isolation can result in other problems and responses. These include anxiety, depression, fear, nutritional alterations, and a threatened self-image.

See also *Anxiety, Alterations in Thought Processes, Powerlessness, Ineffective Individual Coping Related to Depression, Fear, Alterations in Nutrition,* and *Disturbance in Self-Concept.*

## Nursing Goals

Through selected nursing interventions, the nurse will seek to

- Assist the individual in identifying his state as one of social isolation, and help him resolve any feelings associated with this state
- Foster relationships and decrease the sense of isolation; (*e.g.,* with children through play therapy, with psychiatric patients through group therapy)
- Encourage lonely persons to meet other persons with similar problems or needs (*e.g.,* Reach to Recovery, United Ostomy Association, Alcoholics Anonymous, senior centers)
- Encourage physical closeness (touch) for selected individuals
- Provide information for patients and families about a disfigurement or illness to foster understanding and decrease the negative effects of illness on important relationships

## Principles and Rationale for Nursing Care

1. A person does not have to be alone to feel socially isolated. The physically handicapped are frequently ignored, for example.
2. Social isolation can result in intense feelings of loneliness and suffering.
3. The suffering associated with social isolation is not always visible. To diagnose this state, nurses must first be able to identify those persons at risk.
4. The lonely or isolated person often aggravates his condition by suffering alone. The lonely tend to shun each other.
5. The isolated person may resign himself to his situation and never seek companionship. He may deny his own feelings.
6. For the socially isolated, certain times (*e.g.,* nighttime or sundown) are harder to bear than others.

7. Persons who feel isolated may communicate and be communicated with in only the most concrete terms. "Hello, how are you?" "Do you want to eat?"
8. Illness may be the only legitimate way a socially isolated individual can get attention.
9. Hospitalization, which involves separation and isolation from the familiar and the secure, can cause feelings of loneliness.
10. A hospitalized child may have feelings of abandonment.
11. Aging can be an isolating experience.
12. The socially isolated are usually not able to initiate or coordinate various isolation reduction activities on their own behalf.

## Focus Assessment Criteria

The nurse must listen attentively to hear what the patient is telling her. She must also make astute observations of behavior if an accurate nursing diagnosis is to be made and appropriate interventions identified.

### Subjective data

1. Feelings of loneliness
    Does the person feel lonesome (isolated)?
    Why does he think he feels this way?
    Can he describe this feeling of loneliness?
    Are there times (holidays or other occasions) when this feeling is more painful?
    When during a 24-hour period does he feel most alone (morning, afternoon, evening, or during the night)?
    What does he do to relieve this feeling?
2. Desire for more human contact
    Who does the person think could help relieve this feeling of isolation?
    What kind of relationships would he like? (Same sex or opposite sex? Same age? Someone with same situational or maturational problem?)
    Is he willing to make the effort to meet new people and go to new places?
    What kind of group activities does he most enjoy? (Travel? A religious service or activity?)
3. Support system (people, pets)
    Whom does the person turn to in time of need?
    Are there friends or neighbors whom he relies on for such things as meals and transportation?
4. Loss of significant others
    Has divorce or death—of spouse, child, sibling, friend, pet—occurred recently?
    Has the person moved away from vicinity of significant other? (Living alone increases the likelihood of loneliness)
5. Barriers to social contacts
    Does the person lack knowledge of resources available, where to meet others, how to initiate conversation with strangers?
    Is he housebound? (Illness or incapacity—lack of mobility on steps or curbs—and weather hazards can physically isolate the elderly, as does loss of usual transportation, living in dangerous area, and lack of access to public transportation)
    Are there changes in the person's sensory ability (tactile sense, hearing, visual acuity, ability to write letters)?

6. Change in living arrangement

Has the person moved recently (to nursing home or child's home, to an apartment, to a strange location)?

## Objective data

Esthetic problems

Mutilating surgery

Odor (e.g., ulcerating tumor)

Extreme obesity

Incontinence

---

### Outcome Criteria

The person will
- Identify the reasons for his feelings of isolation
- Discuss ways of increasing meaningful relationships
- Identify appropriate diversional activities

---

## Interventions

The nursing interventions for a variety of contributing factors that might be associated with a diagnosis of social isolation are very similar.

## A. Identify causative and contributing factors (see Focus Assessment Criteria)

## B. Reduce or eliminate causative and contributing factors

1. Promote social interaction
   - Support the individual who has experienced a loss as he works through his grief (see *Grieving*)
   - Validate the normalcy of grieving
   - Encourage person to talk about his feelings of loneliness and the reasons they exist
   - Mobilize person's support system of neighbors and friends
2. Decrease barriers to social contact
   - Assist with identification of transportation options
   - Determine available transportation in the community (public, church-related, volunteer)
   - Determine if person must be taught how to use alternate transportation (*e.g.*, drive a car)
   - Identify activities that help keep people busy, especially during times of high risk of loneliness (see *Diversional Activity Deficit*)
   - Assist with the development of alternate means of communication for persons with compromised sensory ability (*e.g.*, amplifier on phone)
   - Assist with the management of esthetic problems (*e.g.*, consult enterostomal therapist if ostomy odor is a problem; teach those with cancer to control odor of tumors by packing area with yogurt or pouring in buttermilk, then rinsing well with saline solution)
   - Assist person in locating stores that sell clothing especially made for those who have had disfiguring surgery (*e.g.*, mastectomy)
   - Refer to *Alteration in Patterns of Urinary Elimination: Incontinence* for specific interventions to control incontinence

3. Identify strategies to expand the world of the isolated
   Senior centers and church groups
   Foster grandparent program
   Day care centers for the elderly
   Retirement communities
   House sharing
   College classes opened to older persons
   Pets
   Telephone contact

## C. Initiate referrals as indicated

Community-based groups that contact the socially isolated
Self-help groups for clients isolated due to specific medical problems (Reach to
   Recovery, United Ostomy Association)
Wheelchair groups

## Bibliography

Burnside IM: Nursing and the Aged. New York, McGraw-Hill, 1976

Carnevali D, Patrick M: Nursing Management for the Elderly. Philadelphia, JB Lippincott,
   1979

Glassman-Feibusch B: The socially isolated elderly. Geriatric Nursing 2(1):28–31, 1981

Lynch JJ: The Broken Heart: The Medical Consequences of Loneliness. New York, Basic Books,
   1979

Roberts SL: Behavioral Concepts and the Critically Ill Patient. Englewood Cliffs, NJ, Prentice-
   Hall, 1976

Roberts SL: Behavioral Concepts and Nursing Throughout the Life Span. Englewood Cliffs, NJ,
   Prentice-Hall, 1978

# Spiritual Distress

*Related to* **Inability to Practice Spiritual Rituals**

*Related to* **Conflict Between Religious or Spiritual Beliefs and Prescribed Health Regimen**

## Definition

Spiritual distress: The state in which the individual experiences or is at risk of experiencing a disturbance in his belief or value system that is his source of strength and hope.

## Etiological and Contributing Factors

Spiritual distress can occur as a response to a variety of health problems, situations, and conflicts. Some common sources follow.

### Pathophysiological

Loss of body part or function
Terminal disease
Debilitating disease

### Situational

Death or illness of significant other
Embarrassment at practicing spiritual rituals
Hospital barriers to practicing spiritual rituals

| | |
|---|---|
| Isolation | Confinement to bed or room |
| Intensive care restrictions | Trauma |
| Surgery | Dietary restrictions |
| Medications | Medical procedures (*e.g.*, IVs) |

Conflicts to belief system

| | |
|---|---|
| Abortion | Surgery or blood transfusion |
| Pain | (when prohibited by religion) |
| Divorce | |

Beliefs opposed by family, peers, health care providers

## Defining Characteristics

Experiences a disturbance in belief system
   Questions credibility of belief system
   Is discouraged
   Is unable to practice usual religious rituals
   Has ambivalent feelings (doubts) about beliefs
   Feels a sense of spiritual emptiness
Expresses concern—anger, resentment, fear—over meaning of life, suffering, death
Requests spiritual assistance for a disturbance in belief system

## Focus Assessment Criteria

### Subjective data
The following questions may be included as part of the psychosocial nursing assessment for individuals and families.
1. "Is religion or God important to you?"
    If answer is yes, "To what religion do you belong?" or "In what do you believe?" If no, "Do you find a source of strength or meaning in another area?"
2. "What effect do you expect your illness (hospitalization) to have on your spiritual practices or beliefs?"
3. "Are there any religious books (statues, medals, services, places) that are especially important to you?"
4. "Do you have a special religious leader (priest, pastor, rabbi)?"
5. "How can I help you maintain your spiritual strength during this illness (hospitalization)?" (*e.g.*, contact spiritual leader, provide privacy at special times, request reading materials)

### Objective data
1. Present practices
    Assess for
        The presence of religious or spiritual articles (clothing, medals, texts)
        Visits from religious leader
        Visits to religious place of worship (chapel)
        Requests for spiritual counseling or assistance
2. Response to interview on spiritual needs
    Assess for the presence of anxiety, doubt, anger, depression

## Nursing Goals
Through selected interventions, the nurse will seek to
  · Promote spiritual integrity
  · Promote spiritual development
  · Assist individual in achieving his spiritual goals

## Principles and Rationale for Nursing Care
1. All people have a spiritual dimension, whether or not they participate in formal religious practices.
2. The practice of nurses should not violate their own moral, ethical, spiritual, or religious values.
3. The nature of the spiritual care an individual receives may directly affect the speed and quality of his recovery from illness.
4. An individual is a spiritual person even when disoriented, confused, emotionally ill, delirious, or cognitively impaired.
5. Religion influences attitudes and behavior related to right and wrong, family, child rearing, work, money, politics, and many other functional areas.
6. The nurse's spiritual and religious background will influence her feelings about the spirituality and religion of her patients.
7. To deal effectively with a person's spiritual needs, the nurse must recognize her own beliefs and values, acknowledge that these values may not be effective for others, and set her own values aside when helping the individual meet his perceived spiritual needs.

8. The value of prayers or spiritual rituals to the believer is not affected by whether or not they can be scientifically "proved" to be beneficial.
9. Do not deny a request to see a spiritual leader except in case of extreme emergency (leader may even be sent to O.R. or treatment room if necessary)
10. The nurse should function as an advocate in recognizing and respecting the individual's spiritual needs, which may sometimes be overlooked or ignored by other health professionals.
11. In order to assist people in spiritual distress, the nurse must know certain beliefs and practices of the various spiritual groups found in this country. Table II-14 provides information on the beliefs and practices that are most directly related to health and illness. It is intended as a quick reference only. Major religions, denominations, and spiritual groups are arranged alphabetically. Denominations with similar practices and restrictions are grouped together. No attempt is made to discuss the broad beliefs and philosophies of the selected groups; see the bibliography for such in-depth information.

(*text continues on page 462*)

Table II–14. **Overview of Religious Beliefs**

---

***Agnostic***

Beliefs
It is impossible to know if God exists (specific moral values may guide behavior)

***Armenian***

*see* Eastern Orthodox

***Atheist***

Beliefs
God does not exist (specific moral values may guide behavior)

***Baptist, Churches of God, Churches of Christ*, and *Pentecostal (Assemblies of God, Four-square Church*)**

Illness
Practices laying on of hands, divine healing through prayer
May request communion
Some prohibit medical therapy
May consider illness divine punishment or intrusion of Satan

Diet
No alcohol (mandatory for most)
No coffee, tea, tobacco, pork, or strangled animals (mandatory for some )
Some fasting

Birth
Opposes infant baptism

Text
Bible

Beliefs
Some practice glossolalia (speaking in tongues)

(*continued*)

Table II–14. **Overview of Religious Beliefs** (*continued*)

---

### Buddhist

Illness

Considered trial that develops the soul

May wish counseling by priest

May refuse treatment on holy days (1/1, 1/16, 2/15, 3/21, 4/8, 5/21, 6/15, 8/1, 8/23, 12/8, 12/31)

Diet

Strict vegetarianism (mandatory for some)

Discourages use of alcohol, tobacco, and drugs

Death

Last-rite chanting by priest

Death leads to rebirth, may wish to remain alert and lucid

Texts

Buddha's sermon on the "eightfold path"

The Tripitaka, or "three baskets" of wisdom

Beliefs

Cleanliness is of great importance

### Church of Christ

*See* Baptist

### Church of Christ, Scientist

Illness

Caused by errors in thought and mind

May oppose drugs; IV fluid; blood transfusions; psychotherapy; hypnotism; physical examinations; biopsies; eye, ear, and blood-pressure screening; and other medical and nursing interventions

Accepts only legally required immunizations

May desire support from a Christian Science reader or treatment by a Christian Science nurse or practitioner (a list of these nonmedical practitioners and nurses may be found in the *Christian Science Journal*)

Death

Autopsy permitted only in cases of sudden death

Text

*Science and Health With Key to the Scriptures* by Mary Baker Eddy

### Church of Christ

*See* Baptist

### Church of God

*See* Baptist

### Confucian

Illness

The body was given by one's parents and should therefore be well cared for

May be strongly motivated to maintain or regain wellness

Beliefs

Respect for family and older persons very important

Table II–14. **Overview of Religious Beliefs** (*continued*)

### *Cults* (variety of groups, usually with living leader)

Illness

Most practice faith healing

May reject modern medicine and condemn health personnel as enemies

Therapeutic compliance and follow-up are generally poor

Illness may represent wrong thinking or inhabitation by Satan

Beliefs

Expansion of cult through conversions important

May depend on cult environment for definition of reality

### *Eastern Orthodox (Greek Orthodox, Russian Orthodox, Armenian)*

Illness

May desire Communion, laying on of hands, anointing, or sacrament of Holy Unction

Most oppose euthanasia and favor every effort to preserve life

Russian Orthodox males should be shaved only if necessary for surgery

Diet

May fast Wednesdays, Fridays, during Lent, before Christmas, or for six hours before Communion (seriously ill are exempted)

May avoid meat, dairy products, and olive oil during fast (seriously ill are exempted)

Birth

Baptism 8 to 40 days after birth, usually by immersion (mandatory for some)

May be followed immediately by confirmation

Greek Orthodox only: If death of infant is imminent, nurse should baptize infant by touching the forehead with a small amount of water three times

Death

Last rites and administration of Holy Communion (mandatory for some)

May oppose autopsy, embalming, and cremation

Texts

Bible

Prayer book

Religious articles

Icons (pictures of Jesus, Mary, saints) are very important

Holy water and lighted candles

Russian Orthodox wears cross necklace which should be removed only if necessary

Other

Greek Orthodox opposes abortion

Confession at least yearly (mandatory for some)

Communion 4 times yearly: Christmas, Easter, 6/30, and 8/15 (mandatory for some)

*Dates of holy days may differ from Western Christian calendar*

### *Episcopal*

Illness

May believe in spiritual healing

May desire confession and Communion

Diet

May abstain from meat on Fridays

May fast during Lent or before Communion

(*continued*)

Table II–14.   **Overview of Religious Beliefs** (*continued*)

---

### Episcopal (*continued*)

Birth
   Infant baptism is mandatory (nurse may baptize infant when death is imminent by pouring water on forehead and saying "I baptize thee in the name of the Father, the Son, and the Holy Ghost")

Death
   Last rites optional

Texts
   Bible
   Prayer book

### Friend (Quaker)

No ministers or priests; direct, individual, inner experience of God is vital

Diet
   Most avoid alcohol and drugs and favor practice of moderation

Death
   Many do not believe in afterlife

Beliefs
   Pacifism important; many are conscientious objectors to war

### Greek Orthodox

*See* Eastern Orthodox

### Hindu

Illness
   May minimize illness and emphasize its temporary nature
   Considered important only as it affects spiritual quest
   Illness or injury may represent sins committed in previous life

Diet
   Various doctrines, many vegetarian; many abstain from alcohol
      (mandatory for some)

Death
   Seen as rebirth; may wish to be alert
   Priest ties thread around neck or wrist of body—do not remove
   Water is poured into mouth, and family washes body
   Cremation preferred

Beliefs
   Self-control, self-discipline, and cleanliness emphasized
   Opposes artificial insemination

Texts
   Vedas
   Upanishads
   Bhagavad-Gita

Worship
   Usually in home
   May involve various images, statues, and symbols of gods
   May include use of water, fire, lights, sounds, natural objects, special postures, and gestures

Table II–14. **Overview of Religious Beliefs** (*continued*)

---

### *Jehovah's Witness*

Illness

Opposes blood transfusions and organ transplantation (mandatory)

May oppose other medical treatment and all modern science

Opposes faith healing

Opposes abortion

Diet

Refuses foods to which blood has been added; may eat meats that have been drained

### *Jew (Judaism)*

Illness

Medical care emphasized

Rabbinical consultation necessary for donation and transplantation of organs

May oppose surgical procedures on the Sabbath (sundown Friday to sundown Saturday); seriously ill are exempted

May prefer burial of removed organs or body tissues

May oppose shaving

May wear skull cap and socks continuously, believing head and feet should be covered

Diet

Fasting for 24 hours on holy days of Yom Kippur (in September or October) and Tisha Bab (in August)

Matzo replaces leavened bread during Passover week (in March or April)

May observe strict Kosher dietary laws (mandatory for some) that prohibit pork, shellfish, and the eating of meat and dairy products at same meal or with same dishes (milk products, served first, can be followed by meat in a few minutes; reverse is not Kosher); seriously ill are exempted

Birth

Ritual circumcision 8 days after birth (mandatory for some)

Fetuses are buried

Death

Ritual burial society members wash body

Burial as soon as possible

Opposes cremation

Many oppose autopsy and donation of body to science

Most do not believe in afterlife

Generally oppose prolongation of life after irreversible brain damage

Texts

Torah (first five books of Old Testament)

Talmud

Prayer book

Religious articles

Menorah (seven-branched candlestick)

Yarmulke (skullcap, may be worn continuously)

Tallith (prayer shawl worn for morning prayers)

Tefillin, or phylacteries (leather boxes on straps containing scripture passages)

Star of David (may be worn around neck)

(*continued*)

Table II–14. **Overview of Religious Beliefs** (*continued*)

### Lutheran, Methodist, Presbyterian

Illness

 May request Communion, anointment and blessing, or visitation by minister or elder

 Generally encourages utilization of medical science

Birth

 Baptism by sprinkling or immersion of infants, children, or adults

Death

 Optional last rites or scripture reading

### Mennonite

Illness

 Opposes laying on of hands

 May oppose shock treatment and drugs

### Methodist

*See* Lutheran

### Mormon (Church of Jesus Christ of Latter-day Saints)

Illness

 Comes from breaking laws of health or failing to keep God's commandments

 May desire Sacrament of the Lord's Supper to be administered by a Church Priesthood holder

 Divine healing through laying on of hands

 May prohibit medical therapy

 Church may provide financial support during illness

Diet

 Prohibits alcohol, tobacco, and hot drinks (tea and coffee)

 Sparing use of meats

Birth

 No infant baptism

Death

 Baptism of dead (mandatory), sometimes with living person as proxy

 May preach Gospel to the dead

 Opposes cremation

Texts

 Bible

 Book of Mormon

Religious articles

 Special undergarment worn by some men should not be removed if possible (seriously ill are exempted)

### Muslim (Islamic, Moslem) and Black Muslim

Illness

 Opposes faith healing

 May be noncompliant due to fatalistic view (illness is God's will)

 Group prayer may be helpful—no priests

 Favors every effort to prolong life

Table II–14.  **Overview of Religious Beliefs** (*continued*)

---

***Muslim* (Islamic, Moslem) and *Black Muslim*** (*continued*)

Diet

Pork prohibited

May oppose alcohol and traditional Black American foods (corn bread, collard greens)

Fasts sunrise to sunset during Ramadan (ninth month of Muslim year—falls different time each year on Western calendar); seriously ill are exempted

Birth

Circumcision practiced with accompanying ceremony

Aborted fetus after 130 days is treated as human being

Death

Confession of sins before death, with family present if possible

Family follows specific procedure for washing and preparing body, which is then turned to face Mecca

May oppose autopsy

Texts

Koran (scriptures)

Hadith (traditions)

Prayer

Five times daily—upon rising, midday, afternoon, early evening, and before bed—facing Mecca and kneeling on prayer rug

Ritual washing after prayer

Beliefs

All activities (including sleep) restricted to what is necessary for health

Personal cleanliness very important

All Muslims: gambling and idol worship prohibited

***Pentecostal***

*See* Baptist

***Presbyterian***

*See Lutheran*

***Roman Catholic***

Illness

Allowed by God because of man's sins but not considered personal punishment

May desire confession (penance) and Communion

Anointing of sick for all seriously ill patients (some patients may equate this with "Last Rites" and assume they are dying)

Donation and transplantation of organs permitted

Burial of amputated limbs (mandatory for some)

Diet

Fasting or abstaining from meat mandatory on Ash Wednesday and Good Friday (seriously ill are exempted); optional during Lent and on Fridays

Fasts from solid food for 1 hour and abstains from alcohol for 3 hours before receiving communion (mandatory) (seriously ill are exempted)

(*continued*)

Table II–14. **Overview of Religious Beliefs** (*continued*)

---

### Roman Catholic (*continued*)

Birth

Baptism of infants and aborted fetuses mandatory; (nurse may baptize in case of imminent death by sprinkling water on the forehead and saying, "I baptize thee in the name of the Father, of the Son, and of the Holy Ghost")

Death

Anointing of sick (mandatory)

Extraordinary artificial means of sustaining life are unnecessary

Texts

Bible

Prayer book

Religious articles

Rosary, crucifix, saints' medals, statues, holy water, lighted candles

Other

Attendance at mass required (seriously ill are exempted) on Sundays or late Saturday and on holy days (1/1, 8/15, 11/1, 12/8, 12/25, and 40 days after Easter)

Sacrament of Penance at least yearly (mandatory)

Opposes abortion

### Russian Orthodox

*See* Eastern Orthodox

### Scientologist

Illness

Believes that "becoming clear" can affect physical and mental health, control weight, etc.

May refuse psychiatric treatment

May request visit by minister, pastoral counselor, or confessor

Text

*Scientology: The Fundamentals of Thought* by L. Ron Hubbard

### Seventh-Day Adventist (Advent Christian Church)

Illness

May desire baptism or Communion

Some believe in divine healing

May oppose hypnosis

May refuse treatment on the Sabbath (sundown Friday to sundown Saturday)

Healthful diet and life-style are stressed

Diet

No alcohol, coffee, tea, narcotics, or stimulants (mandatory)

Some abstain from pork, other meat, and shellfish

Birth

Opposes infant baptism

Text

Bible, especially Ten Commandments and Old Testament

Table II-14. **Overview of Religious Beliefs** (*continued*)

### *Shinto*

Illness

   May believe in prayer healing

   Great concern for personal cleanliness

   Physical health may be valued due to emphasis on joy and beauty of life

   Family extremely important in giving care and providing emotional support

Beliefs

   Worships ancestors, ancient heroes, and nature

   Traditions emphasized

   Esthetically pleasing area for worship important

### *Silva Mind Control*

Type of meditation utilizing various relaxation techniques

Illness

   Believes "sensory projection" can diagnose and cure illness

   All problems are solved through programming the mind for positive action, utilizing dreams and visual exercises

### *Taoist*

Illness

   Illness is seen as part of the health/illness dualism

   May be resigned to and accepting of illness

   May consider medical treatment as interference

Death

   Seen as natural part of life

   Body is kept in house for 49 days

   Mourning follows specific ritual patterns

Text

   *Tao-te-ching* by Lao-tzu

Beliefs

   Esthetically pleasing area for meditation important

### *Transcendental Meditation (TM)*

Form of nonreligious meditation useful in relieving stress

Meditate for 20 minutes once or twice a day using a mantra (special word)

Illness

   Some evidence that TM is useful in treating insomnia, hypertension, obesity

### *Unitarian Universalist*

Illness

   Reason, knowledge, and individual responsibility are emphasized, so may prefer not to see clergy

Birth

   Most do not practice infant baptism

(*continued*)

Table II–14.   **Overview of Religious Beliefs** (*continued*)

---

***Unitarian Universalist*** (*continued*)

Death
   Prefers cremation

***Zen***

Meditation utilizing lotus position (many hours and years are spent in meditation and contemplation); goal is to discover simplicity

Illness
   May wish consultation with Zen master

---

# Spiritual Distress
## Related to Inability to Practice Spiritual Rituals

### Assessment

#### Subjective data
The person expresses one or more of the following feelings related to spiritual belief system

| | |
|---|---|
| Anxiety | Embarrassment |
| Guilt | Sense of loss |
| Depression | Grief |

#### Objective data
Requests spiritual articles, reading materials, sacraments, services, etc.
Questions others about their spiritual rituals
Cannot go to religious services or place of worship
Cannot maintain religious diet or fast
Is separated from religious or spiritual articles, clothing, texts, etc.
Is unable to say prayers or meditate
Is unable to maintain usual contact with spiritual leader or members of spiritual group
Cannot read religious materials
Cannot assume normal position for prayer or meditation

---

**Outcome Criteria**

The person will
  • Continue spiritual practices not detrimental to health
  • Express decreased feelings of guilt and anxiety
  • Express satisfaction with spiritual condition

## Interventions

A. Assess causative and contributing factors

Lack of knowledge of religious restrictions or demands

Fear of imposing upon or antagonizing medical and nursing staff with requests for spiritual rituals

Embarrassment regarding spiritual beliefs or customs (especially common in adolescents)

Separation from articles, texts, or environment of spiritual significance

Limitations related to disease process or treatment regime (*e.g.*, cannot kneel to pray due to traction; cannot vocalize prayers due to laryngectomy)

Lack of transportation to spiritual place or service

B. Eliminate or reduce causative and contributing factors, if possible

1. Fear of imposing upon others
   - Communicate acceptance of various spiritual beliefs and practices
   - Convey nonjudgmental attitude
   - Acknowledge importance of spiritual needs
   - Express willingness of health care team to help in meeting spiritual needs
2. Embarrassment
   a. Provide privacy and quiet as needed for daily prayer, for visit of spiritual leader, and for spiritual reading and contemplation
      - Pull curtains or close door
      - Turn off TV and radio
      - If possible, ask desk to hold phone calls
   b. Contact spiritual leader to clarify religious practices and perform religious rites or services if desired
      - Communicate with spiritual leader regarding person's condition
      - Prevent interruption during visit, if possible
      - Provide table or stand covered with clean white cloth (for most religious statues, etc.; see Table II–14)
      - Chart result of visit
      - Address Roman Catholic, Orthodox, and Episcopal ministers as "Father"; other Christian ministers as "Pastor"; Jewish rabbis as "Rabbi"
   c. Maintain diet with spiritual restrictions when not detrimental to health (see Table II–14)
      - Consult with dietitian
      - Allow fasting for short periods if possible*
      - Change therapeutic diet*
      - Have family or friends bring special food, if possible.
      - Have members of spiritual group supply meals to individual at home
      - Be as flexible as possible in serving methods, times of meals, etc.
3. Separation from articles, texts, or environment of spiritual significance
   a. Question individual about missing religious or spiritual articles or reading material (see Table II–14)
      - Obtain missing items from clergy in hospital, spiritual leader, family, or members of spiritual group

*May require a physician's order.

- Treat these articles and books with respect
- Allow person to keep spiritual articles and books within reach as much as possible, or where they can be easily seen
- Protect from loss or damage (*e.g.*, medal pinned to patient's gown can be lost in laundry)
- Recognize that articles without overt religious meaning may have spiritual significance for individual (*e.g.*, wedding band)
- Utilize spiritual texts in large print, in Braille, or on tape when appropriate

b. Provide opportunity for individual to pray with others or be read to by members of own religious group or member of the health care team who feels comfortable with these activities
- Jews and Seventh-Day Adventists would find Psalms 23, 34, 42, 63, 71, 103, 121, and 127 appropriate
- Christians would also appreciate I Corinthians 13, Matthew 5:3–11, Romans 12, and the Lord's Prayer

4. Lack of transportation
- Take person to chapel or quiet environment on hospital grounds
- Arrange transportation to church or synagogue for individual in home
- Provide access to spiritual programming on radio and television when appropriate

5. Encourage spiritual rituals not detrimental to health (see Table II–14)
- Encourage children to maintain bedtime or before-meal prayer rituals
- Assist individuals with physical limitations in prayer and spiritual observances (*e.g.*, help to hold rosary; help to kneeling position, if appropriate)
- Assist in habits of personal cleanliness
- Avoid shaving if beards are of spiritual significance
- Make special arrangements for burial of limbs or body organs
- Perform baptism for critically ill infant
- Allow family or spiritual leader to perform ritual care of body
- Make arrangements as needed for other important spiritual rituals (*e.g.*, circumcisions, séance)

# Spiritual Distress
## Related to Conflict Between Religious or Spiritual Beliefs and Prescribed Health Regimen

### Assessment

Subjective data

The person expresses one or more feelings related to spiritual beliefs

| | |
|---|---|
| Anxiety | Depression |
| Guilt | Fear of God |
| Grief | Fear of physician |

| | |
|---|---|
| Sense of loss | Dream about angry God or |
| Doubt | minister |
| Sense of powerlessness | Ambivalence in decisions |
| Trapped feeling | |

## Objective data

Questions or refuses therapeutic regimen

Agrees to morally or ethically unacceptable therapy

Frantically seeks advice or support for decision-making

Questions others about their beliefs and values

Experiences insomnia or nightmares

Objects to prescribed or legally required medical procedures (autopsy, blood transfusion, immunization) that conflict with personal spiritual beliefs

Objects to prescribed diet or medication that conflicts with spiritual dietary restrictions

---

**Outcome Criteria**

The person will

- Express religious or spiritual satisfaction
- Express decreased feelings of guilt and fear
- Be supported in his decision regarding his health regimen
- State that conflict has been eliminated or reduced

---

## Interventions

### A. Assess causative and contributing factors (see Table II–14)

Lack of information about or understanding of spiritual restrictions

Lack of information about or understanding of health regimen

Informed, true conflict

Parent conflict regarding treatment of child

Lack of time before emergency treatment or surgery for informed consent

### B. Eliminate or reduce causative and contributing factors if possible

1. Lack of information about spiritual restrictions
   - Have spiritual leader discuss restrictions and exemptions as they apply to those who are seriously ill or hospitalized
   - Provide reading materials on religious and spiritual restrictions and exemptions
   - Encourage person to seek information from and discuss restrictions with others in spiritual group
   - Chart results of these discussions
2. Lack of information about health regimen
   - Provide accurate information about and increased understanding of health regimen, treatments, medications
   - Explain the nature and purpose of therapy
   - Discuss possible outcomes without therapy; be factual and honest but do not attempt to frighten or force person to accept treatment

3. Informed, true conflict
  a. Encourage individual and physician to consider alternate methods of therapy* (*e.g.*, utilization of Christian Science nurses and practitioners; special surgeons and techniques for surgery without blood transfusions)
  b. Support individual making informed decision—even if decision conflicts with own values
  • Consult own spiritual leader
  • Change patient assignments so person can be cared for by nurse with compatible beliefs
  • Arrange for discussions among health care team to share feelings
4. Parent conflict regarding treatment of child
    If parents refuse treatment of child, follow interventions under a and b above
  • If treatment is still refused, physician or hospital administrator may obtain court order appointing temporary guardian to consent to treatment*
  • Call spiritual leader to support parents (and possibly child)
  • Encourage expression of negative feelings
5. Emergency treatment without informed consent
  • Provide as little treatment as possible for Christian Scientists, cult members, etc. (see Table II–14)
  • Delay treatment if possible until spiritual needs have been met (*e.g.*, receiving last rites before surgery)*; send spiritual leader to treatment room or O.R. if necessary
  • Anticipate reaction and provide support when individual chooses to accept or is forced to accept spiritually unacceptable therapy
    a. Depression, withdrawal, anger, fear
    b. Loss of will to live
    c. Reduced speed and quality of recovery

## Bibliography

Ballou RO (ed): The Portable World Bible. New York, Viking Press, 1944

Ellis D: Whatever happened to the spiritual dimension? Canadian Nurse 9(9):42–43, 1980

Fish S, Shelly J: Spiritual Care: The Nurse's Role. Downer's Grove, Intervarsity Press, 1978

Henderson V, Nite G: Worship. In Principles and Practice of Nursing, 6th ed. New York, Macmillan, 1978

Murray R, Zentner J: Religious influences on the person. In Nursing Concepts for Health Promotion, 2nd ed. Englewood Cliffs, NJ, Prentice-Hall, 1979

Pepgras A: The other dimension: Spiritual help. Am J Nurs 68:2610–2612, 1968

Pumphrey JB: Recognizing your patients' spiritual needs. Nursing 7(12):64–70, 1977

Rosten L (ed): Religions of America. New York, Simon & Schuster, 1975

Shannon M: Spiritual needs and nursing responsibility. Imprint 10(12):23, 1980

Smith H: The Religions of Man. New York, Harper & Row, 1958

Stoll RI: Guidelines for spiritual assessment. Am J Nurs 79:1574–1577, 1979

*May require a physician's order.

# Thought Processes, Alterations in

*Related to* **Inability to Evaluate Reality**

## Definition

Alterations in thought processes: A state in which an individual experiences a disruption in such mental activities as conscious thought, reality orientation, problem solving, judgment, and comprehension related to coping (personality and mental) disorders.*

## Etiological and Contributing Factors

### Pathophysiological

Personality and mental disorders related to
Alteration in biochemical compounds
Genetic disorder

### Situational*

Depression or anxiety
Substance abuse (alcohol, drugs)
Fear of the unknown
Actual loss (of control, routine, income, significant others, familiar object or surroundings)
Emotional trauma
Rejection or negative appraisal by others
Negative response from others
Isolation

### Maturational*

Adolescent: Peer pressure, conflict
Elderly: Isolation

## Defining Characteristics

Disoriented in time, place, person
Altered abstraction
Distractibility
Memory deficits
Inaccurate interpretation of stimuli

---

*The diagnosis *Alterations in Thought Processes* describes an individual with cognitive alterations (inaccurate interpretation of the environment) that are the result of personality and mental disorders. This diagnosis differs from the diagnostic category *Sensory-Perceptual Alterations*, which describes an individual with alterations in the amount, pattern, or interpretation of incoming stimuli that are the result of physiological, sensory, motor, or environmental disruptions, not personality and mental disorders.

*These factors should not be considered causative or contributive unless they are present in an individual with a history of coping disorders.

Change in problem-solving abilities
Altered behavior pattern
Regression
Irritability
Fear of others
Fear of losing control
Inappropriate responses
Hallucinations or delusions

## Focus Assessment Criteria

Acquire data from client and significant others

## Subjective data

1. History of the individual
   Life-style

| | |
|---|---|
| Interests | Strengths and limitations |
| Work history | Previous level of functioning and |
| Coping patterns (past and present) | handling stress |

   Support system (availability)
   History of medical problems and treatments (medications)
   Activities of daily living (ability and desire to perform)
2. History of symptoms (onset and duration)

| | |
|---|---|
| Acute or chronic | Continuous or intermittent |
| Sudden or gradual | Time of day |

3. History of unusual sensations and thought productions

| | |
|---|---|
| Precipitating factors | Routine time of occurrence |
| Frequency and duration | Description in individual's own words |

4. Assess for presence of
   Feelings of

| | |
|---|---|
| Extreme sadness and worthlessness | Living in an unreal world |
| Guilt for past actions | Mistrust or suspiciousness of others |
| Apprehension in various situations | Others' making him do and say things |
| Being rejected or isolated | |

   Fears

| | |
|---|---|
| That others will harm him | Of falling apart |
| That mind is being controlled by external agents | Of thoughts racing |
| Of being unable to cope | Of being held prisoner |

   Difficulty concentrating
      Senses difficulty grasping particular circumstances or events
      States he is unable to follow what is being said
   Hallucinations (visual, auditory, gustatory, olfactory, tactile—includes an objective component)
5. Orientation
   Person

| | |
|---|---|
| "What is your name?" | "What is your occupation?" |

Time

"What season is it?"          "What month is it?"

Place

"Where are you?"          "Where do you live?"

6. Problem-solving ability

"What would you do if the phone rang?"

"What is the difference between the doctor and the president?"

## Objective data

1. General appearance

Facial expression (alert, sad, hostile, expressionless)

Dress (meticulous, disheveled, seductive, eccentric)

2. Behavior during interview

| | |
|---|---|
| Withdrawn | Cooperative |
| Hostile | Quiet |
| Apathetic | |

3. Communication pattern

Content

| | |
|---|---|
| Appropriate | Suicidal ideas |
| Rambling | Lacking content |
| Suspicious | Sexual preoccupations |
| Denying problem | Delusionary (grandeur, persecu- |
| Homicidal plans | tion, reference, influence, |
| | control, or bodily sensations) |

Flow of thought

| | |
|---|---|
| Appropriate | Loose connection of ideas |
| Blocking (unable to finish idea) | Jumps from one topic to another |
| Circumstantial (unable to get to | Unable to come to conclusion, be |
| point) | decisive |

Rate of speech

| | |
|---|---|
| Appropriate | Reduced |
| Excessive | Pressured |

Nonverbal behavior

| | |
|---|---|
| Affect appropriate to verbal | Gestures, mannerisms, facial |
| content | grimaces |
| Affect inappropriate to verbal | Posture |
| content | |

4. Interaction skills

With nurse

| | |
|---|---|
| Inappropriate | Shows dependency |
| Relates well | Demanding/pleading |
| Withdrawn/preoccupied | Hostile |

With significant others

| | |
|---|---|
| Relates with all (some) family | Does not seek interaction |
| members | Does not have visitors |
| Hostile toward one (all) members | |

5. Activities of daily living

| | |
|---|---|
| Emotionally capable of self-care | Physically capable of self-care |

6. Nutritional status

| | |
|---|---|
| Appetite | Weight (within normal limits, |
| Eating patterns | decreased, increased) |

7. Sleep/rest pattern

      Recent change               Early wakefulness

      Sleeps too much or too little    Insomnia

8. Personal hygiene

      Cleanliness (body, hair, teeth)    Clothes (condition,

      Grooming (clothes, hair, makeup)    appropriateness)

9. Motor activity

      Within normal limits         Agitated

      Increased                  Repetitive

      Decreased

## Nursing Goals

Through selected interventions, the nurse will seek to

- Improve the individual's ability to define reality
- Teach new methods of coping with stress
- Improve the individual's ability to communicate with others

## Principles and Rationale for Nursing Care

### General

1. Thought is a functioning process of the brain that integrates every individual's daily living experiences.
2. Cognitive processes are the mental processes related to reasoning, comprehension, judgment, and memory.
3. Cognitive function is influenced by physiological functions, stimuli from the environment, and the person's emotional state.
4. The cognitive processes of remembering and perception are influenced by the individual's current needs and interests as well as his fund of knowledge.
5. Development of cognitive abilities follows a systematic pattern of maturational experiences and requires varied perceptual stimulation.
6. A disruption in the quality and quantity of incoming stimuli can affect an individual's thought processes.
7. Psychological equilibrium is enhanced when the individual is able to think clearly and rationally; emotional tension may interfere with rational thinking and behavior.
8. An individual's psychological equilibrium is influenced by his cognitive function, including his perceptions, opinions, attitudes, and beliefs.
9. Actual events frequently become reorganized and reinterpreted individually so that they are substantially changed and distorted during the process of remembering.
10. The ability to conceptualize develops relatively slowly and requires contact with others; the development of concrete concepts precedes the development of abstract concepts.

### Reality

1. Reality testing is the objective evaluation and judgment of the world outside the self, differentiated from one's thoughts and feelings.
2. Reality testing is determined by early life experiences and by significant people in one's life.

3. Delusions—fixed false beliefs—and hallucinations originate during extreme emotional stress when one is unable to cope and reflect underlying feelings.
4. Delusions include those of
> Grandeur: An exaggerated sense of importance of identity or of ability
> Persecution: A sense that one is being harassed
> Reference: Belief that the behavior of others refers to oneself
> Influence: Exaggerated sense of power over others
> Control: Sense that one is being manipulated by others
> Bodily sensations: Belief that one's organs are diseased despite contrary evidence
> Infidelity: Belief, due to pathological jealousy, that one's lover is unfaithful
5. Disorganized thinking often leads to regression in behavior, disturbed communication, and difficulty in interactions with others.

---

# Alterations in Thought Processes
## Related to Inability to Evaluate Reality

---

The inability to evaluate reality is an inability to differentiate one's thoughts and feelings from the actualities of the outside world.

### Assessment

Subjective data

| | |
|---|---|
| Expresses mistrust | Has difficulty concentrating |
| Feels he is being controlled | Accuses others of making him do |
| Fears falling apart | things |

Objective data

| | |
|---|---|
| Delusions | Social isolation |
| Hallucinations | Altered interpersonal |
| Mood alterations | interactions |
| Poor judgment | Poor impulse control |
| Regression (childlike behavior) | Poor hygiene |
| Disturbed communication | |

---

**Outcome Criteria**

The person will
- Identify situations that evoke anxiety
- Describe problems in relating with others
- Differentiate between reality and fantasy
- Describe the rationale for treatment

## Interventions

### A. Promote communication that enhances the person's sense of integrity

1. Encourage open, honest dialogue
   - Approach in a calm nurturing manner
   - Persevere, be consistent
   - Be open and share with the person
   - Discuss expectations and demands
   - Recognize when person is testing the trustworthiness of others
   - Avoid making promises that cannot be filled
   - Explain regular brief contacts (5 to 10 minutes) at first
   - Explain if appointments cannot be kept
   - Verify your interpretation of what person is experiencing ("I understand you are fearful of others")
   - Be an attentive listener; note both verbal and nonverbal messages
   - Help individual verbalize what person indicates nonverbally
   - Utilize terminology that is familiar and evokes little anxiety
   - Recognize the importance of body posture, facial expression, and tone of voice
2. Assist person to clarify his thoughts and avoid misinterpretation
   - Encourage person to assume responsibility for clarifying his thoughts
   - Ask the meaning of communication in an effort to understand what is said or experienced
   - Validate your interpretation of what is said; teach person to do the same
   - Help person gain experience in sharing feelings
   - Recognize that some people mistrust the meaning of words because of past experiences with congruent communication
     a. Help person demonstrate congruence between actions and words
     b. Be congruent in your own verbal and nonverbal messages despite person's distortions
     c. Note trends and themes in the communication and help person understand the messages he imparts

### B. Assist person to define reality and reduce delusions

- Utilize reality therapy
  1. Orient to all three spheres (person, place, time): "What is your name?" "Do you know what today is?"
  2. Encourage individual to check clock or calendar; call him frequently by name
  3. Present information in a matter-of-fact way that is least likely to be misinterpreted
  4. Utilize communication that helps person maintain his own individuality; e.g., "I" instead of "we"
  5. Reduce anxiety-provoking situations that prompt delusional responses
  6. Eliminate whispered comments or incomplete explanations that encourage fantasy interpretation

### C. Assist person to differentiate between reality and delusion

- Direct the focus from delusional expression todiscussion of reality-centered situations
- Encourage person to validate his thoughts by sharing them with significant others
- Avoid derogation or belittling when person misinterprets stimuli or is delusional; do not laugh or make fun of him

- Touch person judiciously to help him identify his separation from others
- Encourage person to identify and focus on his strengths, not his weaknesses
- Encourage differentiation of stimuli arising from inner sources from those from outside (*e.g.*, in respone to "I hear voices," say: "Those are the voices of people on TV" or "I hear no one speaking now; they are your own thoughts")
- Avoid the impression that you confirm or approve reality distortions; tactfully express doubt
- Focus on reality-oriented aspects of the communication; *e.g.*, if person states, "The TV is controlling my mind," the nurse can say, "How does it make you feel when others try to control you?"
- Set limits for discussing repetitive delusional material ("You've already told me about that; let's talk about something realistic")
- Teach person to relearn to focus attention on real things and people
- Help person become aware that his needs are being expressed in fantasy and teach more appropriate ways to meet these needs (*e.g.*, aggression expressed through delusion of persecution can be put into constructive activity such as hammering metal objects)

## D. Encourage a more mature level of functioning

1. Assist person to set limits on his own behavior
   - Discuss alternative methods of coping (*e.g.*, taking a walk instead of crying)
   - Confront person with the attitude that regression is not acceptable behavior
   - Help delay gratification (*e.g.*, "I want you to wait five minutes before you repeat your request for help in making your bed")
   - Encourage person to achieve realistic expectations
   - Pace expectations to avoid frustration
2. Encourage and support person in the decision-making process
   - Help person review options and the advantages and disadvantages of each option
   - Assist in structuring daily living activities (*e.g.*, help schedule bath time before activity hour)
   - Compliment the person who assumes more responsibility
   - Show patience and understanding when a mistake is made
   - Provide opportunity for person to contribute to his own treatment plan
   - Help establish future goals that are realistic; examine problems in achieving a goal and suggest various alternatives
3. Assist person to differentiate between needs and demands
   - Explain the difference between needs and demands (*e.g.*, food and clothing are needs; expectations that others dress and feed him, if he can do it, are demands)
   - Assist person to examine the effects of his behavior on others; encourage a change in behavior if it evokes negative responses
   - Teach negotiation to achieve needs and goals
   - Help person ask for what he wants and tell others how he feels
   - Help person realize that failure of others to meet his needs and demands is not always related to their regard for him

## E. Provide person with opportunities for positive socialization

1. Help him share on a one-to-one basis
   - Be warm, honest, and sincere in interactions
   - Demonstrate that you accept him

- Recognize that some people deny the need for close relationships
- Be sensitive to behaviors that indicate resistance to interpersonal involvement
- Help person know you recognize his uneasiness in social situations ("It must be difficult for you")
- Recognize the person's own use and need for personal space (what he considers his own "turf")
- Use touch judiciously if person fears closeness

2. Help person recognize behaviors that stimulate rejection
   - Identify activities that reduce interpersonal anxiety (*e.g.*, exercise, controlled breathing exercises; see Appendix IV)
   - Set limits firmly and kindly on destructive behavior
   - Allow expression of negative emotions, verbally or in constructive activity
   - Avoid argument, or debate, about delusional ideas or destructive behavior
   - Help person accept responsibility for responses he elicits from others
   - Encourage discussion of problems in relating after visits with family members
   - Help person test new skills in relating to others in role-playing situations

## F. Promote physical well-being and prevent injury

1. Explain and monitor medication regimen
   - Assess person's ability to remember to take medications
   - Assist person to remember to take medications by color coding each bottle with a sticker and writing out the times of the day that medications are prescribed for, with the appropriate color sticker next to the time
   - Teach about the purpose of medications and their side-effects
   - Encourage person to report all physical symptoms

2. Monitor nutritional intake
   - Observe eating habits (amount, selection, frequency, food preferences and dislikes, appetite)
   - Note weight gain or loss
   - Discuss adequate nutrition in relation to activity level
   - Allow person to choose food he especially likes; contract with individual who eats predominantly snack foods (*e.g.*, "If you eat one egg you can order a doughnut")
   - Note delusions regarding food or body that might interfere with nutritional intake
   - Refer to *Alterations in Nutrition* for additional interventions

3. Assess ability for self-care activities
   - Identify areas of physical care for which person needs assistance (sleep and rest, nutrition, bathing, dressing, elimination, exercise)
   - Note person's motivation and interest in appearance
   - Teach skills required to assume responsibility for self-care
   - Assist person in planning his daily routines in order to foster independence and responsibility
   - Refer to *Self-Care Deficit* for additional interventions

## G. Identify a potential for violence

- Be cognizant of physical safety
- Prevent trauma from aggression or suicide; identify harmful or destructive behavior that requires attention

- Identify cues to suicide
    Sudden changes in mood or behavior
    Report of plan to harm oneself
    Report of voices directing person to harm himself or others
- Observe closely for changes in behavior; increase vigilance
- Share with personnel the individual's potential for self-harm
- Note delusions indicative of aggressive impulses ("Those Russian spies are going to attack me tonight")
- Interview family and note approaches that have been beneficial in the past in controlling aggression
- Reduce anxiety and develop a sense of safety through a climate of care and concern
- Remove excessive stimulation and provide a safe environment
- Refer to *Potential for Violence* for additional interventions for suicide precautions

## H. Initiate health teaching and referrals as indicated

- Anticipate difficulties in adjusting to community living; discuss concerns about returning to community and elicit family reaction to individual's discharge
- Provide health teaching that will prepare person to deal with life stresses (methods of relaxation, problem-solving skills, how to negotiate with others, how to express feelings constructively)
- Review signs and symptoms of recurrent illness that indicate impending maladjustment
- Review purpose of medication and how to report side-effects
- Refer to other professions for assistance
    1. To occupational therapist to learn leisure-time activities
    2. To industrial therapist to improve or learn new job skills
    3. To social worker to discuss living arrangements, financial problems, or family negotiations
- Supply phone number and address of local mental health clinic
- Inform individual of social agencies that offer help in adjusting to community living
    1. General social agencies
        Mental health and mental retardation centers
        Mental Health Association
        HELP (alternative to mental health center)
        Family Service (family counseling)
        Drug rehabilitation centers
    2. Specific social agencies
        Alcoholics Anonymous
        Gray Panthers
        Suicide Crisis Intervention Center
        Synanon
        Contact

## Bibliography

Arnold HM: Working with schizophrenic patients. Four A's: A guide to one-to-one relationships. Am J Nurs 76:941–943, 1976

Bayer M: The multipurpose room: A way-out outlet for staff and clients. J Psychiatr Nurs 18(10):35–37, 1980

Dixon B: Intervening when the patient is delusional. J Psychiatr Nurs 7(1):25–34, 1969

Haber J, Leach A, Schudy S et al: Comprehensive Textbook of Psychiatric Nursing, pp 220–245, New York, McGraw-Hill, 1978

Knowles RD: Disputing Irrational Thought. Am J Nurs 81:735, 1981

Kreigh H, Perko J: Psychiatric and Mental Health Nursing: A Commitment to Cure and Concern, pp 195–203. Reston, VA, Reston Publishing, 1979

O'Brien J: Teaching psychiatric inpatients about their medications. J Psychiatr Nurs 17(10):30–32, 1979

Schroeder PJ: Nursing interventions with patients with thought disorders. Perspect Psychiatr Care 17(1):32–39, 1979

Schwartzman ST: The hallucinating patient and nursing intervention. J Psychiatr Nurs 13(6):23–28, 33–36, 1976

Smith JE: Improving drug knowledge. J Psychiatr Nurs 19(4):1916–1918, 1981

# Tissue Perfusion, Alteration in:

*Peripheral:* **Secondary to (specify)**
*Cerebral:* **Orthostatic Hypotension**

## Definition

Alteration in tissue perfusion: The state in which the individual experiences or is at risk of experiencing a decrease in nutrition and respiration at the cellular level due to a decrease in capillary blood supply.*

## Etiological and Contributing Factors

### Physiological

Cardiovascular disorders

    Decreased cardiac output

    Cerebrovascular accident (CVA)

    Transient ischemic attacks (TIA)

    Arteriosclerotic vascular disease (ASVD)

    Atherosclerosis

    Myocardial infarction (MI)

    Angina

    Congestive heart failure

    Pulmonary edema

    Varicosities

    Vasospasm or vasoconstriction

    Hypertension

Diabetes mellitus

Hypotension

    Orthostatic

    Neurogenic

    Hypovolemic

    Drug induced

    Septic shock

    Anaphylactic shock

    Hypoglycemia

    Hyperglycemia

Blood dyscrasias

    Anemia

    Polycythemia

    DIC (disseminating intravascular coagulation)

    Thrombus

    Embolus

    Hemolysis (*e.g.*, transfusion reaction)

    Sickle cell disease

Renal failure

Cancer or tumor

Edema or inflammation

---

*The use of this diagnostic category should not include the treatment of decreased tissue perfusion (which is a medical problem) but focuses on the functional abilities of the individual that are compromised because of decreased tissue perfusion. To represent this relationship, the diagnosis is linked by a colon (:) and not by the phrase "related to." The use of "related to" would label a clinical situation that is more medical than nursing, as with the title "Alteration in Tissue Perfusion: Cardiac, Related to Congestive Heart Failure." The nurse can diagnose and treat certain responses to impaired tissue perfusion, in which case the diagnosis can be structured accordingly. For example, *Alteration in Tissue Perfusion: Cerebral: Orthostatic Hypotension* or *Alteration in Tissue Perfusion: Renal: Fatigue.*

## Situational

Presence of invasive lines, *e.g.*, IVs, Foley catheter (predisposes to thrombi and sepsis)
Prolonged immobility or bedrest
Pressure sites (*e.g.*, decubiti, casts, Ace bandages, tourniquets)
Sudden change from lying or sitting to standing
Dependent venous pooling (predisposes to thrombus formation)
Medications (*e.g.*, diuretics, tranquilizers, insulin)
Anesthesia (causes vasodilation)
Blood vessel trauma or compression
Pregnancy or oral contraception (predisposes to thrombus formation)
Hypothermia (*e.g.*, exposure to cold)
Obesity (poor circulation)
Anorexia or malnutrition

## Maturational

Neonate
  Immature peripheral circulation
  Rh incompatibility (erythroblastosis fetalis)
  Hypothermia
Elderly
  Venous and arterial capillary fragility
  Brittle, hard vessels (due to chronic ASVD)

## Defining Characteristics

### Peripheral

| | |
|---|---|
| Loss of motor function | Flushing |
| Loss of sensory function | Claudication (leg pain on |
| Tissue necrosis (gangrene) | walking, relieved by rest) |
| Coolness of skin | Decreased pulse quality |
| Pallor | Edema |
| Cyanosis | Lack of lanugo hair |

### Cardiopulmonary

| | |
|---|---|
| Tachycardia | Angina (relieved by rest) |
| Tachypnea | Dyspnea |

### Cerebral

| | |
|---|---|
| Restlessness | Memory losses |
| Confusion | Altered level of consciousness |
| Altered thought processes | |

### Gastrointestinal

| | |
|---|---|
| Constipation | Nausea or vomiting |

### Renal

| | |
|---|---|
| Edema | Decreased urinary output |

## Principles and Rationale for Nursing Care

### Blood pressure

1. Blood pressure (necessary for tissue perfusion) is dependent upon two factors: the force of the flow of blood (cardiac output), and the diameter of the blood vessel.

2. Blood pressure is affected by the sympathetic and parasympathetic nervous systems. The *sympathetic nervous system increases blood pressure* by increasing heart rate and ventricular contraction (thereby increasing cardiac output and increasing the force of blood flow) and by controlling the diameter of the arterioles and resistance of blood vessels (*i.e.*, blood vessel constriction). The *parasympathetic nervous system decreases blood pressure* by relaxation of the vessel walls and by vagal stimulation, causing a decreased heart rate (thereby decreasing cardiac output and decreasing the force of blood flow).
3. Blood pressure is dependent upon adequate circulating blood volume (*i.e.*, dehydration predisposes one to hypotension).
4. Constricted vessels cause a rise in blood pressure, while dilated vessels cause a drop in blood pressure.
5. *Systolic blood pressure* is dependent upon cardiac stroke volume (pressure within the vessels while the heart is contracting).
6. *Diastolic blood pressure* is dependent upon the condition of the vessels while the heart is at rest (vessel resistance).

## Cellular perfusion

1. Cellular nutrition and respiration are dependent on adequate blood flow through the microcirculation.
2. Adequate cellular oxygenation is dependent upon following processes:
   The ability of the lungs to exchange air adequately ($O_2$–$CO_2$)
   The ability of the pulmonary alveoli to diffuse oxygen and carbon dioxide across the cell membrane to the blood
   The ability of the red blood cells (hemoglobin) to carry oxygen
   The ability of the heart to pump with enough force to deliver the blood to the microcirculation
   The ability of intact blood vessels to deliver blood to the microcirculation
3. Hypoxemia (decreased oxygen content of the blood) results in cellular hypoxia, which causes cellular swelling and contributes to tissue injury.
4. Obstruction of blood flow can be a result of
   Clot formation (thrombus)
   Embolus (air, fat, thrombi, other)
   Blood vessel injury (*e.g.*, trauma)
   Pressure upon the vessels (*e.g.*, tourniquet, edema)
   Structural changes in the vessels (*e.g.*, arteriovascular disease)
   Vasospasm
5. *Arterial* blood flow is enhanced by a *dependent* position and inhibited by an *elevated* position (gravity pulls blood downward, away from the heart).
6. *Venous* blood flow is enhanced by an *elevated* position and inhibited by a *dependent* position (gravity pulls blood downward toward the heart).
7. Immobility and venostasis predispose one to thrombus and embolus production.

## Hypotension

1. Hypotension causes impaired tissue perfusion of all body organs.
2. The length of time that tissue can survive without adequate blood supply (perfusion) is determined by the tissue type and the metabolic needs of the cell: the heart, brain, lungs, and kidneys may suffer the most catastrophic results, while extremities may tolerate hypotension for quite a long time without problems.
3. Metabolic needs, are reduced by hypothermia and increased by hyperthermia (fever).

4. Decreased tissue perfusion (hypotension) causes cellular hypoxia, resulting in ischemia, cellular swelling, and eventually cellular death.
5. Orthostatic hypotension (a sudden drop in blood pressure when going from a lying or sitting position to a standing position) is frequently seen associated with

> Decreased blood volume or dehydration
> Prolonged immobility or bedrest
> Aging
> Impaired skeletal muscle function
> Severe varicose veins
> Medications (diuretics, antihypertensives, vasodilators, antipsychotics, and anti-Parkinsonian drugs)

6. Prolonged bedrest causes skeletal muscle weakness and decreased venous tone, predisposing the individual to orthostatic hypotension.

## Focus Assessment Criteria

### Subjective data

1. Symptoms
   Complaints of

   | | |
   |---|---|
   | Pain | Numbness |
   | Shortness of breath | Vertigo |
   | Tingling | Headache |

   Onset and duration

   | | |
   |---|---|
   | Location | Precipitated by what? |
   | Description | Relieved by what? |
   | Frequency | Aggravated by what? |

2. Medical history
   Presence of

   | | |
   |---|---|
   | Hypertension | Lung disease |
   | Diabetes mellitus | Kidney disease |
   | Heart disease | Anemia |

3. Risk factors

   | | |
   |---|---|
   | Alcoholism | Sedentary life |
   | Smoking | Overweight |
   | Immobility | |

4. Medications (type, dosage, presence of side-effects)

### Objective data

1. Thought processes

   | | |
   |---|---|
   | Clear | Disoriented |
   | Oriented to time, person, place | Slow |
   | Confused | |

2. Memory

   | | |
   |---|---|
   | For recent events | For past events |

3. Pupils (compare right and left)

   | | |
   |---|---|
   | Size (pinpoint, normal, dilated) | Reaction to light (normal, slow, none) |

4. Respirations (rate, quality)
5. Heart (rate, rhythm)
6. Blood pressure (compare right and left arms)

   | | |
   |---|---|
   | Lying down | Standing |
   | Sitting | Pulse pressure |

7. Peripheral pulse (rhythm, rate, volume*)

    Brachial                  Popliteal

    Radial                     Posterior tibial

    Femoral                Pedal

8. Apical rate compared with brachial, radial, femoral, popliteal, posterior tibial, and pedal pulses

9. Intermittent claudication determination: Number of steps the person is able to climb before feeling pain (pain felt within one minute may be indicative of arterial occlusion)

10. Skin

    Color (normal capillary refill        Turgor

        time is < 3 seconds)           Condition (*e.g.,* lesions)

    Temperature

11. Diagnostic studies (electrolytes, CBC, x-rays, ABGs, BUN and creatinine, Doppler ultrasound)

# Alteration in Tissue Perfusion:
## Peripheral: Secondary to (Specify)[†]

## Assessment

### Subjective data

History of

    Diabetes

    Phlebitis

    Arteriosclerotic heart disease

    Painful extremities (either unrelieved pain or pain brought on by activity and alleviated by rest)

The person reports

    Pain, cramping

    Numbness, tingling, burning

### Objective data

    Decreased or absent arterial pulse equality (radial, femoral, popliteal, pedal, posterior tibial)

    Peripheral edema

    Enlarged, bulging leg veins

---

*A useful method for recording peripheral pulse volume is based on a scale from 0 to +4, as follows:

  0    Nonpalpable: absent pulsations

+1    Thready, weak, fades in and out: marked impairment of pulsations

+2    Difficult to palpate, stronger than +1: moderate impairment

+3    Easily palpable, not easily obliterated with pressure: slight impairment

+4    Strong and bounding: normal pulsations

†For example, *Alteration in Tissue Perfusion: Peripheral: Secondary to Diabetes Mellitus.*

Changes in temperature and color of the involved extremity (coolness or blanching; warmth, erythema accompanied by swelling; cyanosis or pallor; blackening of skin)

---

**Outcome Criteria**

The person will
- Demonstrate improved peripheral circulation
- Relate factors that improve peripheral circulation
- Relate factors that inhibit peripheral circulation

---

## Interventions

### A. Assess causative factors

Inhibited arterial blood flow
Inhibited venous blood flow
Decreased cardiac output
Fluid volume excess or deficit
Hypothermia or vasoconstriction

### B. Promote factors that improve arterial blood flow

1. Keep extremity in a *dependent* position (*i.e.*, extremity lower than the heart if there is not an associated venous problem)
2. Keep extremities warm to increase circulation, but discourage use of external heat sources, since person may have decreased sensation and be prone to burns
3. Eliminate or reduce pressure points
   - Change positions frequently (at least every hour)
   - Discourage leg crossing or sitting for long periods of time
   - Reduce external pressure points (*e.g.*, tight cast edges)
   - Use sheepskins for heels, elbows
   - Encourage person to wiggle fingers and toes every hour or do range-of-motion exercises
   - Use a foot cradle to keep covers off extremities
4. Plan a daily walking program and gradually increase rate and length of walk if person is able
   a. Instruct him to
      - Avoid becoming overly fatigued
      - Stop immediately in the presence of lightness or pain in chest, severe breathlessness, lightheadedness, dizziness, loss of muscle control, or nausea
      - Delay walking for at least 2 hours after meals
      - Refrain from drinking liquids containing caffeine (coffee, tea, chocolate, cola) at least two hours before walking
      - Expect muscle soreness but not pain
   b. Start individual at 1 to 5 blocks a day and increase 1 block or 0.1 mile a week; instruct to lessen length or rate if any of the following occur
      Pulse is 120 beats per minute 5 minutes after stopping exercise
      Pulse is 100 beats per minute 10 minutes after stopping exercise
      Person is short of breath 10 minutes after exercise
      Pain

   c. If person is unable to walk 5 blocks or 0.5 mile without signs of overexertion appearing, decrease length of walking to before signs appear for 1 week and then start to add 1 block or 0.1 mile each week

   d. Have person walk at same rate (use stop watch or second hand on watch); after reaching 10 blocks (1 mile) try to increase speed
  - Increase only rate *or* length of walk at one time
  - Establish a regular time of day to walk, with the goal of 3 to 5 times per week for a duration of 15 to 45 minutes

## C. Promote factors that increase venous blood flow

1. Elevate the extremity *above* the level of the heart (may be contraindicated in congestive heart failure)
2. Consider use of Ace bandages or antiembolus stockings to promote venous return
3. Reduce or remove venous pressure points
   - Do not allow pillows behind knees or Gatch bed elevated at the knees
   - Discourage leg crossing or sitting for long periods of time
   - Instruct person to change positions, move extremity, or wiggle fingers and toes every hour (unless contraindicated)
   - See *Fluid Volume Excess Related to Edema* for additional interventions
4. Use a foot cradle to keep covers off extremity

## D. Initiate health teaching as indicated

1. Instruct to keep dry skin lubricated; use gentle massage for pressure points (do not massage if there is a history of emboli)
2. Keep dressings clean and dry
3. Give special attention to feet and toes
   - Wash and dry feet daily or soak feet in warm water several times a day
   - Inspect feet and legs daily for injuries
   - Wear clean socks
   - Wear shoes that fit comfortably
4. Wear warm clothing (*e.g.*, socks and boots) during cold weather to avoid exposure to cold
5. Eat three balanced meals with sufficient protein and high vitamin C (preferably low cholesterol)
6. See *Impairment of Skin Integrity* for additional interventions

# Alteration in Tissue Perfusion:
## Cerebral: Orthostatic Hypotension

### Assessment

Subjective data

The person reports the following (in association with sudden position change)
    "I black out"
    "I get dizzy"
    "I feel faint"

## Objective data

Supine blood pressure is greater than sitting blood pressure, which is greater on standing

---

**Outcome Criteria**

The person will
- Relate fewer symptoms of vertigo
- Relate methods of preventing sudden decreases in cerebral blood flow

---

## Interventions

A. Identify factors that contribute to orthostatic hypotension

Medications (antihypertensives, diuretics, phenothiazines, barbiturates)
Prolonged recumbent position
Cardiac arrhythmias
Sudden changes in position (from lying to sitting or standing)
Hyperextension of the neck

B. Assess for orthostatic hypotension
- Take a blood pressure reading when person is supine
- Take an immediate blood pressure reading when person sits upright or stands (use assistant to prevent injury in case of fall)

C. Discuss the relationship between blood pressure in a recumbent position and when sitting or standing and its effects on cerebral blood flow; teach techniques to improve cerebral blood flow
- Sleep sitting up or in an elevated position
- Get out of bed slowly (first sit up, then swing legs down; rest a few minutes; then get out of bed slowly, and proceed to walk slowly)
- Use waist-high elastic stockings
    1. While in bed, raise legs for several minutes to promote blood return
    2. Slowly apply stockings evenly, checking for twisting or tightness
    3. Remove stockings when supine and reapply before rising
    4. Remove stockings at least every 8 hours or per physician's advice
        - Avoid straining (lifting; sudden hyperextension of neck; activity immediately after eating)
        - Avoid over-the-counter medications with pressor effects (*e.g.*, cold medications, antihistamines, nasal sprays, diet pills)

D. Encourage person to increase daily activity if permissible
- Discuss the value of daily exercise (increases circulation, decreases the process of osteoporosis, increases energy levels, reduces stress, and contributes to an overall state of well-being)
- Establish an exercise program

E. Teach person precautions to avoid injury
- Discuss the potential hazards of hypotension (drinking, smoking, cooking)
- Teach person to increase fluid intake during periods of excess fluid loss (diaphoresis, exercise)

· Discuss factors that increase vasodilation (alcohol—initially, then followed by vasoconstriction; extreme warmth)

## Bibliography

Adelman EM: When the patient's blood pressure falls: What does it mean? What do you do? Nursing 10(2):26, 1980

Alfaro R: Pneumatic antishock trousers, how and when to use them. Dimensions in Critical Care Nursing 1(1):7–16, 1982

Alwood A: Cerebral artery bypass surgery. Am J Nurs 80:1284–1287, 1980

Bates B: A Guide to Physical Examination. Philadelphia, JB Lippincott, 1980

Dossey B: Pulmonary embolism: Preventing it, treating it. Nursing 11(3):26–30, 1981

Doyle J: If your legs hurt the reason may be arterial insufficiency. Nursing 11(4):74–79, 1981

Hill M: Seeking and finding all those patients with high blood pressure. Nursing 12(2):72–75, 1982

Lamb L: Think you know septic shock? Read this. Nursing 12(1):34–43, 1982

Milazzo V: An exercise class for patients in traction. Am J Nurs 81:1842–1844, 1981

Programmed instruction: New concepts in understanding congestive heart failure. Part I: How the clinical features arise. Am J Nurs 81:119–141, 1981

Programmed instruction: New concepts in understanding congestive failure. Part II: How therapeutic approaches work. Am J Nurs 81:357–380, 1981

Thompson D: Teaching the client about anticoagulants. Am J Nurs 82:278–281, 1982

Tucker P: Ups and downs in septic shock. Nursing 12(1):43, 1982

Wade DW: Teaching patients to live with chronic orthostatic hypotension. Nursing 12(7):64–65, 1982

# Urinary Elimination, Alteration in Patterns of

*Related to* **Enuresis (Maturational)**

*Related to* **Dysuria**

*Related to* **Incontinence**

## Definition

Alteration in patterns of urinary elimination: The state in which the individual experiences or is at risk of experiencing urinary dysfunction.*

## Etiological and Contributing Factors

Pathophysiological

Congenital urinary tract anomolies
|  |  |
|---|---|
| Strictures | Bladder-neck contracture |
| Hypospadias or epispadias | Megalocystis (large-capacity bladder without tone) |
| Ureterocele | |

Disorders of the urinary tract
|  |  |
|---|---|
| Infection | Calculi |

Neurogenic disorders or injury
|  |  |
|---|---|
| Cord injury | Multiple sclerosis |
| Brain tumor | Demyelinating diseases |
| Cerebrovascular accident | |

Prostatic enlargement

Estrogen deficiency
|  |  |
|---|---|
| Vaginitis | Atrophic urethritis |

Situational

Loss of perineal tissue tone
|  |  |
|---|---|
| Scarring of perineal area | Childbirth |
| Obesity | Aging |
| Recent substantial weight loss | Post prostatectomy |

Fecal impaction

Dehydration

Drug therapy
|  |  |
|---|---|
| Antihistamines | Immunosuppressant therapy (chemotherapy) |
| Epinephrine | |
| Anticholinergics | Diuretics |

Irritation to perineal area
|  |  |
|---|---|
| Sexual activity | Diagnostic instrumentation |
| Poor personal hygiene | |

*This diagnostic category pertains to alterations of urine elimination, not urine formation. Nurses can diagnose and treat an alteration in patterns of elimination independently, but they cannot alter polyuria, retention, anuria, and oliguria with independent nursing interventions.

Pregnancy
General or spinal anesthesia
Inability to communicate needs
Lack of privacy
Decreased attention to bladder cues

|                |            |
|----------------|------------|
| Sedatives      | Depression |
| Tranquilizers  | Confusion  |

Foley catheters
Stress or fear
Environmental barriers to bathroom

|                   |             |
|-------------------|-------------|
| Distant toilets   | Bed too high |
| Poor lighting     | Side rails  |

## Maturational

Child: Small bladder capacity, lack of motivation
Elderly: Motor and sensory losses, loss of muscle tone, inability to communicate needs, depression

## Defining Characteristics

|                    |                    |
|--------------------|--------------------|
| Dysuria            | Enuresis           |
| Urgency            | Dribbling          |
| Frequency          | Bladder distention |
| Hesitancy          | Incontinence       |
| Nocturia           |                    |

## Focus Assessment Criteria

### Subjective data

1. History of symptoms
    Complaints of

|                   |                           |
|-------------------|---------------------------|
| Lack of control   | Frequency                 |
| Dribbling         | Pain or discomfort        |
| Hesitancy         | Burning                   |
| Urgency           | Change in voiding pattern |

Onset and duration
Description
Frequency
Precipitated by what?
Relieved by what?
Aggravated by what?
Effects on life-style

|               |                    |
|---------------|--------------------|
| Social        | Sexual             |
| Occupational  | Role responsibilities |

2. Incontinence (adult)
    Onset and pattern (day, night)
    History

|                              |                        |
|------------------------------|------------------------|
| Urinary disorders            | Prostate problems      |
| Kidney or bladder disorders  | Neurological disorders |

Perception of need to void

|             |        |
|-------------|--------|
| Present     | Absent |
| Diminished  |        |

Ability to delay urination after urge
    Present (how long?)               Absent
Sensations occurring before or during micturition
    Difficulty starting stream        Need to force urine out
    Difficulty stopping stream       Lack of sensation to void
    Painful straining (tenesmus)
Relief after voiding
    Complete                  Continued desire to void after
                                    bladder is emptied

3. Enuresis (child)
    Onset and pattern (day, night)
    Toilet training history
    Family history of bed-wetting
    Response of others to child (parents, siblings, peers)

## Objective data

1. Urination stream

| | |
|---|---|
| Slow | Sprays |
| Small | Starts and stops |
| Drops | Slow or hard to start |

2. Urine
    Color

| | |
|---|---|
| Yellow | Yellow brown |
| Amber | Green brown |
| Straw colored | Dark brown |
| Red brown | Black |

    Odor

| | |
|---|---|
| Faint | Offensive |
| Ammoniac | Acetonic (sweet) |

    Appearance (clear or cloudy)
    Reaction (normal—4.6 to 7.5—or alkaline—$> 7.5$)
    Specific gravity

| | |
|---|---|
| Dilute ($< 1.003$) | Concentrated ($> 1.025$) |
| Normal (1.003–1.025) | |

    Negative or positive for

| | |
|---|---|
| Glucose | Bacteria |
| Protein | Red blood cells |
| Ketone | |

3. Voiding and fluid intake patterns (record for 2 to 4 days to establish a baseline)
    What is daily fluid intake?
    When does incontinence occur?
4. Muscle tone
    Abdomen firm, or soft and pendulous?
    History of recent significant weight loss?
5. Bladder
    Distention (palpable)
    Can it be emptied by external stimuli? (Credé's method: warm water over the
        perineum)
    Capacity (at least 300–350 ml)
6. Residual urine

| | |
|---|---|
| None | Present (amount) |

7. Assess for presence of

| | |
|---|---|
| Constipation | Depression |
| Fecal impaction | Mobility disorders |
| Dehydration | Sensory disorders |

8. Diagnostic studies

Urinalysis; culture and sensitivity

Blood (creatinine, urea nitrogen)

Roentgenograms (intravenous pyelogram; kidney, ureters, bladder; cystometrogram)

Electromyography of the muscles of the external urinary sphincter and muscles of the pelvic floor

## Nursing Goals

Through selected interventions, the nurse will assist the individual to
- Alleviate symptoms and prevent complications
- Maintain skin integrity
- Establish (or re-establish) control over micturition

The nurse will assist the child to
- Remain dry during his sleep cycle

The nurse will assist the parents to
- Respond constructively to enuresis

## Principles and Rationale for Nursing Care

### Anatomy and physiology

1. The kidneys produce urine while the rest of the urinary system serves as drainage or storage until the urine is excreted.
2. Innervation of the bladder arises from the spinal cord at the sacral levels of 2, 3, and 4.
3. The bladder is under parasympathetic control.
4. Voluntary control over urination is influenced by the cortex, midbrain, and medulla.
5. The female urethra is 3 cm to 5 cm long. The male urethra is approximately 20 cm long.
6. Continence is maintained primarily by the urethra.
7. Capacity of the normal bladder (without experiencing discomfort) is 250 cc to 400 cc.

### Urination

1. During urination there is simultaneous relaxation of the external urinary sphincter and contraction of the bladder.
2. The sitting position for the female and the standing position for the male allow for optimal relaxation of the external urinary sphincter and perineal muscles.
3. The desire to void occurs when there is 150 cc to 250 cc of urine in the bladder.
4. Stress, anger, and anxiety can inhibit relaxation of the urinary sphincter.
5. Bladder tissue tone can be lost if the bladder is distended to 1000 cc (atonic bladder) or continuously drained (Foley catheter).
6. Mechanisms to stimulate the voiding reflex or Credé's method may be ineffective if the bladder capacity is less than 200 cc.
7. Alcohol, coffee, and tea have a natural diuretic effect and are bladder irritants.

8. Injury to the spinal cord above sacral 2, 3, 4 produces a spastic or reflex bladder tone.
9. Injury to the spinal cord below sacral 2, 3, 4 produces a flaccid or atonic bladder.

## Enuresis (involuntary voiding during sleep)

1. Enuresis before the age of four may be physiological. Causes include a small bladder, structural disorders of the urinary tract, infection, diabetes (mellitus, insipidus), and nocturnal epilepsy.
2. Enuresis after the age of four may be physiological or maturational. Common contributing factors are the arrival of a new sibling and being a deep sleeper.
3. Enuresis is primarily a maturational problem and usually ceases between six and eight years of age. It is more common in boys.
4. There is a high frequency of bed-wetting in children whose parents or other near relatives were bed-wetters.
5. Behavioral problems usually are not the cause of enuresis but may result from lack of understanding or insensitivity to the problem. The child should not be punished or shamed but motivated toward control.

## Infection

1. Stasis or pooling of urine contributes to bacterial growth.
2. Bacteria can travel up the ureters to the kidney (ascending infection).
3. Recurrent bladder infections cause fibrotic changes in the bladder wall with resultant decrease in bladder capacity.
4. Urinary stasis, infections, alkaline urine, and decreased urine volume contribute to the formation of urinary tract calculi.
5. Dilute acid urine helps prevent infection and allows for solubility of inorganic materials.

## The elderly

1. Frequent voiding out of habit may contribute to urgency in the elderly because the bladder is rarely fully expanded.
2. Persons with diabetes mellitus, which can contribute to increased residual urine, frequency, and urgency, may be less aware of bladder fullness.
3. Aging can contribute to urinary incontinence by diminishing the ability of the kidney to concentrate urine (nocturia), decreasing bladder capacity (frequency), and decreasing muscle tone of the pelvic floor (stress incontinence).
4. The diminished vision, impaired mobility, and decreased energy level that may accompany aging mean increased time is needed to locate the toilet, which also requires the person to be able to delay urination.

## Incontinence

1. At least 60% of all incontinence can be reversed if the nurse aggressively assesses for the factors that contribute to it.
2. Incontinence can be either reversible or controllable. Controllable incontinence cannot be cured, but urine removal can be planned.
3. Stress incontinence is the leakage of a small amount of urine when the urethral outlet is unable to control its passage in the presence of increased intra-abdominal pressure (coughing, sneezing, laughing, and bending).
4. In stress incontinence the pelvic floor muscles have been weakened or stretched by childbirth trauma, menopausal atrophy, or obesity.

5. Obstruction of the bladder neck that progresses to bladder distention and overflow (incontinence) can be caused by fecal impactions and enlarged prostate glands.

6. Dehydration can cause incontinence by eliminating the sensation of a full bladder (the signal to urinate) and also by reducing the person's alertness to the sensation.

7. Social isolation of incontinent persons can be self-imposed, because of fear and embarrassment, or imposed by others, because of odor and esthetics.

8. Depression can prevent the person from recognizing or responding to bladder cues and thus contributes to incontinence.

9. Warning time is the amount of time the individual can delay urination after the urge to void is felt.

10. Older persons experience urgency (shortened warning time) owing to the bladder's limited capacity and their decreased ability to inhibit bladder contractions.

11. Diminished warning time can cause incontinence if the person is unable to reach a toilet in time.

12. Factors contributing to urgency include acute urinary tract infections, neurologic impairments (as when CVA causes a decreased ability to inhibit contractions), diuretics, diabetes mellitus, inadequate fluid intake or habitual frequent voiding (which contribute to a limited bladder capacity), and confusion.

## Intermittent catheterization

1. Intermittent self-catheterization is the periodic drainage of urine by the individual by the use of a catheter in the bladder.

2. Intermittent catheterization when performed in a health care facility should follow aseptic technique because the organisms present in such a facility are more virulent and resistant to drugs than organisms found outside. Persons at home can practice clean technique because of the lack of virulent organisms in the home environment.

3. The initial removal of more than 500 ml of urine from a chronically distended bladder can cause severe bladder hemorrhage which results when bladder veins, previously compressed by the distended bladder, rapidly dilate and rupture when bladder pressure is abruptly released. (After the initial release of 500 ml of urine, alternate the release of 100 ml of urine with 15-minute catheter clamps.)

4. An overdistended bladder reduces blood flow to the bladder wall, which makes it more susceptible to infection from normal intestinal flow.

5. Stasis of urine contributes to bacterial growth.

6. The accumulation of more than 500 ml to 700 ml of urine in a bladder should not be permitted.

7. Intermittent catheterization provides for a decrease in morbidity associated with long-term use of indwelling catheters, increased independence, a more positive self-concept, and more normal sexual relations.

# Alteration in Patterns of Urinary Elimination
Related to Enuresis (Maturational)

Enuresis (maturational) is involuntary voiding that occurs in children during sleep and is not pathophysiological in origin.

## Assessment

### Subjective data
Parent reports
    The child is wetting the bed at night
    The child is reluctant (too busy) to visit toilet before going to bed
    The child was toilet trained at a very early age
    The child is a sound sleeper

### Objective data
Small bladder, <300 ml (instruct child to hold off urination as long as possible, then measure and record voided specimen; measure and record at least three specimens)

---

**Outcome Criteria**
  • The child will remain dry during the sleep cycle
  • The child or family will be able to state the nature and causes of enuresis

---

## Interventions

### A. Assess for contributing factors
Small bladder capacity
Sound sleeper
Response to stress (at school or at home; *e.g.*, new sibling)

### B. Promote a positive parent-child relationship
• Explain the nature of enuresis to parents and child
• Explain to parents that disapproval (shaming, punishing) is useless in stopping enuresis but can make child shy, ashamed, and afraid
• Offer reassurance to child that other children wet the bed at night and he is not bad or sinful

### C. Reduce contributing factors if possible
1. Small bladder capacity
    • After child drinks fluids, encourage him to postpone voiding to help stretch the bladder
2. Sound sleeper
    • Have child void prior to retiring
    • Restrict fluids at bedtime
    • If child is awakened later (about 11 p.m.) to void, attempt to awaken child fully for positive reinforcement

3. Too busy to sense a full bladder (if daytime wetting occurs)
   - Teach child awareness of sensations that occur when it is time to void
   - Teach child the ability to control urination (have him start and stop the stream; have him "hold" the urine during the day, even if for only a short time)
   - Have child keep a record of how he is doing; emphasize dry days or nights (*e.g.*, stars on a calendar)
   - If child wets, have him explain or write down, if he can, why he thinks it happened

D. Initiate health teaching and referrals as indicated

1. For children with enuresis
   - Teach child and parents the facts about enuresis
   - Teach child and family techniques to control the adverse effects of enuresis (*e.g.*, use of plastic mattress covers, use of child's own sleeping bag (machine washable) when staying overnight away from home)
2. Seek out opportunities to teach the public about enuresis and incontinence (*e.g.*, school and parent organizations, self-help groups)

# Alteration in Patterns of Urinary Elimination
## Related to Dysuria

Dysuria is the state in which the individual experiences or is at high risk of experiencing painful or difficult urination.

## Assessment

### Subjective data

The person reports

| | |
|---|---|
| Chills | Pain or burning sensation on |
| Nausea | urination |
| Flank pain | |

### Objective data

| | |
|---|---|
| Fever | Cloudy urine |
| Hematuria | Foul-smelling urine |
| Proteinuria | |

---

**Outcome Criteria**

The person will
- Experience a decrease in pain or burning
- Identify practices to prevent recurrence

**Interventions**

A. Assess causative or contributing factors

Infection
Sexual activity (24 to 48 hours before onset of symptoms)
Liquid detergent or bubble bath in bath water

B. Provide comfort measures (sitz baths; warm perineal soaks as needed)

C. Increase the dilution and acidity of the urine
- Increase fluid intake to induce frequent voiding (every 2 to 3 hours)
- Encourage drinking of cranberry juice to acidify urine (children can be given frozen popsicles made from juice)

D. Teach measures to prevent recurrences
- Take showers rather than baths to prevent bacteria from entering urethra
- Instruct women to cleanse the perineum and urethra from front to back after each bowel movement
- Establish the habit of drinking liberal amounts of fluids; void every 2 to 3 hours to flush out bacteria
- If dysuria occurs 24 to 48 hours after intercourse, maintain dilute urine by increasing fluid intake and void soon after intercourse

# Alteration in Patterns of Urinary Elimination
Related to Incontinence

**Assessment**

Subjective data

The person reports
      Inability to control urination
      Lack of sensation or urge to void
      Dribbling

Objective data

      Residual urine ($>50$ cc)
      Reduced bladder capacity ($<350$ cc)
      Reduced sensation in perineal area
      Palpable bladder
      Inability to initiate and stop the urine stream

**Outcome Criteria**

The person will
- Eliminate or reduce incontinent episodes
- Explain the cause of incontinence and the rationale for treatment
- Have a residual urine of 30 cc to 50 cc or 15% of bladder capacity

## Interventions

### A. Assess for causative or contributing factors

1. Physiological

   Infection (urine bacteria above 100,000), *e.g.*
   - Acute cystitis
   - Chronic bacteriuria

   Inflammatory process, *e.g.*
   - Vaginitis
   - Urethritis
   - Atrophic vaginitis or urethritis secondary to estrogen deficiency

   Obstruction of bladder neck, *e.g.*
   - Fecal impaction
   - Enlarged prostate gland
   - Tumor

   Congenital abnormalities

   Loss of tissue and muscle tone (from childbirth, aging, obesity, recent weight loss)

   History of surgery of the bladder and urethra with adhesions to the vaginal wall

   Abdominal binders or girdles

   Postanesthesia

   Diminished bladder capacity

   Cerebral atherosclerosis or vascular accident

   Brain tumor or trauma

   Demyelinating disease (multiple sclerosis, Guillain-Barré syndrome, amyotrophic lateral sclerosis)

   Brown-Sequard syndrome

   Spinal cord disorders (trauma, infection, tumor)

   Polio

   Decreased awareness of sensations involved with normal voluntary micturation

   Barriers to ambulation or use of urinals, bed pans, or toilet (altered hand coordination, visual deficits, vertigo, altered gait, decreased energy)

   Loss of bladder tone with diminished reflex action (overly distended bladder, catheter drainage)

2. Psychological (impaired ability to recognize bladder cues)

   Decreased attention span

   Depression

   Anxiety

   Disorientation

3. Environmental

> Obstacles to toilet (poor lighting, slippery floor, misplaced furniture, inadequate footwear, too far, bed too high, side rails)
>
> Toilet inadequate (too small for walkers or wheelchair, seat too low, no grab bars)
>
> Inadequate signal system for requesting assistance

## B. Reduce or eliminate contributing factors if possible

1. Infection or inflammation
   - Consult with physician for treatment
   - Initiate bladder reconditioning
2. Loss of tissue and muscle tone
   - Explain to person the effect of incompetent pelvic floor muscles on continence (See Principles and Rationale For Nursing Care)
   - Teach person to identify her pelvic floor muscles and strengthen them with exercise
     a. "For posterior pelvic floor muscles, imagine you are trying to stop the passage of stool and tighten your anus muscles without tightening your legs or your abdominal muscles"
     b. "For anterior pelvic floor muscles, imagine you are trying to stop the passage of urine, tighten the muscles (back and front) for four seconds, and then release them; repeat 10 times, 4 times a day (can be increased to 4 times an hour if indicated)"
   - Instruct person to stop and start the urinary stream several times during voiding
3. Environmental barriers
   - Assess path to bathroom for obstacles, lighting, and distance
   - Encourage unstable individual to request assistance with toilet facilities during the day or use bedpan
   - Assess adequacy of toilet height and need for grab rails
4. Impaired ability to recognize bladder cues or to prolong waiting time
   - Determine amount of time between urge to void and need to void (record how long person can hold off urination)
   - For person with difficulty prolonging waiting time, communicate to personnel the need to respond rapidly to his request for assistance for toileting (note on care plan)
   - Teach person to increase waiting time by increasing bladder capacity
     a. Ask the person to "hold off urinating as long as possible"
     b. Discourage frequent voiding which is the result of habit, not need
     c. Refer to the following interventions for bladder reconditioning

## C. Initiate a bladder training or reconditioning program focusing on three components: communication, fluid intake, and voiding patterns

## D. Promote communication between all staff members and between individual, family, and staff

- Provide all staff with sufficient knowledge concerning the program planned
- Assess the staff's response to program
- Assess individual for ability to cooperate
- Provide individual with rationale for plan and acquire his consent

· Encourage individual to continue program through accurate information concerning reasons for success or failure

E. Assess present voiding pattern (see Fig. II–8)
   1. Time
   2. Voluntary or involuntary
   3. Presence of sensation of need to void
   4. Amount voided
   5. Amount of residual urine after voiding
   6. Identify if certain activities precede voiding (*e.g.*, restlessness, yelling)

| | Fluid Intake Type/Amount | Urine Output | | |
|---|---|---|---|---|
| | | Amount | Voided | Incontinent |
| 12m | | | | |
| 1 | | | | |
| 2 | | | | |
| 3 | | | | |
| 4 | | | | |
| 5 | | | | |
| 6 | | | | |
| 7 | | | | |
| 8 | | | | |
| 9 | | | | |
| 10 | | | | |
| 11 | | | | |
| 12 | | | | |
| 1p | | | | |
| 2 | | | | |
| 3 | | | | |
| 4 | | | | |
| 5 | | | | |
| 6 | | | | |

**Figure II–8.** Fluid intake and voiding record form.

F. Maintain optional hydration
   · Increase fluid intake to 2000–3000 ml/day unless contraindicated
   · Space fluids to at least every 2 hours
   · Decrease fluid intake after 6 p.m. and provide only minimal fluids during the night
   · Reduce intake of coffee, tea, and grapefruit juice because of their diuretic effect

G. Maintain adequate nutrition to ensure bowel elimination at least once every 3 days
   · Monitor elimination pattern; check for fecal impaction if indicated
   · Assess daily intake for daily requirements of roughage, basic four food groups, and adequate fluids
   · See *Alterations in Nutrition* and *Alterations in Bowel Elimination: Constipation* for additional interventions

H. Promote micturition
   1. Ensure privacy and comfort
      · Use toilet facilities if possible instead of bedpans
      · Provide male with opportunity to stand if possible
      · Assist person on bedpan to flex knees and support back
   2. Teach postural evacuation (bend forward while sitting on toilet)
   3. Ensure safe access to facilities
      · Provide person with access to urinal or bedpan
      · Provide person with call light
      · Reduce obstacles to toilet facilities (path that is well lighted and free of obstacles, bed at lowest level)
   4. Stimulate the cutaneous surface to trigger the voiding reflex
      · Have person brush or stroke inner thigh or abdomen
      · Pour warm water over perineum
      · Give glass of water to drink while sitting on the toilet

I. Establish a voiding schedule, considering fluid intake, time of day, and past voiding pattern
   1. Provide an opportunity to void approximately eight times a day: upon awakening; about ½ hour after meals, physical exercise, and drinking coffee or tea; before going to sleep
      · Begin by offering a bedpan, commode, or toilet every ½ hour initially and gradually lengthen the time to at least 2 hours
      · If person has an incontinent episode, reduce the time between scheduled voidings
   2. Encourage person to try to "hold" urine until set voiding time if possible

J. Promote skin integrity
   · Identify individuals at risk to develop pressure ulcers
   · Wash area, rinse, and dry well after incontinent episode
   · Use a protective ointment if needed (for area burns, use hydrocortisone cream; for fungal irritations, use antifungal ointment)
   · See *Potential Impairment of Skin Integrity* for additional information

K. Promote personal integrity and provide motivation to increase bladder control

1. Encourage person to share his feelings about incontinence and determine its effects on his social patterns
2. Convey to him that incontinence can be cured or at least controlled to maintain dignity
3. Expect him to be continent, not incontinent (*e.g.*, encourage street clothes, discourage use of bed pads)
4. Use protective pads or garments (incontinent briefs) only after consciousness reconditioning efforts have been completely unsuccessful after 6 weeks
5. Encourage socialization
   - Encourage and assist person to groom self
   - If hospitalized, provide opportunities to eat meals outside bedroom (*e.g.*, dayroom, lounge)
   - If fear of embarrassment is preventing socialization, instruct person to use sanitary pads or briefs temporarily until control is established
   - Change clothes as soon as possible when wet to avoid indirectly sanctioning wetness
   - Advise the P.O. use of chlorophyll tablets to deodorize urine and feces odor
   - See *Social Isolation* and *Ineffective Individual Coping Related to Depression* for additional interventions if indicated

L. Modify the reconditioning program if indicated

1. In persons who are unable to respond to bladder cues
   - Provide opportunity to void prior to person's usual time for incontinence
   - Offer opportunity to void in response to person's usual behavior prior to incontinence (*e.g.*, restlessness, screaming)
   - Wake person during the night and provide an opportunity to void
2. With individuals with residual urines of > 300 ml to 500 ml
   - Institute intermittent catheterization until residual urine quantity decreases*
   - Increase the interval between intermittent catheterizations when the bladder contains less than 500 ml of urine
   - Terminate intermittent catheterization when the bladder is emptied voluntarily or by Credé method with less than 30 ml to 50 ml of residual urine

M. Teach intermittent catheterization to person and family for long-term management of bladder hypertonia (see Principles and Rationale for Nursing Care)

1. Explain the reasons for the catheterization
2. Explain the relationship of fluid intake and the frequency of catheterization
3. Explain the importance of emptying the bladder at the prescribed time regardless of circumstances because of the hazards of an overdistended bladder (*e.g.*, circulation contributes to infection and stasis of urine contributes to bacterial growth)

*May require a physician's order.

N. For incontinent persons, initiate health teaching and referrals as indicated
- Teach person and family the relationship of diet, hydration, socialization, and positive reinforcement to continence
- Teach family how to assess and record person's incontinence pattern for 24 hours (use copy of Figure II–8)
  1. Amount of urine output
  2. Voided or incontinent (estimate amount as small, moderate, large)
  3. Type and amount of fluid intake
- After the assessment, collaborate with person and family to
  1. Maintain optional hydration (2000–3000 ml/day unless contraindicated)
  2. Intervene with an opportunity to void prior to incontinence
  3. Determine if incontinent briefs are needed temporarily until control is established
  4. Teach intermittent catheterization to client and family if indicated
  5. Refer to community nurses for assistance in bladder reconditioning if indicated

## Bibliography

Butts P: Assessing urinary incontinence in women. Nursing 79(3):72–74, 1979

Dufault K: Urinary incontinence: United States and British nursing perceptives. Journal of Gerontological Nursing 4(2):28–33, 1978

Hartman M: Intermittent Self-Catheterization. Nursing 8(11):72–75, 1978

Hickey JV: Clinical Practice of Neurological and Neurosurgical Nursing. Philadelphia, JB Lippincott, 1981

Johnson J: Rehabilitative concepts of neurologic bladder dysfunction. Nurs Clin North Am 15(2):293–307, 1980

Marshall S: Urology in the office. Emergency Medicine 11(9):143–172, 1979

Meadow R: "Problems of micturition in childhood." Nursing Mirror 143(9):59–61, 1976

Napolitano LV (moderator) et al: Enuresis: Passing phase or risk alert. Patient Care 12(7):206–234, 1978

Promoting urine control in older adults. Geriatric Nursing 1(6):236–269, 1980

Spiro L: Bladder training for the incontinent patient. Journal of Gerontological Nursing 4(3):28–35, 1978

# Violence, Potential for

*Related to* **Sensory-Perceptual Alterations**

*Related to* **Inability to Control Behavior**

## Definition

Potential for violence: A state in which an individual experiences aggressive behavior that is or can be directed either at one's self or at others.

## Etiological and Contributing Factors

### Pathophysiological

Temporal lobe epilepsy
Toxic reaction to medication
Toxic response to alcohol or nonprescribed or prescribed drugs
Physical trauma
Physical progressive deterioration (organic brain disease, brain tumor)
Hormonal imbalance
Alteration in biochemical compounds leading to depression or manic depression

### Situational

Increase in stressors within a short period of time
Physical immobility
Suicidal behavior
Environmental controls
Perceived threat to self-esteem
Fear of the unknown
Response to catastrophic event
Rage reaction
Misperceived messages from others
Antisocial character
Response to dysfunctional family throughout developmental stages
Dysfunctional communication patterns
Drug or alcohol abuse

## Defining Characteristics

Hostile threats or rage
History of abuse to self or others
Overt aggressive acts
Fear or anxiety
Suspicion of others
Delusions, hallucinations
Agitation, increased motor activity
Rigid body language (clenched fists, clenched jaw)
Depression
Perception of self as worthless, hopeless
Perception of environment as frightening, hostile

## Focus Assessment Criteria*

### Subjective data

Assess individual, family, or significant others

1. History of emotional difficulties in person or family
2. Coping patterns (past and present)
3. Interaction patterns (note recent changes)

| | |
|---|---|
| Family | Co-workers |
| Friends | Others |

4. History of

    Alcohol or drug use (hallucinogens, amphetamines, barbiturates, marijuana)

    Violence (to self, others)

        Feelings about violence

        Physical or verbal violence

    Exposure to

        Toxic chemicals

        Numerous frequent life stressors

        Catastrophic events

        Violent life-style

    Feelings of

        Hopelessness or helplessness

        Fear of self or others

        Fear of loss of control

        Disorientation to time, place, person

        Suspiciousness or hostility toward self or others

        Hallucinations or delusions

        Flight of ideas or looseness of thoughts

5. Medical history

| | |
|---|---|
| Epilepsy | Therapy |
| Head injury | Hormonal imbalance |
| Brain disease | Alcohol abuse |
| Present medications | Drug abuse |

### Objective data

1. Body language

    Posture (relaxed, rigid)

    Hands (relaxed, rigid, clenched)

    Facial expression (calm, annoyed, tense)

2. Motor activity

| | |
|---|---|
| Within normal limits | Pacing |
| Immobile | Agitation |
| Increased | |

3. Affect

| | |
|---|---|
| Within normal limits | Flat |
| Labile | Inappropriate |
| Controlled | |

4. Aggressive behaviors

| | |
|---|---|
| Abuse of self (*e.g.*, refusal to eat) | Attempt to harm self |

*Refer also to Focus Assessment Criteria for *Ineffective Individual Coping* and *Disturbance in Self-Concept.*

|  |  |
|---|---|
| Threatening others | Possession of or access to |
| Attempting to harm others | destructive means (gun, knife, drugs) |

5. Diagnostic studies

|  |  |
|---|---|
| Electrolyte levels | CT scans |
| Renal function | Blood glucose |
| EEG | Drug levels (blood, urine, gastric) |
| Blood gases | Blood alcohol levels |

## Nursing Goals

Through selected interventions, the nurse will seek to
- Prevent or decrease harm to individual and others
- Decrease or eliminate symptomatology
- Assist the individual to develop alternative coping mechanisms
- Provide the individual with opportunities to maintain self-control

## Principles and Rationale for Nursing Care

### General

1. Each person's capacity to tolerate stress is unique and needs to be individually evaluated.
2. Fear and anxiety can distort the individual's perception of external stimuli.
3. Loss or lack of self-esteem can increase feelings of frustration and anger.
4. The society in which we live defines what is unacceptable violence.
5. A person's normal behavior pattern can be altered by such physiological causes as an alteration in biochemical compounds or exposure or ingestion of toxic chemicals. Examples are lead poisoning, carbon monoxide poisoning, and pesticide poisoning.
6. The caregiver should

   Be cognizant of intuitional sense that client is potentially violent and act accordingly

   Begin to develop self-introspection (*i.e.,* personal fears regarding bodily harm, loss of control, how verbal/physical violence is perceived)

   Be honest and concise during all interactions

   Avoid any challenge or threat to the person's self-esteem or sense of control

   Respect the person's need for personal space

   Assess his tolerance for personal touch

### Suicide

1. Most suicides and suicide attempts are responses to intense feelings of hopelessness, loneliness, and helplessness.
2. People who threaten suicide are trying to express their feelings of hopelessness and helplessness.
3. People attempt suicide because they cannot see a solution to their problem or because their attempts at solving the problem have failed.
4. Situations that can contribute to suicidal feelings include depression, loss (of significant other, job, finances), debilitating disease, and drug and alcohol abuse.
5. The more lethal the method used or planned, the higher the risk. Highly lethal methods include guns, hanging, jumping; less lethal methods include wrist cutting and drug overdose.
6. Adolescents and persons over 45 are the highest risks.

7. Women have a higher rate of attempts than men, but men have higher rates of completion, since they generally use more lethal methods.
8. Persons who are at high risk for suicide are those who have a history of previous attempts, make covert or overt threats ("I won't be a bother anymore"), exhibit sudden changes in appetite, sleep habits, or personality (sudden mood elevation), or make preparations for death (wills, giving away personal possessions, acquiring a weapon).

## Seclusion

1. Seclusion is a temporary measure that allows an extremely disturbed individual to regain control over his behavior. The duration and documentation for seclusion is dictated by institutional regulations.
2. Seclusion provides a means of protecting the person from injuring himself or others, providing time for medication to take effect, or removing the person from stimuli with which he is not able to cope.
3. Safety precautions for staff and individual are the primary concerns for the duration of seclusion. An individual in full restraints is completely helpless; therefore, he must be protected from injury through constant observation or through the use of a seclusion room.
4. The seclusion room should have safety windows and screens, minimal furnishings, recessed lights, and protected outlets. Nothing should be available that could be used as a weapon. It should be possible to observe the individual while he is in seclusion.
5. To protect the individual from injuring self or staff during seclusion, objects that are potentially harmful must be removed (belts, hairpins, jewelry, matches, stockings, pens, pencils, eyeglasses).
6. Fire procedures need to include individuals in restraints or seclusion.
7. Medications, particularly antipsychotics, are useful in controlling agitation. Medications are usually used in conjunction with restraints and seclusion (except in toxic states). Since rapid tranquillization is used, side-effects are likely, including hypotension and extrapyramidal symptoms (*e.g.*, dystonias).

---

# Potential for Violence
## Related to Sensory-Perceptual Alterations

---

The inability to evaluate the environment realistically (*i.e.*, perceiving individuals or objects in the environment as frightening, threatening or hostile), can increase the potential for violence.

## Assessment

### Subjective data

Verbalization of suspicions, paranoid ideation, hearing voices, seeing things not present in external environment

Threatening statements that can or do suggest harm to self or others ("I'm going to hit you"; "I want to kill myself")

Objective data

Abnormal diagnostic studies (thyroid function, EEG, CT scan)
Loud periodic or consistent verbalizations
Rigidity, or increased restlessness
Staring eye contact or avoidance of eye contact
Disorientation to time, place, and person
Inability to remember all or part of recent or past events
Disconnected thoughts

---

**Outcome Criteria**

The person (or family) will
- Begin to describe causation and possible preventive measures
- Explain rationale for interventions
- Experience internal control of behavior (with assistance from others)

---

## Interventions

### A. Assess causative factors

Physiological disease processes (trauma, brain tumor, hormonal imbalance, organic brain syndrome)
Fear derived from misperception of hospital routine or procedures
Unfamiliar environment (hospital)
Sensory overload (hospital personnel, equipment)
Emotional disease process (psychoses, depression)
Toxic reaction to prescribed or nonprescribed drugs (hallucinogens, amphetamines, barbiturates)
Reality deficit

### B. Eliminate or reduce contributing factors if possible

1. Provide and document accurate information concerning the relationship of the physiological alteration and the disturbing feelings or thoughts
2. Reduce or prevent sensory overload
   - Provide short, concise, honest statements concerning hospital routines and procedures
   - Remove excess equipment
   - Decrease noise volume
   - Decrease number of people present at one time
   - Utilize same personnel with individual to promote trust
   - See *Sensory-Perceptual Alterations Related to Sensory Overload* for additional interventions
3. Assess and reduce levels of fear
   - Discuss rationale for fear, if known (if person is able to verbalize)
   - Identify available support systems
   - Allow person to verbalize feelings about hospital environment
   - Allow person to arrange personal belongings to promote a sense of security (see *Fear* for additional interventions)

4. Reduce toxic reaction to medication
   - Eliminate further ingestion of medication that produces this reaction*
   - Begin medical regimen to counteract effects of toxic medication*
5. Reduce reality deficit
   - Reinforce reality; during each interaction, orient individual to time, place, person
   - Provide electric clock and calendar for person's room
   - Set realistic day-to-day goals for person (*i.e.*, recognition of environmental objects or individuals)
   - Give short, consistent statements when explaining care, and be prepared to repeat them frequently
   - See *Impaired Thought Processes Related to Inability to Evaluate Reality* for additional interventions
   - Be aware of the effects of darkness on disorientation and interact with client accordingly

## C. Maintain safety precautions

- Assess client's behavior frequently (every 15 to 30 minutes)
- Eliminate from environment movable stationary objects and objects that could cut or strangle person (belts, ties)
- When person is in bed, provide proper padding for protection
- Use physical restraints if needed*
- Limit setting to protect everyone (*i.e.*, individual may move freely in room area but not in hallway or nurse's station)

## D. Assess for possible suicidal intent

1. Evaluate
   - Level of distress (depression, hopelessness, change in behavior, degree of altered thought processes, impulsiveness, presence of physical illness, alcohol or drug use, recent loss)
   - Intent (statements regarding possessions, what he wants—"I want to die"; "I want to get out of here"—patterns of communicating with support system—anger or an attempt to manipulate family environment—and plan—what it is and whether well-established and thought through or vague)
   - Lethality (prior suicide attempts, method used or planned, present availability of that method
   - Support system (presence of and communication patterns with significant others—rejecting, supporting)
2. Intervene appropriately; for individual with high level of risk, take immediate safety precautions
   - Provide constant monitoring by staff (periodic monitoring—every 15 to 30 minutes—if risk is not acute)
   - Remove potentially harmful objects (razors, sharp instruments, glass objects; person may wear belts and stockings only if constantly monitored)
   - Explain to person why someone is staying with him; provide reassurance that staff will assist in protecting him
   - Encourage person to express his feelings

*May require a physician's order.

- Be aware of own feelings and reactions to suicidal behavior
- If suicidal ideas are suspected, they should be openly discussed ("Have you thought about suicide?")
- Identify and clarify associated problems; focus on precipitating event
- Have individual evaluate what he expects will happen and what other options are
- Assist individual in identifying strengths (*e.g.*, support system, job)

## E. Prevent excessive agitation

- Do not explore cognitive rationale for behavior
- Decrease environmental stimuli
- Allow physical activity in accordance with person's ability
- Interact with person on a one-to-one basis
- Allow him to maintain personal space (do not physically come too close if person moves away rapidly)
- Do not touch person until you explain what the procedure or rationale is for such intervention
- Convey sense of caring, security, reassurance (calm nonverbal behavior, low tone of voice, brief statements that person is in control but at times needs assistance with control that can be provided by staff)
- Administer medication as per physician's order
  a. Monitor effectiveness of the medication at least every 15 minutes
  b. Observe for side-effects of respiratory depression

## F. Initiate seclusion if necessary

1. Remove individual from situation if environment is contributing to aggressive behavior, using least amount of control needed (*e.g.*, ask others to leave and take individual to quiet room)
2. Protect individual from injuring self or others through use of restraints or seclusion*
3. When using seclusion, institutional policy will provide specific guidelines; the following are general
   - Observe individual at least every 15 minutes
   - Search the individual before secluding to remove harmful objects
   - Check seclusion room to see that safety is maintained
   - Offer fluids and food periodically (in nonbreakable containers)
   - When approaching an individual to be secluded, have sufficient staff present
   - Explain concisely what is going to happen ("You will be placed in a quiet room by yourself until you can better control your behavior") and give person a chance to cooperate
   - Assist person in toileting and personal hygiene (assess his ability to be out of seclusion; a urinal or commode may need to be used)
   - If person is taken out of seclusion, someone must be present continually
   - Maintain verbal interaction during seclusion (provides information necessary to assess person's degree of control)
   - When person is allowed out of seclusion, a staff member needs to be in constant attendance to determine whether person can handle additional stimulation

*May require a physician's order.

G. Proceed with health teaching and referrals as indicated

1. Explain to person and significant others
   - Causes and possible sensory-perceptual alterations
   - Interventions that relieve symptoms
   - Factors that increase symptoms
2. When appropriate, refer to outside agencies (day hospital programs, group therapy, support and self-help groups)

# Potential for Violence
## Related to Inability to Control Behavior

The loss of control that results when cognitive abilities are decreased by disturbing experiences (fear, frequent frustration, changes in life-style, or rage) may lead to the person's harming himself or others.

## Assessment

### Subjective data

Series of recent, frequent frustrations
History of violent or potentially violent episodes
History of inability to control behavior following alcohol or drug ingestion
History of impaired communication with others
Recent disturbing changes in life-style
History of temporal lobe epilepsy or brain tumor
Threatening verbalization to self or others
No subjective clues (explosive)

### Objective data

Possession of a weapon (gun, knife)
Abnormal diagnostic studies (*i.e.*, EEG, CT scan)
Staring or lack of eye contact
Hostile affect
Lack of movement, rigid body stance
Clenched fists, throwing of stationary object(s), hostile gestures toward others

---

### Outcome Criteria

The person will
- Experience control of behavior with assistance from others
- Begin to decrease number of violent responses
- Describe causation and possible preventive measures
- Explain rationale for interventions

---

## Interventions

A. Assess causative factors

Physiological disease processes (seizure disorder, brain lesion)

Family or community pattern that uses violence as a way of coping

Poorly developed communication skills or problem-solving methods that result in feelings of frustration and anger

Health personnel, family, and friends confronting person about behavior

Use of alcohol or other drugs.

B. Eliminate or reduce contributing factors, if possible

1. Provide and document accurate information concerning the relationship of the physiological alteration and disturbing feelings and thoughts

2. Provide examples of families or communities that do not use violence to cope with stressful situations and explore these alternatives with person (talking with others, problem-solving about family community difficulties, dealing with one problem at a time)
   - Explore what violence means to the individual
   - Present alternative physical ways to deal with family and community frustration (organize and participate in a group sport such as baseball or basketball; develop boxing skills; plan and assist with building project for family home; utilize occupational therapy, recreational therapy, and physical therapy while hospitalized)

3. Review communication patterns other than verbal or physical abuse (listen closely to others, do not interrupt, think before replying)
   - Have person role-play family communication with personnel and practice problem-solving techniques
   - Discuss with person how communication can be misperceived by others
   - Discuss with person how issues of control interfere with communication and what this means to him
   - Provide frequent short (10-minute) interactions with person rather than one long (30-minute) interaction
   - Comment on positive changes noted in person's communication pattern
   - Be honest during all interactions
   - Refer to appendix VI for crisis intervention guidelines

C. Promote interactions that increase a sense of trust

- Contract with person to spend a certain amount of time together (perhaps 15 minutes three times per shift) and spend *only* this amount of time
- Be honest, clear, and concise during interactions
- Establish short-term goals with person (*e.g.*, to reduce [eliminate] profanity for one hour of one day)
- Establish long-term goals with person (*e.g.*, to reduce [eliminate] profanity during hospitalization)
- Recognize that defensive, manipulative behavior has meaning for person
- Maintain a stable physical environment when possible (*i.e.*, decrease sensory stimuli, do not transfer client from room to room, try to maintain same roommates)

## D. Promote individual control

1. Encourage client to talk rather than act out physically
2. Utilize behavior modification (when client has reduced or not used profanity for one day, reward this positive behavior by complimenting client or spending extra time with him)
3. Function as role model (be calm, quiet, interested in others; discuss the importance of caring about self and other individuals)
4. Do not threaten person's self-esteem or sense of control; assist with external controls when needed
   - Remove easily accessible items that could be used as weapons
   - Do not confront client with issue of control ("If you don't stop this, I'll call Security")
   - When possible, allow person to make the decision
     a. Can choose not to act out *or* can choose to act out
     b. Explain that if acting out occurs, personnel will be requested to assist in reducing client's physical behavior: by being present in room and assisting with medication and restraints, if needed*

## E. Plan for unpredictable violence

1. Assess person's potential for violence and past history
2. Ensure availability of staff prior to potential violent behavior (never try to assist person alone when physical restraint is necessary)
3. Determine who will be in charge of directing personnel to intervene in violent behavior if it occurs
4. Ensure protection for oneself (door nearby for withdrawal, pillow to protect face)

## F. Maintain client safety

1. Assist person to maintain control by discussing frustrations, thus decreasing physical and verbal aggression
2. Utilize seclusion if indicated
   a. Remove individual from situation if environment is contributing to aggressive behavior, using the least amount of control needed (*e.g.,* ask others to leave and take individual to quiet room)
   b. Protect individual from injuring self or others through use of restraints or seclusion.*
   c. When using seclusion, institutional policy will provide specific guidelines; the following are general
     - Observe individual at least every 15 minutes
     - Search the individual before secluding to remove harmful objects
     - Check seclusion room to see that safety is maintained
     - Offer fluids and food periodically (in nonbreakable containers)
     - When approaching an individual to be secluded, have sufficient staff present
     - Explain concisely what is going to happen ("You will be placed in a room by yourself until you can better control your behavior") and give person a chance to cooperate.
     - Assist person in toileting and personal hygiene (assess his ability to be out of seclusion; a urinal or commode may need to be used)

*May require a physician's order.

- If person is taken out of seclusion, someone must be present continually
- Maintain verbal interaction during seclusion (provides information necessary to assess person's degree of control)
- When person is allowed out of seclusion, a staff member needs to be in constant attendance to determine whether person can handle additional stimulation

## G. Utilize restraints when necessary

- Repeatedly tell person what is occurring before control is begun
- Reinforce that you are helping him control himself
- Choose the proper type of restraint and use as little as necessary
- Use leather wrist restraints, which are more comfortable than handmade ones
- Restrain waist and legs along with wrists for an extremely violent person
- Secure restraints to bed frame, not side rails; allow for some mobility
- Apply restraints tightly enough for safety but loosely enough to allow 1 or 2 fingers between restraint and person's skin, so as not to impair circulation; pad bony prominences from the restraint
- Check person in restraints every 15 minutes; check vital signs every 15–60 minutes, as indicated
- Remove or loosen one restraint at a time every 2 hours and perform range-of-motion exercises
- When restraints can be removed, remove one at a time, wrist last; have a second person present in case of problems

## H. Initiate health teaching and referrals as indicated

- Discuss, with individual and family, constructive alternatives to violence caused by stressors (*e.g.*, exercise program, constructive stress management—see Appendix IV—hotlines such as Contact
- Discuss, with individual and family, the importance of seeking assistance before crisis occurs (*e.g.*, in emergency room)
- Refer, if indicated, to psychotherapy, substance abuse groups, group home vocational rehabilitation

## Bibliography

Bennett A: Recognizing the potential suicide. Geriatrics 22:175–181, 1967

Dixon B: Intervening when the patient is delusional. J Psychiatr Nurs 7(1):25–34, 1969

Gluck M: Learning a therapeutic verbal response to anger. J Psychiatr Nurs 19(3):9–11, 1981

Fawcett J (ed): Dynamics of Violence. Chicago, American Medical Association, 1971

Haber J, Leach AM, Schudy SM et al (eds): Comprehensive Psychiatric Nursing. New York, McGraw-Hill, 1978

Knowles RD: Dealing with feelings: Managing angry feelings. Am J Nurs 81:2196–2197, 1981

Misik I: About using restraint. Nursing 11(8):50–55, 1981

Schroeder PJ: Nursing interventions with patients with thought disorders. Perspect Psychiatr Care 17(1):32–39, 1979

Schwartzman ST: The hallucinating patient and nursing intervention. J Psychiatr Nurs 13(6):23–28, 33–36, 1976

Tobachnick N, Farberow N: The assessment of self-destructive potentiality. In Shneidman ES (ed): The Cry for Help, pp 61–77. New York, McGraw-Hill, 1961

# Appendixes

# Appendix I: Data-Base Assessment Guide

This guide directs the nurse to collect data to assess functional health patterns* of the individual and to determine the presence of actual, potential, or possible nursing diagnoses. Should the person have medical problems, the nurse will also have to assess for data in order to collaborate with the physician in monitoring the problem.

As with any printed assessment tool, the nurse must determine whether to collect or defer certain data. The symbol △ identifies data that should be collected on hospitalized persons. The collection of data in sections not marked with △ probably should be deferred with most acutely ill persons or when the information is irrelevant to the particular individual.

As the nurse interviews the person, significant data may surface. The nurse should then ask other questions (focus assessment) to determine the presence of a pattern. Each diagnostic category in Section II has a focus assessment to help the nurse gather more pertinent data in a particular functional area.

For example, the client reports during the initial interview that she has a problem with incontinence. The nurse should then ask specific questions utilizing the focus assessment for *Alteration in Patterns of Urinary Elimination* to determine the possible contributing factors. After the nurse has identified the factors, the plan of care can be initiated.

## Data-Base Assessment Format

1. Health perception–health management pattern

    "How would you usually describe your health?"

    | | |
    |---|---|
    | Excellent | Fair |
    | Good | Poor |

    "How would you describe your health at this time?"

    "What do you do to keep healthy and to prevent disorders in yourself? In your children?"

    | | |
    |---|---|
    | Adequate nutrition | Professional exams |
    | Weight control | (gynecological, |
    | Exercise program | dental) |
    | Self-exams (breast, testicular) | Immunizations |

    △ Reason for and expectations of hospitalization (and previous hospital experiences)

    △ "Describe your illness"

    | | |
    |---|---|
    | Cause | Onset |

    △ "What treatments or practices have been prescribed?"

    | | |
    |---|---|
    | Diet | Surgery |
    | Weight loss | Cessation of smoking |
    | Medications | Exercises |

    △ "Have you been able to follow the prescribed instructions?" If not, "What has prevented you?"

*The functional health patterns have been adapted from Gordon M: Nursing Diagnosis: Application and Process (New York, McGraw-Hill, 1982).

515

△ "Have you experienced or do you anticipate a problem with caring for your-self (your children, your home)?"

| Mobility problems | Financial concerns |
| Sensory deficits (vision, hear-ing) | Structural barriers (stairs, narrow doorway) |

2. △ Nutritional-metabolic pattern

"What is the usual daily food intake (meals, snacks)?"

"What is the usual fluid intake (type, amounts)?"

"How is your appetite?"

| Indigestion | Vomiting |
| Nausea | Sore mouth |

"What are your food restrictions or preferences?"

"Any supplements (vitamins, feedings)?"

"Has your weight changed in the last 6 months?" If yes, "Why?"

"Any problems with ability to eat?"

| Swallow liquids | Chew |
| Swallow solids | Feed self |

3. △ Elimination pattern

Bladder

"Are there any problems or complaints with the usual pattern of urinating?"

| Oliguria | Retention |
| Polyuria | Burning |
| Dysuria | Incontinence |
| Dribbling | |

"Are assistive devices used?"

| Intermittent catheterization | Incontinent briefs |
| Catheter (Foley, external) | Cystostomy |

Bowel

"What is the usual time, frequency, color, consistency, pattern?"

"Assistive devices (type, frequency)?"

| Ileostomy | Cathartics |
| Colostomy | Laxatives |
| Enemas | Suppositories |

Skin

"What is the skin condition?"

| Color, temperature, turgor | Edema (type, location) |
| Lesions (type, description, location) | Pruritus (location) |

4. Activity-exercise pattern

"Describe usual daily/weekly activities of daily living"

| Occupation | Exercise pattern (type, frequency) |
| Leisure activities | |

△ "Are there any limitations in ability?"

| Ambulating (gait, weight-bear-ing, balance) | Dressing/grooming (oral hygiene) |
| Bathing self (shower, tub) | Toileting (commode, toilet, bed-pan) |

"Are there complaints of dyspnea or fatigue?"

5. △ Sleep-rest pattern

"What is the usual sleep pattern?"

| Bedtime | Sleep aids (medication, food) |
| Hours slept | Sleep routine |

"Any problems?"

    Difficulty falling asleep          Not feeling rested after sleep

    Difficulty remaining asleep

6. △ Cognitive-perceptual pattern

    "Any deficits in sensory perception (hearing, sight, touch)?"

        Glasses                 Hearing aid

    "Any complaints?"

        Vertigo

        Insensitivity to superficial pain      Insensitivity to cold or heat

    "Able to read and write?"

7. Self-perception pattern

    △ "What are you most concerned about?"

    "What are your present health goals?"

    △ "How would you describe yourself?"

    "Has being ill made you feel differently about yourself?"

    "To what do you attribute the following?"

        Becoming ill            Maintaining health

        Getting better

8. Role-relationship pattern

    △ Communication

What language is spoken?

Is speech clear? Relevant?

Assess ability to express self and understand others (verbally, in writing, with gestures)

Relationships

"Do you live alone?" "If not, with whom?"

"Who do you turn to for help in time of need?"

Assess family life (members, educational level, occupations)

        Cultural background          Decision-making

        Activities (lone or group)      Communication patterns

        Roles discipline             Finances

    "Any complaints?"

        Parenting difficulties        Marital difficulties

        Difficulties with relative (in-laws,    Abuse (physical, verbal,

           parents)                    substance)

9. Sexuality-sexual functioning

    "Has there been or do you anticipate a change in your sexual relations because of your condition?"

        Fertility               Pregnancy

        Libido                 Contraceptives

        Erections             History

        Menstruation

Assess knowledge of sexual functioning

10. Coping–stress management pattern

    △ "How do you make decisions (alone, with assistance, who)?"

    △ "Has there been a loss in your life in the past year (or changes—moves, job, health)?"

    "What do you like about yourself?"

    "What would you like to change in your life?"

    "What is preventing you?"

    "What do you do when you are tense or under stress (e.g., problem-solve, eat, sleep, take medication, seek help)?"

△ "What can the nurses do to provide you with more comfort and security during your hospitalization?"

11. Value-belief system

"With what (whom) do you find a source of strength or meaning?"

"Is religion or God important to you?"

"What are your religious practices (type, frequency)?"

"Have your values or moral beliefs been challenged recently? Describe."

△ "Is there a religious person or practice (diet, book, ritual) that you would desire during hospitalization (institutionalization)?"

12. △ Physical assessment (objective)

General appearance

Weight and height

Eyes (appearance, drainage)

    Pupils (size, equal, reactive to light)

    Vision (glasses)

Mouth

    Mucous membrane (color, moisture, lesions)

    Teeth (condition, loose, broken, dentures)

Hearing (hearing aids)

Pulses (radial, apical, peripheral)

    Rate, rhythm, volume

Respirations

    Rate, quality, breath sounds (upper and lower lobes)

Blood pressure

Temperature

Skin (color, temperature, turgor)

    Lesions, edema, pruritus

Functional ability (mobility and safety)

    Dominant hand

    Use of right and left hands, arms, legs

    Strength, grasp

    Range of motion

    Gait (stability)

    Use of aids (wheelchair, braces, cane, walker)

    Weight-bearing (full, partial, none)

Mental status

    Orientation (time, place, person, events)

    Memory

    Affect

    Eye contact

# Appendix II: Guidelines for Preparing Diagnostic Categories*

A. The diagnostic category has three parts
- The category label
- Etiological subcategory
- Defining characteristics

B. The criteria for each part are
1. The category label
   a. Clear and concise (2 or 3 words)
   b. Specific enough to be clinically useful
   c. Represents a clinical entity that a nurse can identify and treat
2. Etiological subcategory (if can be identified)
   a. Describes one probable cause of the health problem
   b. Directs interventions when combined with label
   c. Clear and concise, but specificity is vital
3. Defining characteristics
   a. Observable signs and symptoms that are present
   b. Differentiation of critical defining characteristics from others

C. The diagnostic category's rating as to the degree of independent nursing interventions commonly involved in preventing, treating, or resolving the health problem is
1. High
2. Medium
3. Low

D. Cite literature to support category label, etiological subcategory, and defining characteristics (if available)

E. Suggested format
1. Category label
2. Etiological factors
3. Defining characteristics
4. Degree of independent nursing therapy
5. Supportive literature

*North American Nursing Diagnosis Association, St. Louis University School of Nursing, 3525 Caroline Street, St. Louis, MO 63104.

# Appendix III: Guidelines for Play Therapy

Play is a natural means of expression for children and is essential to their mental, emotional, and social well-being. The need for play during stress (*e.g.*, developmental, illness, treatments) is essential in order to provide the child with an outlet for emotional release and a sense of mastery over the situation. Play provides parents and professionals with opportunities to assess the mood, words, and actions of a child and identify the child's present perception of the situation.

## A. General

1. Professionals and parents utilize play to assist the child to
   Recognize his feelings
   Cope with a new concept
   Identify his fears
   Understand threatening or unknown events
   Clarify distortions received from others (parents, peers)
   Gain a sense of mastery
2. Play can be utilized to diagnosis the child's perception of the situation, his perception of caregivers, and his mental responses to events
3. Guidelines for therapeutic play
   Promote spontaneity by reflecting only what the child expresses
   Avoid forcing the child to participate
   Allow sufficient time without interruption
   Identify when it is appropriate to encourage child to share concerns
   Play for the child who cannot play for himself
   Allow child to work freely on his project without direction or adult comment
   Allow child to engage in violent nondestructive acts

## B. Types of play

1. Drawing and painting
   · Supplies: Crayons, paint, brushes, paper
      Artwork usually requires little direction
      Older children can be asked to draw what they like or do not like about the hospital
      An old sheet can cover the bed clothes of a child confined to bed
      Ask child to explain picture when it is done
      Clarify misconceptions
2. Dramatic play
   · Supplies: Puppets, dolls, stuffed animals, replicas of hospital equipment, actual hospital equipment, miniature hospital furniture
      Assign roles to the child and to the doll or puppet ("Mary, you are the nurse and the puppet is you")
      Ask child to administer a treatment to the puppet or doll
      Supervise the child when playing with equipment

3. Needle play (dramatic play)
   - Supplies: Doll, stuffed animals, clean syringes and needles, alcohol wipes, water vial, Band-Aids, miniature IV sets (tubing, tourniquets, tongue blade for arm board)
         Introduce immediately after or in between the child's experiences
         Expect reluctance to touch syringe
         Demonstrate injection and ask the child to help you push the fluid in
         Allow child to give injections on the doll anywhere and however he wants to
         Make appropriate sounds of crying and protest to show child that crying is permitted
         Show child how to give the doll love after the injection
         Encourage child to talk about why injections are needed
         Use group play to encourage participation
         Overly aggressive children should be shown acceptance

## Bibliography

Axline V: Play Therapy. New York, Ballantine Books, 1969

Brooks M: Why play in the hospital? Nurs Clin North Am 5:431–441, 1970

Levinson P, Ousterhout D: Art and play therapy with pediatric burn patients. Journal of Burn Care and Rehabilitation 1(5):42–46, 1980

Oehler J: The frog family books: Color the pictures sad or glad. Matern Child Nurs J 6:281–283, 1981

Petrillo M, Sanger S: Emotional Care of Hospitalized Children, 2nd ed. Philadelphia, JB Lippincott, 1980

Taylor M, Williams H: Use of therapeutic play in the ambulatory pediatric hematology clinic. Cancer Nursing 3:433–437, 1980

## Pertinent Literature for Parents and Children

Books That Help Children Deal with a Hospital Experience (Publication number 017-031-00020-1)

When Your Child Goes to the Hospital (Publication number 793-30092)

A Reader's Guide for Parents of Children with Mental, Physical, or Emotional Disabilities (Publication number [HSA] 77-5290). An annotated reference on basic reading, books on teaching and playing at home, books that deal with particular issues, and books written by parents and children.

The foregoing three titles are available from the U.S. Government Printing Office, Washington, DC 20402.

Preparing Children and Families for Health Care Encounters. A compilation of articles for parents and professionals on various aspects of preparation. Available from the Association for the Care of Children's Health, 3615 Wisconsin Avenue NW, Washington, DC 20016.

# Appendix IV: Stress Management Techniques

The following techniques can be taught to provide an individual with an opportunity to control his response to stressors and thus in turn increase his ability to manage stress constructively. Suggested readings are listed at the end to provide more specific information.

## Progressive relaxation technique

Progressive relaxation is a self-taught or instructed exercise that involves learning to constrict and relax muscle groups in a systematic way, beginning with the face and finishing with the feet. This exercise may be combined with breathing exercises that focus on inner body processes. It usually takes 15 to 30 minutes and may be accompanied by a taped instruction that directs the person concerning the sequence of muscles to be relaxed.

1. Wear loose clothing; remove glasses and shoes
2. Sit or recline in a comfortable position with neck and knees supported; avoid lying completely flat
3. Begin with slow, rhythmic breathing
   a. Close your eyes or stare at a spot and take in a slow deep breath
   b. Exhale the breath slowly
4. Continue rhythmic breathing at a slow steady pace and feel the tension leaving your body with each breath
5. Begin progressive relaxation of muscle groups
   a. Breathe in and tense (tighten) your muscles and then relax the muscles as you breathe out
   b. Suggested order for tension-relaxation cycle (with tension technique in parentheses)
      Face, jaw, mouth (squint eyes, wrinkle brow)
      Neck (pull chin to neck)
      Right hand (make a fist)
      Right arm (bend elbow in tightly)
      Left hand (make a fist)
      Left arm (bend elbow in tightly)
      Back, shoulders, chest (shrug shoulders up tightly)
      Abdomen (pull stomach in and bear down on chair)
      Right upper leg (push leg down)
      Right lower leg and foot (point toes toward body)
      Left upper leg (push leg down)
      Left lower leg and foot (point toes toward body)
6. Practice technique slowly
7. End relaxation session when you are ready by counting to three, inhaling deeply, and saying, "I am relaxed"

## Self-coaching

Self-coaching is a procedure to decrease anxiety by understanding one's own signs of anxiety (such as increased heart rate or sweaty palms) and then coaching oneself to relax.

For example, "I am upset about this situation but I can control how anxious I get. I will take things one step at a time, and I won't focus on my fear. I'll think about what I must do to finish this task. The situation will not be forever. I can manage until it is over. I'll focus on taking slow deep breaths."

## Thought stopping

Thought stopping is a self-directed behavioral procedure learned to gain control of self-defeating thoughts. Through repeated systematic practice, a person does the following:

1. Says "Stop" when a self-defeating thought crosses the mind (*e.g.*, "I'm not smart enough" or "I'm not a good nurse")
2. Allows a brief period—15 to 30 seconds—of conscious relaxation (because of an increased focus on negative thoughts, it may seem at first that self-defeating thoughts increase; however, eventually the self-defeating thoughts will decrease)

## Assertive behavior

Assertive behavior is the open, honest, empathetic sharing of your opinions, desires, and feelings. Assertiveness is not a magical acquisition but a learned behavioral skill. Assertive persons do not allow others to take advantage of them and thus are not victims. Assertive behavior is not domineering but remains controlled and nonaggressive. An assertive person

Does not hurt others
Does not wait for things to get better
Does not invite victimization
Listens attentively to the desires and feelings of others
Takes the initiative to make relationships better
Remains in control or uses silences as an alternative
Examines all the risks involved before asserting
Examines personal responsibilities in each situation before asserting

Refer to suggested readings for specific techniques or participate in an assertiveness training course led by a competent instructor. Assertive behavior is best learned slowly in several sessions rather than in one lengthy session or workshop.

## Guided imagery

This technique is the purposeful use of one's imagination in a specific way to achieve relaxation and control. The person concentrates on the image and pictures himself involved in the scene. The following is an example of the technique.

1. Discuss with person an image he has experienced that is pleasurable and relaxing to him, such as

   Lying on a warm beach
   Feeling a cool wave of water
   Floating on a raft
   Watching the sun set

2. Choose a scene that will involve at least two senses
3. Begin with rhythmic breathing and progressive relaxation

4. Have person travel mentally to the scene
5. Have the person slowly experience the scene; how does it look? sound? smell? feel? taste?
6. Practice the imagery
   a. Suggest tape-recording the imagined experience to assist with the technique
   b. Practice the technique alone to reduce feelings of embarrassment
7. End the imagery technique by counting to three and saying, "I am relaxed" (if the person does not utilize a specific ending, he may become drowsy and fall asleep, which defeats the purpose of the technique)

## Suggested Readings

Alberti RE, Emmons L: Your Perfect Right: A Guide to Assertive Behavior, 2nd ed. San Luis Obispo, CA, Impact, 1974

Benson H: The Relaxation Response. New York, Avon Books, 1976

Bloom L, Coburn K, Pearlman J: The New Assertive Woman. New York, Dell, 1976

Chenevert M: Special Techniques in Assertiveness Training for Women in the Health Professions. St. Louis, CV Mosby, 1978

Gridano D, Everly G: Controlling Stress and Tension. Englewood Cliffs, NJ, Prentice-Hall, 1979

Herman S: Becoming Assertive: A Guide for Nurses. New York, D Van Nostrand, 1978

McCaffery M: Nursing Management of the Patient with Pain, 2nd ed. Philadelphia, JB Lippincott, 1979 (especially Chapter 10, Imagery; Chapter 9, Relaxation)

# Appendix V: Noninvasive Pain Relief Techniques

Noninvasive pain relief techniques are external measures that influence the person internally.

## General principles

1. Convey to the person that you believe that the pain is present.
2. Explain the relationship of stress and muscle tension to pain.
3. Explain the various methods of relief and allow the person to choose one or two.
4. Attempt to teach the method when the pain is absent or mild.
5. Perform the technique with the person to coach him and encourage him to focus on details of the distraction.
6. Encourage the person to practice the technique when the pain is mild.
7. Teach the person to use the technique before feeling pain (if the pain can be anticipated) and to increase the complexity of the distraction as the pain increases in intensity (*e.g.*, increase the volume of music via earphones as discomforts increase during a bone-marrow aspiration).
8. Inform others (staff, family) about the technique and its purpose.
9. Explain that noninvasive pain relief can be utilized with medications and usually increases their effects.

## Specific techniques

- Distraction
- Cutaneous stimulation
- Relaxation

## Distraction

Distraction is the deliberate focusing of attention on stimuli other than the pain sensation. The ability to be distracted from pain does not denote that the pain is nonexistent or mild. Even persons with severe pain can choose to be distracted from their pain.

Distraction can be taught to children. (Caution parent not to confuse this therapeutic distraction technique that the child chooses to practice with the surprise distraction of a child prior to painful events. This latter technique serves only to produce feelings of mistrust and fear in children.)

Distraction cannot usually be practiced for very long periods. After the distraction ends, the person may have an increased awareness of the pain and fatigue.

1. Examples of distraction methods
   a. Visual distractions
      - Counting objects (flowers on wallpaper, spots on wall, animals in picture, someone's blinks)
      - Describing objects (pictures, slides)
   b. Auditory distractions (songs, tapes)

    c. Tactile kinesthetic distractions (holding, stroking, rocking, rhythmic breathing)

    d. Guided imagery (see Appendix IV)

2. Breathing techniques

    a. Slow rhythmic
- Have person take slow deep breaths through nose and exhale through mouth
- Try to slow rate to nine breaths a minute if possible
- Instruct person to take extra breaths if needed

    b. Heartbeat breathing (McCaffery). Teach person to
- Take a slow deep breath
- Count pulse on wrist
- Inhale as you count two beats
- Exhale as you count the next three beats

    c. He-who breathing (McCaffery). Instruct person to
- Take a slow deep breath
- Inhale and say *he* on inhaling
- Exhale and say *who* on exhaling
- Rate can be increased (should not exceed 40 per minute) if pain increases

## Cutaneous stimulation

Cutaneous stimulation is stimulation of the skin's surface. Examples of methods follow.

1. Massage

    Rub with warm lubricant over painful part or over the opposite adjacent part if the actual painful part cannot be massaged (*e.g.*, if a fractured left leg is casted, the person can massage the fracture site on the right leg)

2. Application of cold

    a. The therapeutic effects of cold are (Lehmann et al)

        Reduces small-diameter nerve conduction, which lessens the perception of pain

        Decreases the inflammatory response of tissues

        Decreases blood flow

        Decreases edema

    b. The use of cold is indicated with

        Trauma (first 24–48 hours)

        Fractures

        Insect bites

        Hemorrhage

        Muscle spasms

        Rheumatoid arthritis (if relief is acquired)

        Pruritus

        Headaches

    c. The use of cold is contraindicated

        With Raynaud's disease

        With cold allergy

        48 hours after trauma

    d. Guidelines for use of cold
- Protect skin from cold burn (*e.g.*, layers of cloth between skin and cold source)

       · Caution its use with persons with limited communication ability or decreased sensorium (infants, sedated persons)

       · Caution its use on areas with impaired sensation (*e.g.,* diabetic's foot)

  e. Examples of cold application methods

      Towel or washcloth soaked in ice water and wrung out

      Ice bags (Zip-loc plastic bag filled with ice water or frozen)

      Reusable gel pak (stored in refrigerator or freezer)

      Massage of painful site with ice

3. Application of heat

  a. The therapeutic uses of heat are

      Slows small-diameter nerve conduction, which lessens the perception of pain

      Increases the inflammatory response of stress

      Increases blood flow

      Increases edema

  b. The use of heat is indicated with

      Trauma (past 48 hours)

      Cystitis

      Hemorrhoids

      Backache

      Arthritis (if relief is attained)

      Bursitis

  c. The use of heat is contraindicated with

      Trauma (first 24–48 hours)

      Edema

      Hemorrhage

      Malignant sites

      Pruritus

  d. Examples of heat application methods

      Towel or washcloth soaked in warm water and wrung out (cover cloth with plastic around area to trap heat longer)

      Heating pads (moist or dry)

      Warm bath or shower

      Sunbathing

      Moist heat pack (commercially available)

4. External analgesic preparations (McCaffery)

  External analgesic preparations—ointments, lotions, liniments—produce a sensation (usually warmth) that may persist for several hours

  a. Guidelines for use

      · Do not use on broken skin

      · Do not apply to mucous membranes (anus, vagina)

      · Always skin-test each product before using

      · Follow directions and use sparingly or painful burning may occur

  b. Examples of external analgesic preparations

      Products with methyl salicylate (oil of wintergreen)

      Products with menthol

## Relaxation

Relaxation is a state of relief from skeletal muscle tension that the person achieves through the practice of deliberate techniques.

1. The therapeutic effects of relaxation are
       Decreases anxiety
       Provides the person with some control over pain
       Decreases skeletal muscle tension
       Serves as a distraction from pain
2. Examples of relaxation techniques
       Biofeedback
       Yoga
       Meditation
       Progressive relaxation exercises (see Appendix IV)

## Bibliography

Benson H: The Relaxation Response. New York, Avon Books, 1976

Breeden SA, Kondo C: Using biofeedback to reduce tension. Am J Nurs 75:2010–2012, 1975

Brown B: Stress and the Art of Biofeedback. New York, Bantam Books, 1977

Donovan M: Relaxation with guided imagery: A useful technique. Cancer Nursing 3(1):27–32, 1980

Lehmann JF, Warren CG, Scham SM: Therapeutic heat and cold. Clin Orthop 99:207–245, 1974

McCaffery M: Pain relief for the child: Problem areas and selected non-pharmacological methods. Pediatric Nursing 3(4):11–16, 1977

McCaffery M: Technique to help a patient relax. Am J Nurs 77:794–795, 1977

McCaffery M: Nursing Management of the Patient with Pain, 2nd ed, Chapters 7 and 8. Philadelphia, JB Lippincott, 1979

McCoy P: Further proof that touch speaks louder than words. RN 40(11):43–46, 1977

Mennell JM: The therapeutic use of cold. American Osteopathic Journal 74:1146–1158, 1975

Michelsen D: Giving a back rub. Am J Nurs 78:1197–1199, 1978

Petrello JM: Temperature maintenance of hot moist compresses. Am J Nurs 73:1050–1051, 1973

Simonton C, Mathews-Simonton S, Creighton J: Getting Well Again: A Step-by-Step Self-Help Guide to Overcoming Cancer for Patients and Their Families. Los Angeles, JP Tarcher, 1978

Wilson RL: An introduction to yoga. Am J Nurs 76:261–263, 1976

# Appendix VI: Guidelines for Problem Solving and Crisis Intervention

The two basic coping behaviors in response to problems are emotion-focused behaviors and problem-focused behaviors.*

## Emotion-focused behaviors

1. *Minimization* occurs when the seriousness of a problem is minimized. This may be useful as a way to provide needed time for appraisal, but it may become dysfunctional when it precludes appraisal.
2. *Projection, displacement, and suppression of anger* occur when anger is attributed to or expressed toward a less threatening person or thing, which may reduce the threat enough to allow an individual to deal with it. Distortion of reality and disturbance of relationships may result, which further compound the problem. Suppression of anger may result in stress-related physical symptoms.
3. *Anticipatory preparation* is the mental rehearsal of possible consequences of behaviors or outcomes of stressful situations, which provides the opportunity to develop perspective as well as to prepare for the worst. It becomes dysfunctional when the anticipation creates unmanageable stress, as, for example, in anticipatory mourning.
4. *Attribution* is the finding of personal meaning in the problem situation, which may be religious faith or individual belief. Examples are fate, the will of the divine, luck. Attribution may offer consolation but becomes maladaptive when all sense of self-responsibility is lost.

## Problem-focused behaviors

1. *Goal-setting* is the conscious process of setting time limitations on behaviors, which is useful when goals are attainable and manageable. It may become stress-inducing if unrealistic or short-sighted.
2. *Information-seeking* is the learning about all aspects of a problem, which provides perspective and, in some cases, reinforces self-control.
3. *Mastery* is the learning of new procedures or skills, which facilitates self-esteem and self-control: for example, self-care of colostomies, insulin injection, or catheter care.
4. *Help-seeking* is the reaching out to others for support. Sharing feelings with others provides an emotional release, reassurance, and comfort, as, for example, with Weight Watchers and other self-help and support groups.

## Problem-solving techniques

1. Identify the problem
   What is wrong?
   What are the causes?
   Refer to pertinent literature, individuals, and organizations for more knowledge about the problem, if indicated

*Lazarus RS, Folkman S: Analysis of coping in a middle-age community sample. J Health Soc Behav 21(9):219–239, 1980

2. Find the cause
    Who or what is responsible for the problem?
    How have you contributed to the problem?
    Put yourself in the place of each person and consider the problem from their
        perspective
3. Discover the options
    What are your goals?
    What do you want to accomplish?
    What are the goals of the others involved in the problem?
    List all possible options for dealing with the problem (including not doing
        anything)
4. List advantages and disadvantages for each option
    What will happen if you do nothing?
    What is the worst thing that could happen with each option?
5. Choose an option and a plan
    What preparation do you need before implementing the plan?
    How do others fit into the plan?
    How will you know if the plan is working or not?

## Guidelines for crisis intervention

1. Assist the victim to confront reality (*e.g.*, encourage viewing of dead body)
2. Encourage persons involved to display emotions of crying and anger (within
   limits)
3. Do not encourage the person to focus on all the implications of the crisis at once
   —*e.g.*, divorce, death—for they may be too overwhelming
4. Avoid giving false reassurances such as "It will be all right" or "Don't worry"
5. Clarify fantasies with facts; encourage verbalization to assist with catharsis and
   to identify misinformation
6. Avoid encouraging person or family to blame others but allow ventilation of
   anger (*e.g.*, rape)
7. Encourage person or family to seek help and validate its acceptability (*e.g.*, "A
   friend of mine found the American Cancer Society very helpful")
8. Assist person or family to identify resources (agencies, people) to help with
   everyday tasks of living until resolution is attained

# Appendix VII: Age-Related Developmental Needs

## General guidelines for nurses and parents

1. Practice open, honest dialogues. Never threaten (*e.g.*, "If you are bad I will not take you to the movies").
2. Don't lecture. Tell the child he was wrong and let it go. Spend time talking about pleasant experiences.
3. Compliment children on their achievements. Make each child feel important and special. Especially tell a child when he has been good; try not to focus on negative behavior.
4. Do not be afraid to hold and hug (boys as well as girls).
5. Set limits and keep them. Expect cooperation. Encourage the child to participate in activities that conform to your values. Do not be trapped by "But everybody else can."
6. Let the child help you as much as possible.
7. Discipline the child by restricting his activity. For a younger child, sit him in a chair for 3 to 5 minutes. If the child gets up, spank him once and put him back. Continue until the child sits for the prescribed time. For an older child, restrict bicycle riding or movie-going (pick an activity that is important to him).
8. Make sure the discipline corresponds to the unacceptable behavior. Children should be allowed opportunities to make mistakes and to verbally express anger.
9. Spank only once (the first spank is for the child, the rest are for you). Stay in control. Try not to discipline when you are irritated.
10. Remember to examine what you are doing when you are not disciplining your child (*e.g.*, enjoying each other, loving each other).
11. Never reprimand a child in front of another human being (child or adult). Take the child aside and talk.
12. Never decide you cannot control a child's destructive behavior. Examine your present response. Are you threatening? Do you follow through with the punishment or do you give in? Has the child learned you do not mean what you say?
13. Be a good model (the child learns from you whether you intend it or not). Never lie to a child even when you think it is better; the child must learn that you will not lie to him, no matter what.
14. Children learn to be responsible adults by having responsibilities as children. Give each child a responsibility suited to his age, such as picking up toys, making beds, or drying dishes. Expect the child to complete the task.
15. Share your feelings with children (happiness, sadness, anger). Respect and be considerate of the child's feelings and of his right to be human.

## Age-Related Developmental Needs

*1½ to 2½ years*

| Child's Developmental Stage | Parental Guidance | Implications for Nursing |
|---|---|---|
| **Personal/Social** | Provide child with peer companionship | Allow child to take liquids from a cup including medicines |
| Extremely curious, prefers to do things for himself | Allow for brief periods of separation under familiar surroundings | Allow child to perform some self-care tasks |
| Plays independently alongside other children (parallel play) | Practice safety measures that guard against child's increased motor ability and curiosity (poisoning, falls) | Wash face and arms<br>Brush teeth |
| Negativistic | | Expect resistant behavior to treatments |
| **Motor** | Tell the truth | Use firm, direct approach and provide child with choices only when possible |
| Walks alone | Discipline child for violation of safety rules | Restrain child when needed |
| Runs well | Running in street | Reinforce that treatments are not punishment |
| Can drink from cup | Touching electrical wires | Explain to parents methods for disciplining child |
| Developing fine-motor control | Allow child some control over fears | Slap hand once |
| Can open doors, gates | Favorite toy | Sit in chair for 2 minutes (if child gets up, put him back and reset timer) |
| Climbs | Night light | |
| **Language/Cognition** | | |
| Uses symbolic language | | |
| Cannot understand time | | |
| **Fears** | | |
| Strangers | | |
| Dark | | |
| Loud noises | | |

*2½ to 3½ years*

| Child's Developmental Stage | Parental Guidance | Implications for Nursing |
|---|---|---|
| **Personal/Social** | Explain why things happen as simply as possible | Praise child for helping you |
| Imitates | Allow child to explain why he thinks things are happening | Holding still<br>Holding the Band-Aid |
| Frequently asks why, how, what, where | Correct misconceptions | Give child choices whenever possible |
| Eager to please | Include child in domestic activities when possible | Tell child he can cry or squeeze your hand but you expect him to hold still |
| Strong fantasy world | Dusting | |
| Short attention span | Cleaning spoons | |
| **Motor** | Discuss differences in opinion (between parents) in front of child | Have parents present for procedures when at all possible |
| Holds cup by handle | Discipline child | Explore with child his fantasies of the situation |
| Jumps | Sit in chair 3–5 minutes | Use play therapy. Explain the procedure immediately beforehand if short (*e.g.*, injection) and two hours before if longer or intrusive (*e.g.*, x-ray, IV insertion) |
| Climbs | Do not threaten child with what will happen if he doesn't behave | |
| Pedals tricycle | Always follow through with punishment | |
| **Language/Cognition** | | |
| Talks a lot | | |
| Use 4 or 5-word phrases | | |

Age-Related Developmental Needs (*continued*)

### 2½ to 3½ years

**Child's Developmental Stage**

**Fears**

Separation from parents
Dark
Monsters

### 3½ to 5 years

| Child's Developmental Stage | Parental Guidance | Implications for Nursing |
|---|---|---|
| **Personal/Social** | Provide child with regular contact with other children (*e.g.*, nursery school) | Explain to child how he can cooperate (*e.g.*, hold still) and expect he will |
| Boasts, brags | Explain that TV movies are make-believe | Use play therapy to allow child free expression |
| Has feelings of indestructibility | Practice definite limit-setting on behavior | Explain all procedures |
| Quarrels | Offer child choices | Use equipment if possible |
| Reports fantasies as truth | Allow child to express anger verbally but limit motor aggression ("You may slam a door but you may not throw a toy") | Encourage child to ask questions |
| Enjoys visiting, helping with chores | | Tell child the exact body parts that will be affected |
| May attempt things that are too difficult | | Explain when procedure will occur in relation to daily schedule (*e.g.*, after lunch, after bath) |
| Shares better as ages | Discipline | |
| Imaginative group play | Sit in chair 5 minutes | |
| Assumes sex roles | Forbid a favorite pastime (No bicycle riding for 2 hours) | |
| Establishes friendships (4–5) | | |
| May arbitrarily exclude a child from group play | Be consistent and firm | |
| Uses aggressive language and motor activity | Teach safety precautions about strangers | |

**Motor**

May ride bicycle with training wheels (over 4)
Climbs
Throws ball but has difficulty catching

**Language**

Speech has highly emotional content
Uses complex phrases

**Fears**

Castration, mutilation
Dark

### 5 to 11 years

| Child's Developmental Stage | Parental Guidance | Implications for Nursing |
|---|---|---|
| **Personal/Social** | Teach what foods are needed each day and provide choices when possible; allow child to keep record of intake | Explain illness is not a punishment |
| Has strong food preferences | | Always involve child in care and in unit activities |
| Has erratic mood changes | | |
| Likes to complete a task | | |

**Age-Related Developmental Needs** (*continued*)

*5 to 11 years*

| Child's Developmental Stage | Parental Guidance | Implications for Nursing |
|---|---|---|
| Enjoys helping<br>Likes privacy<br>Develops a strong sense of right and wrong<br>Group play (established as child ages)<br>Peer relationships important | Encourage interaction outside home<br>Include cooking and cleaning in home activities<br>Teach safety (bicycle, street, playground equipment, fire, water, strangers)<br>Maintain limit-setting and discipline<br>Prepare child for body changes of pubescence and provide with concrete sex education information<br>Expect fluctuations between immature and mature behavior<br>Respect peer relationships but do not compromise your values (*e.g.,* "But Mom, all the other girls are wearing makeup") | Always prepare child and perform a painful procedure in private away from other children<br>Expect cooperation but encourage verbal expression of fears and concerns<br>Reason with child<br>Prepare for procedure<br>  As soon as scheduled<br>  Use diagrams and simple anatomic drawings<br>  Allow child to handle equipment<br>  Be specific about body part affected<br>Determine what child thinks will happen and why<br>Correct misconceptions |

**Motor**

Moves constantly
Swims
Draws more representatively
Accident-prone

**Language/Cognition**

Enjoys telling stories
Uses thought processes
Understands cause and effect (over 8)
Perceives future and past
Concentrates on concrete reality

**Fears**

(See nursing diagnosis *Fear* for specific age-related fears)
School failure
Loss of status
Disability

*11 to 15 years*

| Child's Developmental Stage | Parental Guidance | Implications for Nursing |
|---|---|---|
| **Personal/Social**<br><br>Peer group very important<br>Desires to be "grown up"<br>Wants authority over himself<br>Wants privacy<br>Likes popular music<br>Desires independence from family<br>Chooses career | Be available when needed<br>Compliment child's achievements<br>Expect unpredictable behavior<br>Allow increasing independence but maintain limit setting for safety<br>Assist in selection of career but avoid pushing<br>Respect privacy | Allow visiting from peers<br>Provide telephone for peer contacts<br>Explain and prepare for procedures separate from parents<br>Encourage other children of same age to share similar experiences<br>Explain procedures<br>  Use diagrams<br>  Correct terminology in private |

**Age-Related Developmental Needs** (*continued*)

*11 to 15 years (adolescence)*

Child's Developmental Stage

Sexual identity fully ma-
tures

**Motor**

Well developed

Rapid physical growth

**Language/Cognition**

Uses problem-solving techniques randomly

Gradually draws inferences
from general principles

Uses slang and obscene
words and symbols exces-
sively

Frequently sterotypes others

**Fears**

Being alone

Intruders

Being unsuccessful (school)

Parental Guidance

Provide with concrete information concerning: sexu-
ality, sexual function,
body changes

Teach about
    Automobile safety
    Drug abuse
    Alcohol abuse
    Tobacco hazards
    Mechanical safety (*e.g.*,
    tools, appliances)

Implications for Nursing

Respect privacy and fear of
embarrassment

Determine what child
thinks will happen and
why

Correct misconceptions

# Index

Terms in *italics* following *See* or *See also* cross references represent nursing diagnostic categories and are followed by the appropriate textual page numbers. Terms not in *italics* following *See* or *See also* cross references are entries found elsewhere in the Index and are not followed by page numbers. The letter *t* following a page number represents tabular material.

accidents. *See also Injury, Potential for,* 238–253
    automobile, 247, 250
Ace bandages, 273, 276
activity
    diversional deficit, 160–161
        monotony of confinement and, 162–163
        postretirement inactivity and, 164–165
    intolerance to, 71–77
    physiological response to, 73t
adolescence, developmental needs of, 534–535
aggression. *See also* anger
    assessment of, 474–475
aging
    sensory–perceptual alterations and, 400–404
    sexuality and, 410–411, 411t
airway, ineffective clearance of, 346–347, 361–364
allergy. *See Respiratory Function, Alterations in, Related to Chronic Allergy,* 357–360
amputations. *See Self-Care Deficit,* 374–388
    self-concept with. *See Self-Concept, Disturbance in,* 389–396
anger
    anxiety and, 86
    grieving and, 208
    principles of, 83–84
    violence and, 508–511
anorexia. *See Nutrition, Alterations in: Less Than Body Requirements, Related to Anorexia,* 296–298
anthropometric measurements, 293t
anxiety, 78–87
    learning and, 261
    noncompliance and, 280–282
aphasia. *See also Communication, Impaired Verbal, Related to Aphasia,* 139–142
    principles of, 136
assertiveness, 523
assessment, 24–31
    of coping patterns, 517
    data collection format, 25–26, 515–518
    of decision-making abilities, 391
    of edema, 198
    of endurance, 266
    of family function, 232–233
    of hazards in the home, 241–242

of health practices. *See Health Maintenance, Alterations in,* 215–229
of housing, 233
of independence–dependence patterns, 392
of individual functional abilities, 231–233
of learning needs, 256–257
of pain, 113–114
of perception of control, 333
of peripheral circulation, 481
physical, 26–27, 28t
of physical capabilities, 240
of response to illness, 391
of role responsibilities, 390
of sexual knowledge in children, 409
of stress-related symptoms, 146
of support systems, 318
attachment. *See Parenting, Alterations in,* principles of, 320

bathing difficulties, 381–383
bedwetting. *See* enuresis; incontinence
behavior modification, obesity and, 304–305
bladder retraining. *See Urinary Elimination, Alteration in Patterns of, Related to Incontinence,* 486–500
blood pressure, 478
body image. *See Self-Concept, Disturbance in,* 389–396
body part loss, sexual dysfunction and, 417–418
bonding. *See Parenting, Alterations in,* 317–331
boredom. *See Diversional Activity Deficit,* 160–166
braces, leg, 272
breast-feeding. *See Parenting, Alterations in, Related to Breast-Feeding Difficulties,* 328–330
breathing exercises, 353, 371
breathing patterns, ineffective, 346–347, 365–367

cancer
    and home care, 234
    and nutrition, 291
canes, 246
cardiac output, decreased, 104–110
care planning
    components of, 35
    documentation and, 47–49, 48t, 50t
    evaluation and, 46–47
    goals and, 41–43
    nursing orders and, 43–44
    samples of, 54–56, 58–61
casts, 272, 276
catheterization, intermittent, 491, 499–500
chewing difficulties, 293–296
child abuse. *See Parenting, Alterations in, Related to Child Abuse/Neglect,* 325–328